PSYCHOSOCIAL ASPECTS
OF DEAFNESS

Nanci A. Scheetz
Valdosta State University

PEARSON

Boston   New York   San Francisco
Mexico City   Montreal   Toronto   London   Madrid   Munich   Paris
Hong Kong   Singapore   Tokyo   Cape Town   Sydney

To Richard
and my four daughters
Melissa, Marie,
Megghan, and Monique

Executive Editor and Publisher: Stephen D. Dragin
Editorial Assistant: Barbara Strickland
Production Administrator: Joe Sweeney
Editorial-Production Service: Walsh & Associates, Inc.
Composition and Prepress Buyer: Linda Cox
Manufacturing Buyer: Andrew Turso
Cover Administrator: Kristina Mose-Libon
Electronic Composition: Publishers' Design & Production Services, Inc.

For related titles and support materials, visit our online catalog at www.ablongman.com.

Library of Congress Cataloging-in-Publication Data

Scheetz, Nanci A.
  Psychological aspects of deafness / Nanci A. Scheetz.
      p.   cm.
  Includes bibliographical references and index.
  ISBN 0-205-34347-3
    1. Deaf—Psychology.   2. Deaf—Mental health.   3. Deaf—Counseling of.
  4. Self-esteem in people with disabilities.   I. Title.

HV2380S34 2003
305.9′08162—dc21

                                                                  2003041817

Printed in the United States of America

10   9   8   7   6   5   4   3   2   1   09   08   07   06   05   04   03

Contents

Preface

Psychosocial Aspects of Deafness has been written to provide the reader with a broad overview of topics discussed in the fields of psychology, sociology, and deafness. It is also intended as a resource text for educators, psychologists, sociologists, vocational rehabilitation counselors, interpreters, parents, and other professionals who come in contact with the Deaf community. Included in the chapters are issues that lie at the heart of Deaf culture and provide the reader with information pertaining to the impact of deafness on psychosocial development.

The text highlights contemporary mental health issues, including the development of identity, the emergence of the healthy personality, and the establishment of mental health services for deaf and hard-of-hearing individuals. In addition, it provides the reader with a review of assessment instruments, counseling techniques, and therapeutic models. Family dynamics are discussed from a multiplicity of ethnic backgrounds reflecting the cultural diversity that is evident within the Deaf community. Furthermore, strategies for classroom management are included that focus on enhancing the emotional growth of deaf and hard-of-hearing children. The broad scope of the subject matter presented allows flexibility and provides fresh material for new approaches to courses related to this topic within the field of deaf education.

This book is designed as a teaching–learning vehicle. For this reason, basic concepts recur in varying situations, and some concepts are repeated in diverging contexts to promote comprehension and enhance retention. It is a source book on the many dimensions of psychosocial aspects of deafness. It is dedicated to a panoramic view of a complex field rather than an in-depth analysis of each major dimension. The chapters are intended to provide the reader with insights into crises that occur and intervention techniques that can be implemented. Topics pertaining to sexuality, social issues, eating disorders, and chemical dependency are addressed. Through a discussion of these topics the reader is provided insights regarding the impact of deafness on psychosocial development.

This book is addressed to future and current educators, beginning with those who work with infants and continuing on to those who are faced with the challenges of adult learners. Counselors who work with these diverse populations are uniquely aware of the complexities of providing quality services to both deaf children and deaf adults. This text is designed to furnish them with additional insights into the developmental process of those who are deaf. The intention is to provide a foundation for those students entering the field of interpreting, psychology, and social work. In addition, information for parents and educators who want to gain insights and under-standing into the complexities surrounding psychosocial issues is included.

The author wishes to acknowledge Ms. Kristy Strong, and Ms. Kimberly Mus-grove Williams for their assistance with the research and Mr. Daniel M. Smith for his computer expertise. Special thanks are also extended to Dr. Phillip L. Gunter for granting release time and offering support to this project and to Dr. Evelyn E. Dodd for taking time to read the manuscript and offer so many constructive suggestions. Her advice and suggestions have been very beneficial. The author would also like to acknowledge Ms. Vanessa Brunston for her many words of encouragement through-out the duration of this project. Input and feedback from the following reviewers is also gratefully acknowledged: Richard C. Nowell, Indiana University of Pennsylvania, and James C. Blair, Utah State University. Special thanks are also extended to the author's husband for his support, encouragement, and the many hours he devoted to reading the chapters and for the suggestions he offered for enhancing the content. And finally, thanks are extended to Steve Dragin, Barbara Strickland, and the staff at Allyn and Bacon for making this an enjoyable experience.

1

The Emerging Self: A Lifelong Process

In a society brimming with diversity and shrinking cultural boundaries we find ourselves entwined with others in a tapestry of human existence. Each thread represents our beliefs, attitudes, perceptions, and dreams, and portrays an image of who we are. As we interact with others and our surroundings, the threads become woven together and thus represent a unique picture of how we as individuals interface with society. Where do these individual beliefs come from? What events occur to color one person's perceptions and not another's? How do daily experiences contribute to the way one's self-image is shaped? And what factors are instrumental in influencing development as infants emerge into childhood, then adolescence, and later into adulthood?

From the moment of birth infants are endowed with the legacy of their family unit. The environment in which they are raised, the history and origins of family members, their language, beliefs, religious preference, and their relative position to the larger society all contribute to the molding of each new being. Throughout life, these elements continue to influence individuals as their personalities are formed and a sense of belonging to the larger group is established. As children mature into adulthood, their self-identities are fashioned and a sense of group belonging is instilled.

Through the years the scientific study of our behavior and mental processes has provided psychologists with a wealth of information. Human behavior has been and continues to be studied from biological, cognitive, psychoanalytical, behavioral, and phenomenological perspectives. Neurobiological processes that underlie behavior and mental functions are explored; stimulus-response approaches are examined; thought processes, both conscious and unconscious, are analyzed; and those factors that influence our ability to make choices, become motivated, and achieve self-actualization are studied. Emphasis is placed on those behaviors and mental processes that individuals engage in through the course of their lifetime.

Another discipline that probes the study of human behavior is sociology. Whereas psychology focuses on the individual, sociology explores interpersonal relations, and the study of human behavior within the many groups that comprise a society. Individuals are examined to see how well they comprehend and interact in complex social settings.

Aspects of interpersonal relations that sociologists study include interactions that occur as one person provides a stimulus to which another person responds. Furthermore, they examine social organizations to discern the recurring and interrelated patterns of interaction among the members, and the actual behavior involved in interpersonal relations: social groups, cultures, social institutions, socialization, demography, and social problems. Through inspecting these complexities, the socialization process is explored and social problems are scrutinized.

A subdivision of both sociology and psychology focuses on the way in which individuals interact in social groups, and on social and cultural influences on personality development. Termed "social psychology," it is in part the study of how any individual's thoughts, feelings, and behaviors are influenced by the actual, imagined, or implied presence of others. In this context, the term "implied presence" refers to the multitude of activities individuals engage in based on their position (role) in a complex social structure and membership in a cultural group (Atkinson et al., 1990, Allport, 1985). This field developed from the recognition of human diversity within cultural uniformity. The social psychologist views the individual as "the intersection point of a variety of pressures: immediate situational demands, conflicting social expectations, and internalized beliefs and values" (Jones, 1985, p. 53). The task of the social psychologist is to understand how the conflict among these pressures is resolved.

Based on the assumption that we identify with and encounter many diverse groups, the social psychologist studies the roles individuals assume in various social settings. Attention is directed toward how the persons involved think, influence, and relate to each other. The structure and functioning of groups, both large and small, are studied. Individuals are viewed in regard to how they think about other people, are influenced by them, and relate to them. Thus, the social psychologist wants to ascertain how groups affect individual people, and sometimes how an individual can affect a group (Myers, 1987).

By examining the situations in which these interactions occur, one can gain insights into how our self-identity is formed, the role society plays, and the effect these interactions have on the way the individual responds to his or her community. Recognizing that each person experiences life equipped with his or her own beliefs, perceptions, and attitudes, it becomes apparent that upon entering any given situation our reaction to the stimuli may differ somewhat from those around us. By obtaining an understanding of those factors that contribute to the shaping of our responses, further insights can be gained into the way members of society interact with one another.

Perspectives in Psychology

Psychology can be defined as the science of mental processes and behaviors that probes the emotional and behavioral characteristics of individuals, groups, or activities. It touches upon almost every aspect of our lives as it attempts to explain where our ideas originate, why we behave the way we do, and why people respond differently when confronted with the same situation. In order to understand the complexities of human behavior, psychologists have examined the relationship of various aspects that contribute to these processes and behaviors.

Psychology delves into the areas of the brain, investigating intelligence, aptitudes, and emotional disturbances while analyzing the mental processes involved in the intricate activities undertaken. It also explores intellectual functioning capabilities, researches the method in which sensory impulses are interpreted, and defines emotions and thoughts. Becoming familiar with psychological perspectives provides us with a clearer understanding of how individuals relate to those around them.

The extent to which we internalize our beliefs and express ourselves is contingent upon many factors. Explanations abound of how our personalities are formed and the reasons why we respond and react the way we do. Although these theories focus on the same problems, their perspectives are diverse as they attribute the unique characteristics of our behavior to a multiplicity of causes. By examining the various perspectives, one can obtain greater insights into the manner in which individuals internalize their thought processes and behaviors. These perspectives can work independently or in tandem with one another. However, they all comprise a part of the complex phenomenon occurring within the field of psychology.

Biological

The biological approach to the study of human behavior attempts to relate overt actions to electrical and chemical events that take place in the body, particularly within the brain and the nervous system. This approach focuses on the "neurobiological processes that underlie behavior and mental processes" (Atkinson et al., 1990). The biological perspective studies learning and memory as they relate to nerve cells and chemicals produced by the brain.

Our biological processes provide information that enables us to be aware of and adjust to our environment. Our sense organs detect stimuli, which then are relayed to the brain where the information is interpreted. The brain is extremely complex. It is responsible for deciphering signals that alert us to signs of physical stress. In addition, it provides us with a storehouse for language, memory, and the ability to solve problems. The intricate thought processes individuals engage in result from the specific patterns of electrical and chemical events that occur in the brain.

Behavioral

The origins of behaviorism as a field of scientific study can be traced to the early 1900s. During that time, an American psychologist, John B. Watson, proposed the idea that individuals' mental abilities could be studied by examining their behaviors. He further suggested that the study of those behaviors become the sole subject matter of psychology. In addition, Watson ascertained that by studying and noting the verbal expressions exhibited in human behavior, one could gain insights into the individuals' perceptions and feelings.

The offspring of behaviorism, stimulus-response psychology, is still influential today (Atkinson et al., 1990). This branch of psychology examines the interplay of external stimuli, responses, and rewards and punishments that occur in the environment. In the beginning strict behavioral psychologists chose to refrain from speculating about any mental activity that transpired in this process. Although there are only a few today that adhere to a strict behavioral approach, this theory has provided the groundwork for the development of many of the modern tenets in psychology.

Cognitive

The modern study of cognition combines attributes from both the biological or mental process internal in the individual with one's observable external behaviors. Specific behaviors are viewed and then interpreted in terms of our underlying mental processes. Psychologists who ascribe to the theory of cognition study the processes involved in perception, memory, reasoning, decision-making, and problem solving.

Cognitive psychologists analyze the way the individual processes information. Particular attention is paid to how the individual acquires new knowledge, combines it with existing information, and applies it, as evidenced in his or her behaviors.

Psychoanalytic

Another branch of psychology that explores human behavior is embedded within the field of psychoanalysis. The name most frequently associated with it is Sigmund Freud. Freud based his theory of psychology on the premise that many of our behaviors stem from processes that are unconscious. In this respect, the term "unconscious" was used to refer to those beliefs, fears, and desires that, unbeknownst to the individual, influence his or her behaviors.

Freud believed that all of us are born with instincts. He felt that many of these inherent impulses were negative in nature and therefore had to be suppressed. He theorized that throughout childhood these impulses surface, are punished, and are later stored in the unconscious. They remain there and influence our actions, beliefs, and behaviors. Although many psychologists today do not completely embrace this theory, they do concede that individuals engage in activities and experience feelings without understanding the underlying causes for their reactions.

Phenomenological

The field of phenomenological psychology focuses on the development of the inner self as one relates to one's environment. Psychologists who espouse this theory tend to reject the concept that behavior is controlled by external stimuli (behaviorism), the processing of information in perception and memory (cognitive psychology), or by unconscious impulses (psychoanalytic theories) (Atkinson et al., 1990). Rather, they believe that individuals have the ability to control their actions, act upon their environment, and contribute to the shaping of their own destinies. One of the basic tenets of this theory is that the individual's principal motivating force is toward growth and self-actualization. Phenomenological psychologists believe that we are "free agents," capable of making choices, setting our own goals, and being responsible for our decisions.

This approach to psychology examines human growth and development from a very subjective standpoint. Also referred to as humanistic psychology, it explores the obstacles we encounter in our environment while attempting to develop to our fullest potential.

Social Psychological

Social psychology can be defined as the scientific study of how people think about, influence, and relate to each other (Myers, 1987). In addition, it studies how others influence our actions. Social psychology emphasizes that human behavior is a "function of both the person and the situation" (Atkinson et al., 1990, p. 719).

Focus is placed on the individual as he or she interacts in a variety of social situations. Social situations are considered to have a profound influence on individual persons. Likewise, the individual is thought to influence the social situation. The interaction between these two provides the area for the social psychologist's study.

Social interactions are influenced by three factors. First, our minds do not see reality identically; hence each situation affects people somewhat differently. Each person responds to any given circumstance as he or she perceives it. Second, people can choose to be a part of certain situations. While some become engaged in particular events, others do not. Furthermore, while involved in the event the interaction between the individual and the experience will influence how he or she responds to others in the environment. Third, people frequently create their own situations. As the individual enters a group or social gathering, the behavior the group expects the newcomer to project may become evident. Thus, if the group expects someone to be extraverted, hostile, or belligerent, the actions toward the person may induce the behavior that is anticipated (Snyder & Ickes, 1985). By examining these factors one can obtain insights into the dynamics involved in the socialization of the individual. Table 1.1 provides a summary of the various perspectives in psychology.

Perspectives in Sociology

Just as psychologists endeavor to learn about the mental processes of the individual, sociologists research, compare, and analyze the behavior of persons within the numerous groups that comprise a society. They study these groups within the context and confines of their environment. Particular attention is paid to those agents that affect the socialization process. Social structures, such as the environment and the individual's experiences, are explored. By analyzing these situations, the sociologist gains insights into the formation of the personality (Kornblum, 1991).

TABLE 1.1 *Summary: Perspectives in Psychology*

Biological	• Relates actions to electrical/chemical events within the body (brain/nervous system). • Studies learning and memory as they relate to nervous cells produced by the brain. • Provides information enabling us to adjust our environment.
Behavioral	• Proposed by John B. Watson's studies of verbal expressions exhibited in human behavior. • Stimulus-Response Psychology examines the interaction between external stimuli, responses, rewards, and punishment within the environment.
Cognitive	• Examines specific behaviors and interprets them in terms of mental processes. • Explores how an individual acquires new knowledge, combines it with existing schemata, and applies such knowledge in their behaviors.
Psychoanalytical	• Comprises Sigmund Freud's theories that "unconscious" thoughts and feelings are repressed unpleasant or misunderstood childhood experiences. • Not fully supported by psychologists today.
Phenomenological	• Focuses on the development of the inner self as one relates to his or her environment. • Believes that we are "free agents," capable of making choices, setting our own goals, and being responsible for our decisions. • Also referred to as humanistic psychology; explores the obstacles encountered in our environment while attempting to develop to our fullest potential.
Social Psychological	• Examines how people think about, influence, and relate to each other. • Claims social interaction is influenced by three factors: our minds do not see reality identically, people choose to participate in certain situations, and people often create their own situations.

Several institutions within the environment are of particular interest to the sociologist. Those studied encompass the family, peer group, schools, the media, and all other agents whose messages are responsible for influencing people's behaviors.

Defining Environment

In sociological terms the word "environment" can be employed to refer to sets of people, groups, and organizations, all with their own ways of thinking and acting. It encompasses all of the expectations and incentives that are established by other people in a person's social world (Kornblum, 1991).

The environment is responsible for contributing to the shaping of human behaviors. It sets the stage for interactions to occur and provides circumstances that delimit the range of our choices. Further, the environment institutes the objectives and standards by which individuals make choices (Shils, 1985).

Societies or groups of people form communities in the environment. Here they share common goals and carry out certain responsibilities as they interact with each other. The common goals they share and the behaviors they reflect originate in their culture. One's cultural identity is characterized by the "way" a group of people believes and is therefore transmitted into how they behave.

Establishing Cultural Identity

A culture is comprised of a "set of learned behaviors of a group of people who have their own language, values, rules for behavior, and traditions" (Padden, 1989). These modes of thought are handed down from one generation to the next by communicative interaction. Through gestures, speech, writing, and other channels, ideas are shared. Culture is conveyed to its members by sharing beliefs, rather than transmitting them through genetics or heredity.

Culture has three major dimensions: ideas, norms, and products. Ideas are the ways of thinking that organizes human consciousness. Norms are the accepted ways of doing or carrying out ideas, and material culture refers to the pattern of possessing and using the products of a culture (Bierstedt, 1963).

Culture is learned through language. It consists of a large, unpublished code that addresses how one should behave in any given situation. It provides us with a storehouse of ways of believing and behaving. Ideas of good and bad are transferred and positive or negative behaviors are respectively rewarded or punished in cultural ways (Lasswell, Burma, & Aronson, 1986).

Each culture provides the framework for the development of folklore, myths, and heroes. Within the realm of one's cultural heritage customs are shared, norms are established, and values are instilled. The knowledge and beliefs individuals cherish are passed down to successive generations with the hope of preserving those traits that characteristically represent the cultural group. This process by which culture is transmitted from one generation to the next is termed "socialization."

A Look at the Socialization Process

Socialization occurs throughout one's lifetime. It endows us with the knowledge needed in order to exhibit appropriate behaviors in accordance with our cultural norms. As members interact in the community and cultural knowledge is transmitted and acquired, the process of socialization ensues.

Early in life the newborn begins to be molded into a social being. This primary phase of socialization occurs as children continue to grow and interact with family members and other intimate groups in their social environment. During this time, children are told whom they can interact with, and what society expects of them.

The secondary phase of socialization occurs later in childhood and in adolescence. As children reach school age they leave the family for schooling and come under the influence of adults and peers outside the household and the immediate family. This is followed by the third phase of socialization, which takes place later in life. During this time individuals learn the norms associated with new statuses such as wife, husband, journalist, grandparent, worker, nursing home patient, and so forth (Danziger, 1971).

Agents of Socialization

Throughout these three primary phases, certain institutions provide environments and experiences that shape the individual's personality. These institutions are viewed as agents of socialization and include the family, schools, social agencies in the community, the individual's peer group, and the mass media. The messages they transmit influence the roles people play and are instrumental in influencing people to behave in characteristic ways. All of these socializing agents use what sociologist's term "anticipatory socialization." This is a technique applied for the purpose of instilling norms and developing the person's identity.

Children become involved with anticipatory socialization at an early age. As they begin playing house, school, or assuming the role of a parent at work, they are imitating adult behaviors. The roles are played with the assumption that they will obtain a similar position in society later in life.

The family unit is the primary agent of socialization. It functions as a "microenvironment" into which the child is born and where his or her earliest experiences with other people occurs. These initial experiences have a lasting influence on the individual's personality development (Kornblum, 1991).

Personality Development

What is personality? How does it develop? Why do we find some people's personalities more endearing than others? What role does personality play in establishing one's sense of identity?

Personality has been described as being complex and multifaceted. Psychologists tend to agree that it is comprised of those distinctive and enduring thoughts, emotions, and behaviors that are reflected in the way an individual interfaces and adapts to the world and its inhabitants. Through the years, several theories of personality development have been proposed. Although each is unique in approach, all attempt to explain how our personalities unfold and why we behave the way that we do. Four of these theories merit discussion.

Psychoanalytic Approach

The key architect in the development of the psychoanalytic theory was Sigmund Freud. He believed that our personality develops in stages and the majority of what we think is unconscious rather than conscious. He stressed that our early experiences with our parents play a critical role in our development and that our external behaviors are merely symbolic reflections of the inner workings of the brain.

Freud described the structure of personality in terms of the id (our instincts), the ego (the demands of reality, the executive branch of personality), and the superego (the moral branch of personality). He felt our lives were filled with tension and conflict and to reduce both our unconscious mind would revert to dreaming while we slept. Furthermore, he placed a great deal of emphasis on defense mechanisms and felt these were used to reduce anxiety by unconsciously distorting reality.

His theory of personality development revolved around five stages, each of which focused on a specific part of the body where we experience intense pleasure. The stages can be delineated as follows:

1. Oral stage (birth to 18 months of age): The infant finds pleasure in the mouth.
2. Anal stage ($1^{1}/_{2}$–3 years): The greatest pleasure comes from eliminative functions.
3. Phallic stage (3–6 years): Pleasure focuses on the genitals as children discover self stimulation.
4. Latency stage (6 years): The child represses all interest in sexuality and develops social and intellectual skills.
5. Genital stage (puberty on): This is a time of sexual reawakening.

In essence, Freud felt that we progress through the stages as our id, ego, and superego struggle among themselves to produce acceptable behavior. As a result, what we observe externally is only the "tip of the iceberg" when compared with what is being resolved internally.

Behavioral and Social Cognitive Theories

Behaviorism and personality development can be linked to B.F. Skinner, who felt that the environment is instrumental in shaping the personality. In essence "he took the person out of personality" (Santrock, 2000, p. 412). He equated one's behavior with one's personality and felt it was not contingent upon any internal traits or thoughts. When determining a person's personality one need only focus on overt behaviors, recognizing that the individual has the capacity for change if new experiences are encountered.

While Skinner is associated with behaviorism and personality development, Albert Bandura and Walter Mischel are considered key figures in the contemporary theory of social cognitive personality development. Both recognized the importance of behavior and environment but felt cognitive factors were equally important. They stressed that although the environment can determine a person's behavior, the individual can also work to change the environment. Bandura felt that three key person/cognitive factors could be influential in influencing a person's behavior or vice versa. These factors are self-efficacy (I can master the situation and produce positive outcomes), plans, and thinking skills. He also felt that observational learning is a key aspect associated with how we learn.

Humanistic Theory

Psychologists closely affiliated with the humanistic theory of personality development are Carl Rogers and Abraham Maslow. They believed individuals had the capacity for personal growth, freedom to choose their own destiny, and the ability to develop positive qualities. Rogers, as well as the other humanistic psychologists, placed emphasis on one's self-concept as a central theme in personality development. He defined self-concept as individuals' overall perceptions of their abilities, behaviors, and personality. His definition of personality included the real self, the self as it really is as a result of our experiences, and our ideal self, the self we would like to be. He further stressed that the larger the discrepancy between the real self and the ideal self, the more maladjusted we would be.

Trait Theory

Theorists who support a trait theory of personality development believe that our personalities consist of broad dispositions, called traits, and that these traits tend to lead to characteristic responses. They further ascertain that traits are the fundamental building blocks of personality. Gordon Allport, one of the leading proponents of the trait theory, believed each individual has a unique set of personality traits, which Allport grouped into three main categories. Cardinal traits are the most powerful and pervasive of the traits and when present dominate the personality. Central traits are limited in nature and can be used to describe most people's personalities. Secondary traits are limited in frequency and are the least important in understanding the individual's personality.

Today most psychologists in the field of personality are interactionists. They believe that both trait variables (person and situation) are necessary to understand the personality. They also feel that the narrower and more limited a trait is the more likely it will predict behavior. Furthermore, they portend that personality traits exert a stronger influence on an individual's behavior when situational influences are less powerful.

Our personalities are complex and multifaceted. While some theorists believe they are innately determined, others feel our personalities are controlled by external situations. Furthermore, some stress that our unconscious is responsible for our personality development, while others emphasize the importance of the internal workings of the mind as one reacts to and with the environment.

What role does personality play with the development of self-identity? Are the two entities related? How do children begin to discover who they are and where they ultimately fit in society? See Table 1.2 for a summary of the various theories of personality development.

TABLE 1.2 *Summary: Theories of Personality Development*

Psychoanalytic Approach	• Sigmund Freud described the structure of personality in terms of the id (our instincts), the ego (the demands of reality, the executive branch of personality), and the superego (the moral branch of personality).
	• Personality development involves five stages: oral (Birth–18 months), anal (1½–3 years), phallic (3–6 years), latency (6–puberty), and genital (puberty on).
Behavioral and Social Cognitive Theories	• B.F. Skinner felt that the environment is instrumental in shaping the personality.
	• Contemporary figures in social cognitive personality development include Albert Bandura and Walter Mischel.
Humanistic Theory	• Carl Rogers and Abraham Maslow felt that individuals have the capacity for personal growth, the freedom to choose their own destiny, and the ability to develop positive qualities.
	• Emphasis is placed on one's self-concept, real-self and ideal-self.
Trait Theory	• Our personalities consist of broad dispositions, called traits, that lead to characteristic responses.
	• Gordon Allport grouped personality traits into three categories: cardinal (most powerful), central (limited in nature), and secondary (limited in frequency).

Establishing a Sense of Identity

By imagining themselves in various roles and assuming the appropriate characteristics, children begin to form a sense of self-identity. They begin to learn who they are and what they are like by comparing themselves to others and by observing how others respond to them. They tell themselves how to behave, how they should have behaved, and how they think others should act in response to their actions.

They begin to identify with those who share the same values, symbols, and common histories, and frequently view members of other cultural groups as strange or different. In this manner individuals begin to establish roots within the ethnic group with which they are the most comfortable. They assimilate their behaviors and strive to gain full membership into the group.

Ethnic Identity, Ethnicity, and Ethnocentrism

An ethnic group is a reference group established by people who share a common historical style (which may only be assumed), based on overt features and values, and who through the process of interaction with others identify themselves as sharing that style (Royce, 1982). One assumes an "ethnic identity" by embracing the symbols, values, and beliefs that belong to that distinct group.

Ethnic groups establish their own norms and expectations. Knowledge is shared and members are expected to become familiar with, and engage in, appropriate cultural behaviors. Individuals seeking membership in the group are judged by their ability to assimilate the required roles rather than by the doctrine to which they claim to ascribe. Birthright alone does not guarantee acceptance by the group. Individuals must be willing to make their identity viable. They must affirm and reaffirm their identity in order for it to remain a salient feature of their personalities (Royce, 1982).

Language lies at the core of one's ethnic identity. It provides the vehicle whereby knowledge, values, and information are transmitted. It quickly becomes apparent if two groups do not share the same communication base. Members are readily identified and grouped with those with whom they can freely and easily communicate.

Language is responsible for the shaping of ideas, and is instrumental in guiding mental activities. It provides a channel allowing for the expression and reception of ideas. Although it is a highly visible indicator of ethnic identity, it is not the sole determiner that distinguishes groups.

Ethnic identity is designated by ethnic boundaries that reflect social differences between groups. These differentiations mark the edge of each social system where they interface with each other. The unique intrinsic characteristics associated with each structure assist in the identification of members (Wallman, 1983).

As individuals become aware of their own identities they also begin to gain insights into how their beliefs differ from nonmembers—those who reside in the larger confines of society. Members begin to identify with an ethnic consciousness and perceive themselves as part of the "we-group," while those who emulate the philosophies of the wider world are considered the "them" or the "out-group" (Patterson, 1983). As individuals differentiate groups and identify with the beliefs of select social structures, they engage in the process of ethnicity.

Ethnicity occurs when there is interplay of two types of social concourses. It is initiated when the inner, intersubjective concourse involving an individual and a we-group interacts with a structured organization involving the wider world or out-group. Three domains of experience within the inner group contribute to the process of ethnicity: consciousness, grouping, and symbolizing (Patterson, 1983).

During their lifetimes individuals become attuned to their own sense of being and their proclivity for belonging. This generates their need to discover and identify with a group whose members share similar experiences and emotions. Through these cultural experiences a kinship is formed and commitments are made. As a sense of belonging is achieved, feelings of group superiority may arise. Members have a tendency to begin comparing and evaluating their group with the cultural groups that surround them. They scrutinize other groups and evaluate the norms and values held by them. Through this process they frequently judge others to be inferior and see themselves as superior. This process of comparing the cultural standards of two groups and considering one's own to be superior is referred to as ethnocentrism.

Stereotyping: An Offshoot of Ethnocentrism

In an attempt to establish ethnic boundaries, individuals seek to categorize groups of people whose behaviors appear to be similar. Generalizations are made and the behavior of one group member is transferred to the anticipated behavior of the group's totality. This process is due in part to the individual's attempt to simplify the world by clustering people into two categories: those who are similar to us and those who are different from us.

Once individuals are categorized, their behaviors are scrutinized. If these behaviors contradict cultural norms, there is a tendency to label these individuals as peculiar or inferior, because they exhibit beliefs and behaviors that are foreign to us. Situations recalled involving such distinctive behaviors, people, or events trigger the formation of opinions, and judgments are formed. Therefore, the less knowledge one has about a group and its behavior, the more likely the person will be influenced by a vivid case or two (Myers, 1987).

When individuals outside the group, consciously or unconsciously, oversimplify a person's behavior and attribute the cause of the action to that person's cultural group rather than to the person himself or herself, stereotyping occurs. Stereotypes develop as those on the outside select some conspicuous attribute or attributes and allow it or them to represent the whole. The person, group, event, or issue is considered to typify or conform to an unvarying pattern or manner, lacking any individuality. Stereotypes assume a sense of relative permanence and inflexibility (Royce, 1982).

Stereotyping directs our interpretations of other's behavior. Whenever we observe a member of a group behaving in the manner that is expected, the fact is noted, and the prior belief is confirmed. However, when a member of the group behaves inconsistently with the observer's expectation the behavior may be explained away as due to special circumstances, or it may be misinterpreted, leaving the prior belief intact (Crocker & McGraw, 1983).

Attribution: Linking an Event to Its Causes

Our interpretation of others' behaviors influences the way we perceive them and the way that we respond to them. This perception affects our decisions regarding how we relate to people. The process whereby we attempt to interpret and explain the behavior of other people is referred to as attribution.

Fritz Heider is widely regarded as the originator of the attribution theory. Termed "common sense psychology," it analyzes how we make judgments about people. People's actions are analyzed and attributed to either internal or external causes (Myers, 1987).

Attributions enable us to understand and react to our surroundings. Situations and events are considered and explanations are provided for why people behave the way they do in various situations. The goal of this theory is to describe how the average person comes to attribute events to one or more of their possible causes (Ross & Fletcher, 1985).

Frequently people tend to attribute other's actions to their dispositions (internal causes) rather than realizing the full impact of the situation (external causes). This becomes particularly evident when people attempt to explain the actions of groups with whom they are unfamiliar. One reason for this lies in the fact that we focus our attention on the people themselves and fail to gain the full perspective encompassing their situation.

When members of a group become angry or behave in a manner we deem inappropriate, we tend to attribute the behavior to the group, rather than to the mitigating circumstances that surround it. Termed "attributional error," it is the mistake individuals make when the explanation for the cause is found in the individual at the risk of underestimating the impact of the situational factors.

Evidence of attributional error can be found within groups, as well as when evaluating the behaviors of those residing outside of the member's "in-group." The error within the in-group occurs when members close to us exhibit inappropriate behaviors and we give them the benefit of the doubt—attributing their behaviors as simply a response to the situation. However, when we are examining the behaviors of those who are not part of the in-group, we tend to assume the worst.

Perspectives in Deafness

One group that falls victim to the error of attribution consists of members of the Deaf community. Because their disability is invisible and the ramifications of it are far reaching, their mannerisms and behaviors are frequently misunderstood and mislabeled. The Deaf community is a sociolinguistic community as intricate and complex as any other sociolinguistic community (Lucas, 1989). It is a small community and membership is gained through the acquisition of American Sign Language (ASL), identification with the collective needs expressed by the group, and a desire to embrace the values of Deaf culture. Membership or inclusion in the Deaf ethnic group is not based solely on one's degree of hearing loss, or because one has deaf parents. Rather, the person must "act like a Deaf person," according to the expectations and evaluations made by group members.

When discussing the topic of deafness it is important to view it from three different perspectives. First, how do outsiders view deafness and the Deaf community? Second, how do those from within the community view their deafness, their language, and their culture? And third, what impact does deafness have on the emerging self as one forms an individual sense of self-identity?

Within the professional sector (medical, audiological, educational, and rehabilitative settings) hearing loss is classified according to the physiological site of the hearing dysfunction. Categories of hearing loss are conductive loss, sensorineural loss, mixed losses, and central auditory processing dysfunction. The term "conductive" loss is used to identify those abnormalities that occur in the external or middle ear. When a blockage occurs in this part of the ear, airborne sound is not heard, or is heard poorly. Other common causes of conductive losses are attributed to middle ear infections or their residual effects, congenital abnormalities in the structure of the ear, middle ear tumors, and otosclerosis, whereby movement of the ossicular chain is restricted. Furthermore, trauma to the head can cause damage to the structures of the ear.

Sensorineural deafness occurs when there is a dysfunction in the inner ear or damage to the auditory nerve. This type of loss may also be due to disease, maldevelopment, or trauma, occurring either prenatally, at birth, or at some point in one's lifetime. Those who experience a mixed loss have concurrent conductive and sensorineural losses in the same ear (Bradley-Johnson, & Evans, 1991).

The term "central auditory processing dysfunction" refers to problems in the auditory neural network. This may involve a dysfunction with the integration and interpretation of auditory stimuli. Auditory processing involves complex functioning that appears to take place in various sites in the brain.

There are in excess of 100 clearly delineated genetic syndromes involving deafness. These are of particular interest to professionals because approximately half of these hereditary syndromes contain evidence of secondary disabilities. Some of these involve the central nervous system and thus have direct psychological correlates (Vernon, 1976).

Although heredity is responsible for approximately one-third of all childhood deafness, the remaining two-thirds can be attributed to disease, drug-induced ototoxicity, prematurity, and complications of the RH factor. Many of these diseases are responsible for neurological damage and other organic pathologies that directly affect behavior (Karchmer, 1985).

When exploring the ramifications of deafness the etiology of the loss is only one factor that merits consideration. Attention is also given to the age of onset at which the loss occurred, and its impact on language development. A distinction is made between individuals who are born deaf or lose their hearing prior to the age of three (prelingually deaf) and those who lose their hearing after their auditorily based speech and language patterns have been established (postlingually deaf). In addition, labels refer to mild hearing loss (27–40 dB loss), moderate loss (41–55 dB loss), moderately severe loss (56–70 dB), severe loss (71–90 dB) or profound loss (91+ dB). Further, the group of individuals who lose their hearing later in life are referred to as the deafened population or late deafened adults. From a medical perspective these groups all reflect characteristics relative to the degree of hearing loss. Table 1.3 illustrates the various categories of hearing loss and the implications for spoken communication.

TABLE 1.3 *Categories of Hearing Loss and Implications*

Degree of Hearing Loss	Label	Implications
27 to 40 dB	Mild	Typically placed in regular education program; preferential seating is important; may benefit from a speech reading program.
41 to 55 dB	Moderate	Has the ability to understand conversational speech at a distance of 3 to 5 feet. Can benefit from a hearing aid, auditory training, and speech therapy; preferential seating is beneficial. Group activities can be challenging.
56 to 70 dB	Moderately severe	Conversation will not be heard unless it is loud. The person will benefit from all of the above and should also receive enhanced language instruction.
71 to 90 dB	Severe	May identify environmental noises and loud sounds. May be able to distinguish vowels but not consonants; special education classes designed for deaf children may be beneficial. Speech is not always intelligible.
91dB+	Profound	Does not rely on hearing for primary means of communication; may hear some loud sounds—special education services are beneficial. Speech may be difficult to understand, or may not be developed.

Adapted from Turnbull et al. (2002).

Hearing Loss

The term "hearing loss" is broad and is applied to anyone who experiences difficulty receiving stimuli through the auditory channel. The term refers to those who are hard of hearing as well as to senior citizens who have lost their auditory acuity due to the aging process. Within the medical and educational domains classifications are made and labels are attached. These labels reflect the degree of loss and the effect it has on the individual's ability to function auditorily in his or her environment.

In the past the term "hearing impaired" has been used to describe individuals with varying degrees of hearing loss. Although some hard-of-hearing and deaf individuals continue to use the term today to describe their hearing loss, others who are deaf may find the use of the term offensive. These individuals frequently prefer to be referred to as deaf or hard of hearing.

Hard of Hearing

Professionals frequently categorize a person who experiences a slight to moderate loss as hard of hearing. Oftentimes their hearing can be enhanced through the use of hearing aids. By incorporating communication strategies they are able to access the mainstream of the larger hearing society and function as hearing individuals. The label "hard of hearing" can be misleading. For some, it implies the inability to hear high-frequency sounds such as the high notes projected by a musical instrument, a whistle, or a bird chirping. For others, its impact is within the range of hearing responsible for the understanding of speech. Although some may be able to understand these sounds, they may be prevented from conversing with those who are soft spoken, and may be prevented from comprehending messages expressed over the telephone.

Those wishing to be identified as members of the larger hearing society may inwardly deny the ramifications of their hearing loss. Their acceptance of what they can and cannot hear is influenced by this desire. Others who experience similar patterns of hearing loss may find solace within the realm of the Deaf community, preferring to communicate through American Sign Language (ASL). Although the medical profession classifies both as hard of hearing, one may opt to become hearing while another chooses to become a member of the Deaf community.

deaf

Audiologists use the term "deaf" to identify individuals who have varying degrees of hearing loss. Educators also use this term to label those whose hearing loss necessitates the provision of special services. In essence, the use of the word with a lowercase "d" refers to those who, with or without amplification, receive fragmented acoustic messages or no message at all (Paul & Jackson, 1993). Although they may hear some loud sounds, they do not rely on their auditory mechanism as their primary channel of communication.

Within the professional sector, the labels hard of hearing, moderate hearing loss, and severe to profound deafness can serve in a very useful capacity. They provide practitioners with terminology that can be employed for identification purposes, allowing for placements to be made and services to be rendered. However, these labels can be misleading and must be used with caution.

Classifications of hearing loss are based on an audiological evaluation. The audiologist determines how well the individual can hear and identify sounds at varying frequencies. Speech reception threshold and discrimination tests are administered, focusing on the person's ability to hear and understand speech sounds. This in turn is coupled with the individual's capability to function socially in everyday settings.

Additional factors influence how well the person is able to respond to auditory cues within his or her surroundings. Environmental sounds, educational background of the individual, and ability to speechread all influence the degree to which the person functions audiologically as a "deaf" individual.

The medical model evaluates hearing loss and searches for ways to alleviate the "problem" so the person can function "as close to a hearing person" as possible in a hearing society. The focus is on "fixing" the individual through capitalizing on residual hearing, promoting hearing devices, and offering communication strategies that can be used while interacting with those who can hear. However, not all individuals who experience a loss view themselves as needing to be "fixed."

Deaf

In 1972 the term "Deaf" began appearing in the literature pertaining to deafness. During that time, James Woodward proposed the idea that the word "deaf" be capitalized when referring to "a particular group of deaf people who share a language—American Sign Language (ASL)—and a culture" (Padden & Humphries, 1988). Since that time the term has been used to identify those who have some degree of hearing loss, who identify with and behave like other Deaf people, and who share the same cultural values of the Deaf ethnic group (Wilcox, 1989).

Hearing loss alone does not guarantee membership into this group, nor is it strictly dependent on Deaf parentage. If a person is profoundly deaf and has Deaf parents, but does not "act" or "behave" like a Deaf person, he or she is not viewed by group members as a member of the group (Lucas, 1989). The peer group within the Deaf community determines the rules for behavior. From these communities, values are instilled and cultural characteristics are personified.

Deaf Communities

The Deaf community is very small. Roughly one in a thousand children is born deaf or becomes deaf prior to the age of three. And less than 10 percent of these children are born to Deaf parents (Bienvenue & Colonomos, 1992).

Deaf communities are located in cities throughout the United States, and each is uniquely affected by its location. Within the community members share common goals and work toward achieving them. A Deaf community may include persons who are not themselves Deaf but who actively support the goals of the community. These individuals work with Deaf people to achieve these goals (Padden, 1989).

The Deaf community is a microcosm, similar to any hearing community, wherein members pursue a variety of interests, activities, and intellectual pursuits (Garretson, 1991). Those who are Deaf embrace the group because they sense a feeling of acceptance and belonging with those who share similar concerns. Within the community they do not feel self-conscious about their deafness, and can relate to each other as people, without the stigma of a disability being attached. Within this domain they thrive, not in a subculture, a subsociety, or a ghetto, but as a composite part of a whole. Those who elect to become members view themselves as members of a distinct linguistic and cultural group rather than as disabled people (Garretson, 1991).

Deaf Culture

Upon entering the Deaf community, members bring with them their own sense of cultural identity. These identities reflect the heritage of the individuals, and are an outgrowth of their roots, ancestry, religious beliefs, families, and upbringing. These factors contribute to the shaping of the person's values, and are reflected in what the individual cherishes. Values vary from person to person and provide insights into who people are, where they came from, what they believe in, and frequently where they are going (Gannon, 1991).

Each of us has several cultural identities. Our beliefs and values form a composite and influence the manner in which we respond to our surroundings. Deaf individuals possess the cultural identity bestowed upon them by their family unit and enter the Deaf community bringing these beliefs and values with them. These ideas are then shared, modified, and transformed into the fabric that represents the culture of the Deaf community.

Within this culture there is folklore, history, song, poetry, art, and a growing collection of plays. There are puns in sign language and deaf jokes (Gannon, 1991). Language lies at the heart of the Deaf community and one's hands are thought of as sacred because they provide the communication link with other members. However, sign language is only one of the cultural features displayed by this group.

The ability to come together and share in the companionship with those who are like-minded, to communicate concerns, ideas, and beliefs, provides the foundation for Deaf culture. In this social setting, the stories and literature of the people are handed down, heroes are created, and support is given. Within this cultural setting a need is met, and those who are Deaf are provided with the opportunity "to communicate deeply and comfortably in their own language" (Padden, 1989, p. 10).

Some deaf individuals elect membership in the Deaf community while others do not. Some form a Deaf identity while others prefer blending into the mainstream of the larger hearing society. How is one's Deaf identity formed and what relationship, if any, does this identity have on self-concept and personality development?

Establishing a Deaf Identity

This chapter has focused on how one's identity emerges throughout the duration of a lifetime. Personality theories have been examined and group affiliations have been explored. Based on the premise that a Deaf community does exist and that there is a Deaf culture, we can begin to examine the age when deaf children recognize they are deaf, equate their deafness with differentness, and include this characteristic as an identifying feature when describing themselves.

Significant people, events, and environmental conditions all contribute to the self-identity process. By viewing the individual as he or she emerges from childhood into adolescence and on into adulthood, we can trace how our identities are shaped and formed.

A Deaf Identity Development Model

The first theory of Deaf identity development is attributed to Neil Glickman (1993). Based on the assumption that Deaf individuals can be viewed as a minority group, he ascertained that the same psychological processes involved in minority identity development can be applied to Deaf individuals.

Glickman's Deaf Identity Model proposes four developmentally related Deaf cultural identities: Culturally Hearing, Culturally Marginal, Immersed, and Bicultural (Glickman & Carey, 1993). Each identity type is considered a potential stage that affords the individual the opportunity to acquire a Deaf identity. Where the person begins the developmental process is influenced by various factors. These include the hearing status of the person's family, the age of onset when the hearing loss occurred, and the individual's social and educational experiences (Melick, 1998).

The Culturally Hearing stage can be described as people who use the hearing world "as their reference point for normality and health, and the Deaf world for abnormality, disability, and deviance" (Glickman & Carey, 1993, p. 276). In this instance deafness is viewed as a disability, hence the medical model, as something that is to be overcome. Culturally Hearing deaf individuals seek out hearing people, identify themselves as experiencing a hearing loss, rather than being deaf, and avoid deaf people in general. They search for ways to become more "hearing like" so they can function as a member of the dominant hearing society.

The Culturally Marginal stage encompasses those deaf individuals who experience life by trying fit between the Deaf and hearing worlds, but who never become comfortable in either. Characteristics of individuals in this stage include their confusion regarding their identity, their demonstration of inappropriate social behaviors in either culture, a sense of being a misfit in both cultures, a weakened command of both English and ASL, and a sense of isolation (Glickman, 1993).

Another stage in this model has been termed Immersion identity. These individuals immerse themselves totally in the Deaf world. During the initial part of this stage the Deaf world is idealized, ASL is thought to be superior to English, and hearing people are viewed as malevolent and oppressive toward the Deaf. Hearing values such as using one's voice, wearing hearing aids, or signing in English word order should not be endorsed (Glickman, 1993; Glickman & Harvey, 1996a). Toward the end of this stage "one's vision of affirmative Deafness grows and becomes more inclusive. One becomes more concerned with supporting other Deaf people than with attacking Hearing people" (Glickman, 1993, p. 100).

The final stage Glickman describes is Bicultural. Those functioning within this stage have achieved a "personal and balanced perspective on what it means to be Deaf" (Glickman, 1993, p. 100). These individuals affirm deafness as a cultural difference and feel strongly connected to other Deaf people.

At this stage the person is able to ascertain and appreciate the differences between the Deaf and the hearing worlds. A value is placed on both English and ASL and alliances with supportive Hearing people are maintained.

Glickman's Deaf Identity Development model has provided us with insights into the way deaf/Deaf individuals perceive themselves fitting into hearing and Deaf communities.

At what point do deaf children become aware of their deafness as a physical difference? Once this physical difference is recognized, what affect does it have on self-concept and self-esteem? And at what point do deaf children assume a Deaf identity?

Childhood Deafness and Self-Identity

When attempting to answer the question "How do deaf children develop an understanding of themselves and their deafness?" it is essential to examine factors in their social environment that are likely to influence their self-understanding. As Padden and Humphries (1988) have so succinctly stated, "Being able or unable to hear does not emerge as significant in itself; instead it takes on significance in the context of other sets of meaning to which the child has been exposed" (Padden & Humphries, 1988, p. 22).

One of the contexts that impacts significantly on child development is the family unit. For it is in this setting that the socialization process begins. From the time infants enter the world they become part of a family unit. This unit can be characterized as consisting of hearing or Deaf family members, married or single mothers, parents with or without other children, parents from diverse ethnic and socioeconomic backgrounds, and parents with shared communication systems. As they begin to interact with these significant others, bonds of varying degrees are formed and the developmental process is initiated.

Central to this core of development is communication. At a very young age the child becomes part of the "feedback loop." This loop allows for early expression and reinforcement and is instrumental in assisting children in developing an understanding of who they are. Later as they make the transition from home to school and they form associations with peers this "feedback loop" grows and children begin to develop their own sense of unique identity.

Communication conveys a sense of caring and acceptance, and thus becomes the vehicle for establishing one's concept of self-identity. When deaf children are born to Deaf parents a shared communication system exists and from the onset the child becomes an interactive player who can fully utilize the feedback loop. However, when children are faced with the reality that they cannot freely access the communication surrounding them, they can become painfully aware of what "deafness" means. Countless stories have been recited in the literature reflecting the isolation felt from being cut off from familial exchanges. As deaf adults reflect back on their experiences of deafness, many share similar stories of anger and frustration:

> At home, dinner was absolutely the worst time; I couldn't understand the jokes. Everyone was laughing and I'd say, "What's so funny?" And they'd sort of shrug it off and say "Nothing" I couldn't follow the conversations my parents and sister had either, though sometimes I could tell they were talking about me.
>
> It made me mad growing up . . . I mean always being left out. It didn't have to be that way. But my parents felt that if I ever learned fifty signs I'd be contaminated. So I can say, I never relaxed. Every sentence was an effort, all day long (Lane, Hoffmeister, & Bahan, 1996, p. 219).

In addition to stories such as these, there are also numerous tales of children who assumed that deafness was unique to them and that there was no one else like them. Because of the low incidence of deafness, deaf children born into families with all hearing members may never encounter another deaf individual until they attend school. Even then, depending where they are raised (in an urban or a rural area), where they attend school (in a residential or a mainstreamed setting), will determine if they will have several deaf peers, only one or two peers, or remain the only deaf child in the school.

Recently several studies have been conducted on school-aged deaf children to determine the effects of communication, family background, peers, and school setting on the development of self-concept.

Developing a Positive Self-Concept

However, before embarking on a review of the studies that pertain specifically to deafness, it is helpful to examine the origins of theories regarding self-development. For it is from these early beginnings that contemporary research studies have been grounded. Although the early psychologists and sociologists differed in their individual views of self-development, they all stressed the importance of social/environmental experiences and how they impact on the formation of one's self-concept.

From the initial works of William James (1890–1983) to the recent writings of Ulric Neisser (1993), the development of the self has been described through the eyes of the psychoanalyst, the behaviorist, and the cognitive psychologist (Prout, 1998). While the psychoanalysts have placed emphasis on cognition and on the developmental nature of the self, the behaviorists have stressed the importance of the social environment to human growth and self-actualization.

Early theorists postulated that children progress through stages or steps as they become aware of their self-identities in relation to others (Baldwin, 1894–1968; Kohlberg, 1987; Mead, 1934; Cooley, 1909–1956). Although they differed as to how many stages or steps there were and what transpired in each one, all of them concurred that the shaping of the self emerged through social interaction. Later theorists recognized the value of stages; however, they also emphasized the importance of studying the self as both an "object" and as a "subject" (Mahler, Pine, & Bergman, 1975; Kegan, 1982; Stern, 1985). In this respect the object (me), refers to the part of the self that is involved in interpersonal relations, and the subject self (I) is viewed as the internal component of the self.

Theorists such as Kegan (1982) and Stern (1985) have examined how the individual differentiates himself or herself from the world while establishing boundaries for the self as a unique entity. Both believe that self-development begins in infancy and continues to grow throughout childhood. According to Kegan, as children grow and develop, they are engaged in self-reflection. Self-reflection becomes an integral part in development and leads to an understanding of both the self and an understanding of others. He conceptualizes the child as progressing through six stages as his or her identity is formed. In his analysis, cognitive development and social experiences are described as being the two major forces that drive self-development.

Stern (1985) shared similar views with Kegan. He hypothesized that there are four senses of self that emerge at varying times during infancy (the emergent self, the core self, the subjective self, and the verbal self); and that once formed, they remain with us throughout our lifetimes. He felt strongly that our "sense of self and its counterpart, the sense of other, are universal phenomena that profoundly influence all our social experiences" (Stern, 1985, p. 5). By dealing with others as subject-subject, rather than subject-object, the child develops a sense of intersubjectivity. Furthermore, when the child enters the final stage of verbal development, he or she "demonstrates competence in the language of the community and learns how to organize the world accordingly" (Prout, 1998, p. 19).

These theorists, as well as others, have set the stage for contemporary research. Damon and Hart (1988), Harter (1990), and Neisser (1993) are three of the contemporary researchers who merit particular discussion. Although all of them have retained some of the basic ideas of earlier writers, they have each added their own important insights.

Damon and Hart (1988) felt that self-understanding needed to be studied qualitatively rather than quantitatively. So they developed an interview protocol that could be adapted and used at various grade levels. Throughout a six-year time span they interviewed children. The results of their study confirmed several trends found in previous research:

1. An early awareness of self is based on the activities one becomes engaged in and the contingencies that arise from these activities.
2. Children develop an early awareness of physical self (size and gender).
3. Children progress through an age-related shift where they initially define themselves through external characteristics (physical, material, active) to a point in time when they identify themselves in terms of internal characteristics (psychological, spiritual).
4. There is an age-related tendency when children integrate these diverse aspects of self into a coherent system (Prout, 1998).

Based on these trends, Damon and Mast defined and provided a detailed description of four developmental levels children traverse while forming and shaping their self-identity. In essence, their research reflected the following: in early childhood the child identifies the self by categories; in middle and late childhood their ability to engage in comparatives and assessments emerge; in early adolescence they become aware of the implications of interpersonal relations; and in late adolescence they develop an understanding of the self that includes both systematic beliefs and plans. Furthermore, these researchers stressed that the child experiences all the various selves: physical, social, and psychological throughout each of the stages.

Susan Harter (1990) is another contemporary theorist who is sensitive to the multidimensional nature of the self. Within her work she examines self-concept through five domains: scholastic competence, athletic competence, physical appearance, peer social acceptance, and behavioral conduct. Harter has postulated that children's self-concepts show increasing differentiation and integration with age. Her research indicates that children between the ages of 4 and 7 are unable to differentiate between cognitive and physical competence; however, children between the ages of 8 and 12 can distinguish between mathematical and reading competence. She supports the premise that children develop an understanding of themselves based on the various roles and membership categories that define who they are. Her findings are significant when examining how school-aged children develop their sense of self within the educational setting.

One final theorist bears mentioning before examining the research that pertains to self-identity and deaf children. Ulric Neisser (1993) has focused on the ecological nature of self-development. He describes five selves that come to fruition from five different sources of information that is available to us. He states that the "ecological self" is the initial self that develops. This emerges as a result of the individual's action in the environment. Another self that develops early in life is the "interpersonal self," resulting from the infant's interactions with others. Neisser states that these early selves are perceived but not constructed or imagined. The actual "conceptual self" where the self is viewed as an object of thought is perceived near the end of the first year. The "private self" emerges at age four or five; at this time children become aware of their minds and realize that their thoughts are private. The fifth self that Neisser refers to is the "narrative self," resulting in an individual's inclination to construct a life story or a narrative (Prout, 1998, p. 26).

From the early writings to the contemporary schools of thought, recurring themes of self-development have been noted. Some of these include the self being viewed in components, the importance of social experience and social interaction to self-development, the self being viewed from the dimensions of the self and the other, and the self developing through stages. In addition, recent theorists have ascertained that the mind constructs a self that is not exclusively dependent on social environment, but that it is a self reflective of strong cognitive capabilities.

How do these theories relate to deaf children? What research has been conducted in the area of self-development and self-identity with those who are deaf? Do children who experience a hearing loss parallel the same stages as hearing children seeking to establish a self-identity? At what point do children recognize that their deafness makes them different? Then, after this realization occurs, how do they develop an understanding of what deafness means to them, thus allowing the child to integrate the physical attributes of deafness into the total self? How is a deaf child's self identity affected by his familial unit, communication mode, and educational setting? And at what point does the deaf individual transition from identifying deafness in terms of physical attributes posing a barrier to social interaction and begin to view it as a positive identifying feature granting him or her access to the Deaf community?

Establishing a Deaf Identity: A Lifelong Process

Beginning in the late 1980s and continuing into the twenty-first century, the field of deaf education has seen a proliferation of articles that examine the cultural aspects of Deafness based on those who seek affiliation with the Deaf community. The majority of these publications focus on Deaf adults and their role in preserving the language, customs, and values of this particular community. Research indicates that those most instrumental in keeping the "spirit" of the Deaf community alive reflect these beliefs: they embrace the language (ASL), traditionally receive their education in a residential school setting, support and promote the social activities initiated from within the group, and have assimilated a Deaf identity. How do deaf children progress through the developmental stages to arrive at adulthood with a positive self-concept and a healthy Deaf identity?

The Early Years

From the time a child is conceived until the time he or she is born, parents assume they will produce a healthy child complete with all of its "working parts." However, when this does not occur and a diagnosis of deafness is made, the parents may experience feelings of guilt, sorrow, anger, and depression. While some deny the medical findings, others consult an array of professionals in an attempt to find a cure. Although a small percentage of deaf babies are born to deaf parents (approximately 10 percent), the majority enter the world and find themselves as members of the larger hearing community. Initially hearing parents may be relieved to discover their child has only a hearing impairment, only to realize later the significance of this as they attempt to draw their child into dialogues that hinge on spoken communication.

From these early beginnings, parental frustrations can mount and be projected onto the child, thus planting the seeds for inadequacy and inferiority to develop. For it is through our interactions with others that our self-concept begins to form and take shape. Tom Humphries (1991) has written extensively about learning to be deaf. He reminds us that the view deaf children have of themselves is "unmarked" until they discover others' definition of them. This definition is conveyed through spoken communication that begins in infancy and continues throughout a lifetime. In some homes parents embrace a method of manual communication and attempt to include their child in daily conversations and the discussions involved in planning family activities. In these instances family members accept deafness as another dimension that must be accommodated through alternative communication avenues. When this occurs, the child has the opportunity to interact through sign language, and a signal is sent that the child's deafness is accepted. This is similar to the signal conveyed by Deaf parents as they interact with their children through sign communication.

However, this is not the case in most homes. The majority of hearing families (approximately 90 percent) embrace spoken communication as they interact with their deaf child. When this is used as the sole mode of communication, the child can infer that his or her deafness is being rejected (Bat-Chava, 1994). Furthermore, the child may sense that the spoken mode of communication embraced by the family unit is superior to one involving signed exchanges.

Although a plethora of research studies stress the positive effects of early sign communication, the studies themselves may remain in the professional sector and never find their way into the parents' hands. Therefore many parents are oblivious to the literature. This in turn impacts the approach they will take as they raise their child. The majority of parents tend to rely on communication skills and parenting strategies that they were subjected to as children. As a result they may not be sensitive to the special needs of their children, and expect them to function as if they could hear normally. However, when difficulties arise and breakdowns in communication occur, the parents then find themselves feeling very unsettled and wondering what is wrong with their child:

> In a Deaf-hearing exchange, the hearing person does not accept any breach or difference in communication and is uncomfortable when that breach occurs. Rather than approaching the interaction as one of mutual misunderstanding the hearing person typically blames the Deaf "other" for the communication failure (Rose & Smith, 2000).

The breakdown is a shared problem, and it accentuates both the parents' and the child's inability to communicate. However, when this occurs hearing parents may become extremely uncomfortable with their inadequacies and seek validation for their actions by placing the blame on their "dysfunctional" child. In those instances where a form of manual communication is needed but is not employed, this can signal to the child that a visual form of communication is substandard and can be construed by the child to mean that he or she is inferior.

Many parents and significant others feel that communicating in sign disrupts the expected behavior of everyday life in the larger society:

> It sets the user off as someone who is not following the rules and is not behaving, as one ought to. Moreover, this inability to listen and/or speak disrupts what are perhaps the most fundamental assumptions of what should happen in face-to-face conversations. Differences of this sort are devalued by the larger group as an undesired characteristic, that is, they are stigmatized (Goffman, 1963).

Hence, this sets the stage for the early underpinnings of feelings of being different and inferiority that can be internalized by the deaf child who is raised in the home with hearing parents.

Frequently parents of deaf children underestimate the impact they have on the early development of their child (Altshuler, 1974; Meadow, 1969). When children feel accepted by their families, especially by their parents, this feeling will positively affect their self-esteem. However, when communication is nonexistent or breakdowns occur, the child may internalize his or her feelings of frustration (Schlesinger & Meadow, 1972).

When an appropriate communication outlet for these feelings does not exist, they can remain internalized for an extended period of time. Then when the child enters school these feelings may begin to surface and manifest themselves in a negative manner. At that time, he or she may display problem behavior that is evidence of a psychological impairment (Marschark & Clark, 1993–1998). However, it is essential to realize that it is not the deafness itself that is directly causing the problem, but rather the inability to communicate (Schlesinger & Meadow, 1972). Therefore, the problem behavior is an external representation of a breakdown in the communication process that can be correlated with the child's sense of low self-esteem.

Communication, or lack thereof, influences the way we perceive ourselves, especially in relation to other people. It equalizes the playing field while enhancing our self-identity. It provides us with a means of self-expression through which we reveal who we are. In addition, it supplies us with a springboard whereby we assess other's reactions and responses to us and determine where we fit in. This self-expression can be equated with a sense of empowerment. However, the absence of a sense of communication contributes to a depressed understanding of social and cultural knowledge, because "very little we know is not filtered through our everyday experiences" (Humphries, 1991, p. 215).

Furthermore, communication serves other critical functions. It provides the vehicle through which language is developed and later opens our minds to the vast richness locked within the meaning of words. Deaf children denied access to a mutual form of communication face barriers as they try to grasp an understanding of meaningful spoken messages. As a result they see the spoken English language itself as "an object instead of a source of meaning." This realization is often compounded when deaf children enter school and attempt to engage in academic tasks that assume and require competence in the English language (Finn, 1995).

Some deaf children become aware of their linguistic handicap early as they embark on their academic career. For others the realization comes at a much later time. However, it is critical to note that from these initial endeavors into communication, children begin to weave the perceptions of how others assess their persona, including their self-identity.

Establishing an Identity within the Educational Arena

Gail Finn has poignantly described the effect and the impact of early communication on the development of her self-concept. Through her recollection of one of her early school experiences we gain insights into the significance of a shared language:

> The particular moment of my first perceived self-concept, which I can remember vividly. I was seven and at a deaf/oral residential school (having been there since the age of three), I had no concept of time, therefore I had no idea of my birthday, my age, or the meaning of the clock's hands. As I was sitting in the communal dining room, I "overheard" older deaf children talking with excitement about birthdays. (We communicated through lipreading and homemade local gestures.) Although my parents gave me a birthday party every year before the age of seven, I had not the slightest idea what the intention of a birthday celebration was, nor the meaning of birthday. However, at seven I began to perceive my "existence" and became gradually motivated to find out more about myself—my age, birth date, month, and year (Finn, 1995, pp. 4–5).

At this point she experienced what the Russian linguist Lev Vygosky refers to as a "dialectic leap." She began to realize that the word "birthday" did not refer to a single object but a group of objects, in this case individuals. The connection was made between what she saw (sensory perception) and what she thought, and a generalized reflection of reality was formed. This experience provided her with the opportunity to begin developing the internal component of her inner self.

Numerous studies have examined the development of self-concept in deaf children and adolescents. While many have compared those who are deaf with those who are hearing, others have examined the positive and negative implications of the educational settings (mainstreamed versus residential). We know that communication and social interaction are two of the key variables that impact the internalization of one's self-concept. We also know that family background plays a significant role in this developmental process.

Recent studies have begun to compare the developmental process deaf individuals engage in as they form their self-identity, with the developmental process that ethnic minority group members experience when they seek to clarify their identities. The early work provided by Neil Glickman and his Deaf Identity Model (1993) has provided the impetus for additional studies. Three of these merit particular discussion:

the works of Teresa Prout, Robin Gordon, and Amy Melick. While each of their studies has a slightly different focus, they all examine how deaf individuals arrive at an understanding of what it means to incorporate a Deaf identity.

The Work of Teresa Prout

Prout's dissertation (1998) examined how deaf children develop both a general understanding of themselves and a specific understanding of deafness. She interviewed nine children with severe to profound hearing losses ranging in age from 5 to 14. All of the students involved in her study had hearing parents and all of them signed with the exception of one of the fathers. They were all from middle-income families, and all had been involved in a parent-infant program and received home services throughout their child's first three years.

All the students entered a center-based program when they were either 3 or 4 years old; and at the time of the study they spent between 50 and 90 percent of their school day in regular classes with support services. These services included sign language interpreters and support teachers. Furthermore, they associated with hearing rather than deaf peers. All the students wore hearing aids and they used sign combined with speech as their main mode of communication.

Prout questioned whether the children's perceptions of themselves varied with age, whether deafness was a key factor in the children's general understanding of the self, and how the social environment was related to the children's understanding of themselves and their deafness. Data from her study revealed strong age trends with regard to how the children viewed both themselves and their hearing loss. In general, the deaf students' general development of self-understanding was similar to that of normally hearing peers. However, the responses made by students at various ages suggested there was a difference in one respect—the awareness of their deafness was a key aspect of their self-understanding, especially during the adolescent years. In addition, the data collected from the interviews indicated that the children's specific understanding of deafness also followed a developmental pattern.

The very young children (ages 5 and 6) who were interviewed appeared to equate their hearing loss with external indicators, such as their hearing aids and their sign mode of communication. Children in the middle age group (ages 10 and 11) were able to go beyond the external indicators and define terms associated with deafness such as "deaf, hearing, and hard of hearing." However, at this age they still lacked a precise understanding of the effects of hearing loss. It is interesting to note that this group only mentioned their deafness when they were asked about it. Then they alluded to the fact that they had a special knowledge (sign language) and wisdom (the experience of being different and deaf) that was valued by their hearing peers (Prout, 1998).

Those interviewed in the oldest group (ages 12 to 15) were able to discuss the impact of deafness on their lives. They also shed insights into how they felt their hearing losses made them different from their peers. Through their comments the researcher was able to gain insights into their perceptions of being the sole deaf member among their hearing classmates. When questioned what they would ask for if they could have three wishes, they gave Prout responses such as, "Communicate better (read lips—not be separate from others)." Also, when asked, "What made you what you are?" a student responded, "Being with people. That's how to make friends with people." These responses indicate that deaf adolescents are on par with their hearing counterparts (Prout, 1998, p. 78).

Responses from the interviews suggested that deaf children progress through a development pattern similar to that of hearing children, with two significant qualifications. First, because of the communication delay experienced by the young children, it was difficult to ascertain their understanding of their self-concept. Second, deafness appeared to be a major issue in a child's self-concept beginning in early adolescence.

Although hearing loss seemed to be an integral aspect of a deaf child's self-understanding at all ages, it was more salient to the older children. These adolescents were more aware of the negative aspects of deafness, although their awareness never included a totally negative evaluation of their own hearing loss (Prout, 1998, pp. 67–68).

Research conducted with hearing children suggests that within the first few years of life children develop a general sense of self. By the time they are 3 or 4 they can use categorical identifications to describe themselves, and by the time they are 8 or 9 they become involved with social comparisons. The answers given by the deaf children in this study reflect that they progress through the same levels of general development. Their responses further suggest that deafness, especially its role in inhibiting communication, becomes a focal point for their self-concept during adolescence when interpersonal relationships become critical.

Interview results from this study contradict the findings of studies that conclude that deaf students attending public school programs demonstrate impaired self-concept (e.g., Farrugia & Austin, 1980; Loeb & Sarigianai, 1986, as cited in Prout). Rather, this study supported earlier findings of Bozik (1985) and Cates (1991) that suggested deaf students' self-concept was at the very minimum on par with their hearing peers. This may be due in part to the degree of parental involvement, the mode of communication used both within the home and within the school environment, and the educational support services (Prout, 1998).

Although this study reflected that deaf student's self-concept development runs parallel to their hearing peers, it is important to note that the older students' comments suggested a desire to have a deaf peer group. These findings support previous research of Stinson and Whitmore (1992) that indicated that deaf students who spend the majority of their time in mainstreamed programs need special consideration with regard to their social needs and desire for a deaf peer group.

Prout's study is limited in sample size and in number of interview questions. However, the results indicate that "deafness did not warp the development of self-understanding, that it was different from that of hearing peers, but not necessarily inferior, and in some cases, more complex" (Prout, 1998, p. 113).

Robin Gordon is another researcher who has explored self-concept and identity patterns of deaf adolescents. Her research study focused on a cross-cultural comparison to identify and investigate the ways female and male deaf adolescents view the world and perceive themselves in relation to it.

The Work of Robin Gordon

Participants in Gordon's study (1997) included male and female Deaf adolescents ranging in age from 14 through 21. Forty-eight of the students attended private schools, of these, 29 were residential students and 19 were day students. Additional subjects involved in the study included 42 residential students who all attended the state-operated school for the deaf. Thirty-seven females and 53 males participated in the study; 12 of them had at least one parent that was deaf and 78 of them had hearing parents. The mean age of the participants was 16.82 years, and those involved represented diverse ethnic backgrounds, with Caucasian (66) and African American (17) being in the majority.

The purpose of Gordon's study was to investigate the ways male and female Deaf adolescents viewed themselves in relation to the world. She wanted to ascertain how they identified with their culture and how they perceived their sense of self. Furthermore, she wanted to determine how this sense of self influenced their view of the daily activities that were required of them (Gordon, 1997).

Gordon developed a Deaf Cultural Identity Scale (DCIS) to measure how deaf individuals identify with the Deaf community and Deaf culture. Her scale was adapted from the original Deaf Identity Development Scale developed by Glickman and Carey (1993) and the Racial Identity Attitude Scale developed by Helms and Parham (1996). The scale consisted of 40 items and questions were presented using a Likert scale format. A few sample statements representative of the questionnaire are included below:

1. Deaf people should use ASL.
3. Deafness is a terrible disability.
18. I do not fit in with either hearing or deaf people.
30. I remember my pride as a deaf person when I am with hearing people.
40. Deaf people should only socialize with hearing people. (Gordon, 1997)

The scores from the DCIS were used to assign participants to different cultural identity categories. These categories reflect those found in Glickman's (1993) DID Scale, and are labeled Hearing, Marginal, Immersion, and Bicultural. Upon completion of the questionnaire, each individual's highest score was used to place him or her in one of the designated cultural identity categories. This study presented evidence indicating that there is a significant difference between the ways adolescents with different Deaf cultural identities evaluate their real and ideal sense of self within the time orientation subcategory Present. "Deaf adolescents with a bicultural identity appear to evaluate Real Self, Ideal Self, and Present more positively than Deaf adolescents with other cultural identities" (Gordon, 1997, p. 73).

Results from Gordon's study further indicate that Deaf adolescents with a bicultural identity:

- Evaluate themselves more positively and feel better about themselves than those Deaf adolescents whose scores reflect membership in the other cultural identity categories.
- Rate their present lives more positively than other cultural identity groups.
- View their activity in life as an integrated being of self that is interfaced with external factors.

These findings confirm previous studies found in the literature that correlate one's bicultural identity with higher and more positive levels of self-esteem (Bat-Chava, 1993; Glickman & Carey, 1993). Those who reflected a marginal cultural identity tended to:

- Feel that they were currently not moving forward in a positive direction. This could be attributed to them feeling less satisfied with their current life situation.
- Feel like they did not fit with either the Deaf community or the hearing majority.
- Feel uncomfortable in both groups.
- Have a tendency to interpret the world around them as more hostile and bad natured (Gordon, 1997).

Further results from Gordon's study reflected how gender influences the way Deaf adolescents view the present and the future, and their perceptions of themselves. There was a striking difference between how males and females viewed the world and their relation to it. Males regarded the larger hearing society as a place where they would attend postsecondary education and find employment, and thus perceived it as an important factor in their lives. One the other hand, females tended to feel more responsible for the home and family and therefore felt less of a need to interact with the larger hearing society.

Although Gordon's study is limited in scope and in geographic location, it does shed light on the importance of supporting bicultural programs whereby deaf children can begin to establish a positive Deaf self-identity. Furthermore, the research clearly illustrates that without a strong cultural identity base, Deaf individuals will experience difficulty venturing into and negotiating with the hearing world (Rutherford, 1988).

As Corson (1995) has so aptly concluded:

> Culturally different children deprived of the everyday reinforcers of values that are central to their culture's worldview have less understanding of who they are, where they are going, and their value as group members (Corson, 1995, p. 19).

In essence, we must know who we are (our self-concept) and where we belong (our cultural affiliation) before we can freely mingle in and out of groups that are both similar to and different from us.

The Work of Amy Melick

Amy Melick (1998) has also conducted research in the area of deafness and the development of self-identity. She conducted a qualitative study involving Deaf adults to determine how this group of individuals learned about and became connected with Deaf culture. Within her study she explored the relevant and influential factors that contributed to the shaping of a Deaf cultural identity of Deaf adults who had been born into hearing families.

Melick (1998) used a semi-structured interview with ten deaf adults (five men and five women, between the ages of 19 and 64) who had all attended school in a mainstreamed setting. She wanted to determine if they shared common patterns of enculturation, and how they experienced the enculturation process. She also wanted to ascertain if they fell into one of the four types of cultural identity proposed by Glickman's DID model.

Based on previously held beliefs that one's Deaf cultural identity stems from having Deaf parents and/or attending a residential school, she wanted to determine how this same identity was developed by those who had hearing parents, who experienced a hearing loss from an early age, and who received their education in mainstream programs.

Results of her analyses yielded a model reflecting four phases involved in developing a deaf identity that were relative to the Deaf community. The four phases can be identified as follows:

Phase One: Being an Outsider

Phase Two: Encountering/Connecting

Phase Three: Transitioning from an Outsider to an Insider

Phase Four: Self-Definition

Melick identified one central theme that ran throughout the entire process of establishing a Deaf cultural identity: the sense of being different from others and thus feeling that one is an outsider. From the early stages of experiencing feelings of isolation, frustration, confusion, and rejection in the hearing world to similar feelings as one enters the boundaries of the Deaf world, a level of self-acceptance is formed. Each of these phases provides insights into the formation of one's Deaf identity.

Phase One: Being an Outsider.   Deaf children born into hearing families begin their lives as outsiders in a hearing world, and thus their first role models project an image that is different from them. During this initial stage they may attempt to model hearing behaviors even though they may struggle with speech as they endeavor to communicate with those around them.

The awareness that they are different from those in the hearing community can be heightened when children attend a mainstreamed program. In this setting they may encounter one or two others who experience some degree of hearing loss; however, the majority of their peers will be hearing. Unlike deaf children who attend a residential school where they have daily contacts with Deaf adults and Deaf culture, most of those who attend a mainstreamed program are not privy to these contacts or this environment. Therefore, their awareness and understanding of this community may be virtually nonexistent.

Phase Two: Encountering/Connecting.   This phase is used to describe a life event or events when a deaf person encounters the world of Deaf culture. Melick stresses that encountering is not synonymous with assimilating, and that contact with the culture and the language does not automatically equate with one wanting to belong. The encountering process can occur for different individuals at various times throughout their lives.

Phase Three: Transitioning from an Outsider to an Insider.   The encountering process can be a time of both excitement and tribulation for the deaf individual. Those who have experienced a lifetime struggling to communicate with the larger hearing world may see this group as a respite from their daily frustrations. They may sense a feeling of community and shared communication, thus prompting them to transition into the Deaf world. However, they are quick to realize that membership is not automatically granted. In order to become part of the group the individual must learn ASL; learn and adopt Deaf cultural norms, behaviors and beliefs; and change the perceptions he or she holds about what deafness means and about Deaf persons. This is an active process, a time of learning and change for the person. It is also a time when members from the "inside" question the individual's desire to become part of the group.

Phase Four: Self-Definition.   Moving through the transition period, one begins to develop a comfort level with the role and identity he or she has formed. At this point the person has developed a sense of self-acceptance and is proud to be called a Deaf person. He or she feels a sense of belonging, and identification and connection with the Deaf community. Even though some within the community may still view the person as an "outsider," the individual in his or her own mind becomes an insider, assumes a Deaf identity, and feels that he or she finally belongs to a group with others like him or her (Melick, 1998).

Interviews conducted by Melick determined that Deaf individuals do experience a common pattern of enculturation that is both sequential and for individuals cyclical. Furthermore, it is viewed as a lifelong process that is influenced and shaped by changes in personal and societal events. While each of the participants experienced their enculturation in an individualistic way, overall they all described it in terms of a struggle.

Deaf adults who participated in this study described how they struggled to fit in throughout their early years while functioning as minority members in a hearing society. They also defined the inner turmoil they experienced as they transitioned from one culture to the next and the difficulty they encountered while trying to gain acceptance in the Deaf community. Furthermore, they expressed how they felt as they entered the final phase of enculturation whereby they experienced a sense of "belonging, connectedness, fulfillment, and acceptance" (Melick, 1998, p. 168–169). In turn, this connectness allowed them to be proud of their membership in the Deaf community while they continued to interface with the larger hearing society. According to Melick, this identity-building process is developmental in nature and is contingent upon the experiences and changes that occur in each phase.

Although there are limitations to any study, Melick's research heightens our awareness and understanding of the process deaf children of hearing parents go through in their quest to determine who they are, where they belong, and how they want to relate to others. Comments received from those who were interviewed reiterate the impact that a shared communication base and the opportunity to freely interact with others have on us as we internalize and develop a sense of our own self-identity.

Impact of the School Setting on Deaf Identity

The studies cited above are only three of the many research projects that have been designed to examine peer relationships, self-identity, self-esteem, and socialization in the school setting. Mainstream classrooms and included environments have been compared with residential settings in an attempt to determine the optimal learning environment for deaf children. These learning environments encompass academic as well as social and emotional development, whereby educators take into account both the curriculum that is taught in the classroom and the unwritten curriculum (Garretson, 1977). This includes informal or spontaneous interactions, extracurricular activities, sports, clubs, and an assortment of other activities that transpire outside the classroom.

Communication, both formal and informal, lies at the heart of these studies. For it is through communication that students develop friendships and peer groups, share their thoughts, and shape their identities. As common interests are discovered, bonds are formed and boundaries are distinguished between those who belong to the "in-group" and those who remain on the outside.

Through this social interaction students learn how to listen as well as participate, how to assume leadership roles, and how to express personal feelings. Furthermore, they learn how to handle confrontation, rejection, and acceptance. These experiences afford students the opportunity to discover who they are (self-identity) and develop positive feelings about themselves (self-esteem).

School placement decisions greatly impact the opportunities for peer interaction and involvement in extracurricular activities. The number of available activities and the ease with which one can communicate will directly impact the child's self-confidence and self-esteem. These activities vary from residential schools to mainstream settings.

Residential School Setting

Individuals who have attended residential schools have commented on the following:

- Many felt they were very fortunate to attend school with so many of their peers, for here they developed close, long-lasting friendships (Foster & Emerton, 1991).

- Some felt that being a full and equal participant in student organizations, clubs, sports, and other extracurricular activities was a plus (Stinson & Foster, 2000).
- Some students commented on their feelings of being fundamentally separated—culturally, academically, socially, and physically—from hearing society.
- Students also noted a lack of experience with hearing people, not knowing what to expect in dealing with them or how to engage effectively in interaction with them (Foster, 1989b).
- Some mentioned they missed going home from school every day and associating with neighborhood friends.

Mainstream and Included Classrooms

Students who have received their education in these types of settings have commented:

- Interpreters usually function solely in classroom settings, thus students are not privy to hallway comments, lunchroom discussions, or dialogues that occur on the bus.
- Even though their support services might be good, by the time they receive questions via the interpreter the hearing students have already responded (Stewart & Kluwin, 1996).
- Because of the communication difficulties experienced between themselves and their hearing classmates, they had limited opportunities for peer interaction and frequently experienced social isolation.
- Some felt they benefited from attending mainstreamed settings because they believed they received a better education and learned how to interact with hearing people.

What the Research Shows

Since the 1970s the face of deaf education has undergone a significant transformation. Research indicates:

- Seventy percent of deaf and hard-of-hearing children are educated in local schools.
- Twenty-two percent are educated in residential schools.
- Eight percent are educated in local, separate day schools (Schildroth & Hotto, 1994, 1996).
- Students educated in public schools suggest that students with a range of hearing loss experience an absence of close friendships (Antia, Kreimeyer & Eldredge, 1994; Stinson, Whitmore, & Kluwin, 1996; Tvingstedt, 1993).
- Deaf adolescents consistently feel more emotionally secure and more accepted in relationships with deaf peers than with hearing peers (Foster, 1989a; Stinson & Whitmore, 1991).
- Quantitative studies with questionnaires or rating scales designed to tap self-esteem indicate that self-esteem is not related to educational placement (Cohen, 1991; Gans, 1995; Jacobs, 1989).

- Higher self-esteem is associated with greater academic achievement (Desselle, 1994; Joiner, Erickson, Crittenden, & Stevenson, 1966; Koelle & Convey, 1982).

Factors That Influence Self-Identity

Research indicates that family hearing status, degree of hearing loss, onset of loss, educational environment, and communication all contribute to the formation of one's self-identity. While researchers may vary in their opinions of which educational settings may be the most beneficial, almost all agree that communication is essential for development to occur.

Communication can be viewed from two distinct perspectives: first, the communication exchange that occurs when individuals interact with others and their environment (external factors); second, the process that occurs when we reflect on these interactions and from our perception of what has transpired. Both processes are instrumental in shaping our self-identity. However, there is a third factor that also plays a significant role in this developmental process: our personality traits. Those attributes that influence how we respond to life's situations add another dimension that must be considered when we examine self-identity.

Personality traits contribute to why one individual feels lonely in one situation while another person feels content. These traits are associated with our temperament, and are linked to those characteristics that describe our internal feelings (introverted, extroverted, happy, malcontent, hostile, gregarious, and so forth) that are expressed in our external behaviors. Therefore, the personality we bring into any given situation, the events that occur at that point in time, and our perception of what transpired are all instrumental in shaping who we are and what we will become. Figure 1.1 illustrates the interaction that transpires.

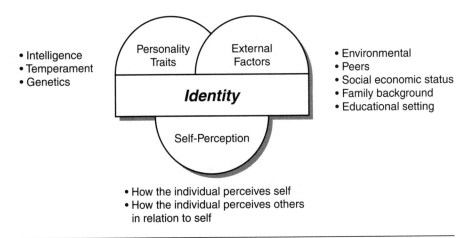

FIGURE 1.1 *Factors that influence self-identity.*

Strategies for Enhancing the Deaf Child's Self-Concept: Enriching Self-Identity

Current trends indicate the majority of deaf and hard-of-hearing children are educated in mainstream/inclusion settings rather than residential schools. Recent research has also revealed that children and adolescents who assimilate a bicultural identity tend to evaluate themselves more positively and feel better about themselves. What can be done to encourage a positive sense of self within deaf and hard-of-hearing children? The following strategies represent only a few examples of what can be implemented:

- Ensure communication occurs at all levels. Particular attention should be paid to individual differences. Create opportunities for effective communication exchanges so the child can effectively interact with you, thus eliciting feelings that he or she is making a contribution to the discussion.
- Make sure all activities (both formal and informal) are accessible to the child. Encourage and structure small group work where the deaf and hard-of-hearing child can participate and begin to develop communication and socialization skills.
- Include both informal and formal instruction in sign language and Deaf culture. All children need the opportunity to learn about both Deaf and hearing cultures.
- Be open to flexible scheduling. While some children may grasp subject matter in one setting, they may struggle in the same setting with different material.
- Structure activities so the child can succeed and then reinforce positive behavior.
- Emphasize the positive side of cultural diversity and accentuate how each of us has something to contribute.
- Be prepared to explain what is entailed in appropriate social behavior. Give students the opportunity to role-play these behaviors and reinforce them.
- Provide students with forced-choice decisions whereby they are compelled to make decisions. This will set the stage for developing an internal locus of control.
- Provide children with the opportunity to meet and socialize with positive Deaf adult role models. This will assist them in forming their own self-identity.
- Provide children with leadership training at all levels so they can assume these roles when called upon to do so.

Summary

The composite of who we are can be traced to our early beginnings. Through a life-time of experiencing, interacting, and communicating, our identity is woven into the mosaic it represents. A multitude of factors contribute to the design, allowing each of us to develop into the unique individuals that we are.

By providing all children, especially those who are deaf and hard of hearing, with the tools they need for social interaction, we promote growth and foster self-development. This in turn allows children to form their own identities and, once established, provides them with a foundation as they continue on their journey through life.

2

Family Dynamics and Deafness

The evolution of American families can be viewed through a kaleidoscope of diversity. Characterized by a multitude of structural relationships, socioeconomic backgrounds, and ethnic identities, today's families represent a unique contrast of social entities. From the onset, children are exposed to the rich cultural heritage of their parents. Here, they are steeped in a predetermined set of values, beliefs, and expectations. Expected to conform to the norm, they are molded by those around them and emerge with an identity reflective of their parentage. By examining the structure of the family unit, ethnic diversity, and economic variability, one can gain insights into the environments where deaf and hard-of-hearing children grow and develop.

Variations in Family Structures

In 1989 the Massachusetts Mutual Life Insurance Company conducted a survey of 1,200 randomly selected adults. They were asked to check the definition that best described what "family" meant to them. Of those surveyed, fewer than one in four (22 percent) selected the traditional definition: "a group of people related by blood, marriage or adoption" (Seligmann, 1989). This is indicative of the changes evidenced in the present-day structure of family units. The nuclear family of the past is being replaced with single-parent families, extended families, blended families, subfamilies, augmented families, families with secondary members, and nonblood extended families.

Single-Parent Families

Recent statistics indicate that the average duration of a marriage in the United States is just over nine years (Santrock, 2000). Of those who divorce, many will remarry. However, others will remain single and raise their children in single-parent families. According to Norton and Glick (1986) fewer than 10 percent of all U.S. families live in their original nuclear families and over 80 percent of children under the age of 18 will spend a portion of their school years in a single-parent family. Currently 23 percent of children under the age of 18 live in single-parent families.

Divorce is not the sole contributor to this family structure. Other single-parent family units occur as the result of problems that have been experienced historically, as well as what is occurring today: children born out of marriage, spousal desertion, and death of a spouse (Epanchin, Townsend, & Stoddard, 1994).

Approximately 90 percent of deaf and hard-of-hearing children are born to hearing parents (Moores, 2001; Scheetz, 2001; Vernon & Andrews, 1990). Research suggests that more than half of these children might spend part of their childhood being raised by only one parent. These children, like their hearing counterparts, respond to being members of single-parent households in a variety of ways. For some it creates economic hardships and can contribute to parental depression. For others the new living arrangements facilitate reduced levels of stress, and provide for a more amiable home environment.

It is critical to keep in mind that all single-parent families are not alike, nor are they all dysfunctional or pathological (Hetherington & Stanley-Hagan, 1995). For many the role the extended family creates, as an alternative to the traditional nuclear structure, affords children the opportunity to be raised in a warm, nurturing environment.

Extended Families

Extended families have traditionally provided support to adolescent and never-married mothers, as well as nuclear families involved in a crisis such as incarceration, drug and alcohol dependence, or spousal abuse. However, more recently this role has been expanded to provide support to family members who are pursuing higher education, purchasing housing, or encountering serious eldercare and childcare difficulties.

There is considerable variation within the framework of the extended family structure (Epanchin, Townsend, & Stoddard, 1994). While some rely only on parental support, other family units are comprised of larger kinship networks that include aunts and uncles. Cross-cultural variations account for the diversity in this family structure.

Stepfamilies and Blended Families

The number of remarriages involving children increased steadily until the early 1990s, when it began to stabilize. Currently, stepfather families, where the woman has primary custody of the children from a previous marriage, comprise the majority of the stepfamilies, although in some instances the father has custody of his children from a previous marriage. When both parents bring children into their marriage from previous relationships, a blended family unit is formed.

Many variations occur in step- and blended families. As new roles are created a sense of boundary ambiguity may ensue while family members attempt to ascertain their roles and responsibilities within the newly formed family system (Santrock,

1999). Although research on stepfamilies has lagged behind studies that focus on divorced families, those that do exist indicate that children of all ages show a resurgence of behavior problems following a remarriage of their parents (Freeman, 1993).

Subfamilies

Billingsley (1968) has defined three primary variations of subfamilies. These occur when two or more individuals become involved in: (1) the "incipient extended family" where a married couple with no children of their own take in other relatives; (2) the "simple extended family" where a married couple with their own child or children take in other relatives; and (3) the "attenuated extended family" that consists of a single, abandoned, legally separated, divorced, or widowed mother or father with his or her children, who are taken into the household of other relatives. Each of these structures develops patterns of interaction between family members.

Families with Secondary Members

These family units are designed to "take in" relatives, primarily children and elderly persons during a time of crisis or transition in the family life cycle. Established to provide a haven for refuge, these units can include nieces, nephews, parents, and grandparents (Hill, 1993). When examining the family structure from the perspective of the extended family, it is imperative to consider the secondary stressors that may be introduced into the home.

Augmented Extended Families

Augmented extended families refer to those family structures where children are cared for by parents who have no biological relationship to them, and they are not related by marriage, ancestry, or adoption (Hill, 1972). In these instances children may have been neighbors, church members, or playmates of their children at school. Those situations frequently occur when families attempt to provide these children with a better home environment.

When engaging in a discussion of family dynamics, each of these structural groups needs to be taken into consideration. It is critical that these units be viewed both from within the context of the historical experiences that surround them, and from the perspective of the current circumstances that embody them. This understanding, coupled with an awareness of the characteristics that distinguish one ethnic group from another, and an appreciation for the varied socioeconomic backgrounds that they represent, helps to provide a more in-depth look at the complexities surrounding contemporary American families.

The Diversity of Families

Kumabe, Nishida, and Hepworth (1985) as cited in Epanchin (1994) describe family ethnic groups as "a collection of people who conceive of themselves as being alike by virtue of their presumed common ancestry and cultural heritage (race, religion, or national origin) and who are regarded by others to be part of such a group" (Epanchin, Townsend, & Stoddard, 1994, p. 77). The U.S. Census Bureau affords citizens the opportunity to identify with race based on categories established by the federal government. Based on the response to this survey a portrait can be presented that reflects the diversity of the American people.

When the 2000 census was conducted, two significant changes were made in the form. First, the questions on race and Hispanic origin were changed and delineated as two distinct concepts. The question on Hispanic origin asked if someone were Spanish, Hispanic, or Latino. The question on race asked the respondents to indicate what race or races they considered themselves to be. Second, respondents were given the option of selecting one or more race categories to indicate their racial identities. This is the first time an attempt has been made to identify the biracial/bicultural population. Table 2.1 provides a description of the categories that were used in the 2000 Census.

Table 2.2 reflects the data that was compiled from the survey regarding the percent of the total population that identified with each of the categories by race or by the Hispanic or Latino population.

Members who ascribe to each of these distinct groups embrace the values, beliefs, and traditions that are cherished by that specific collective whole. Furthermore, they adhere to the communication patterns and the child-rearing practices that are established by the group. Through interactions with respected group members they form in-group loyalties as well as perceptions of the larger, dominant group.

How do the lifestyles of these cultural groups differ from the one held as "the ideal" by the middle-class Anglo-European white segment of society? How does each of these ethnic groups view the family unit and child development? And finally, how do these various groups view their offspring who are born with a disability?

TABLE 2.1 *Categories by Race as Defined by Census 2000 (Based on information from the U.S. Census Bureau, Census 2000a)*

CATEGORY	DEFINITION
White	Origins of any of the original peoples of Europe, the Middle East, or North Africa
Black or African American	People having origins in any of the black racial groups of Africa and including people who indicated they were Nigerian or Haitian
Asian	Origins in any of the original peoples of the Far East, Southeast Asia, or the Indian subcontinent
Native Hawaiian and other Pacific Islander	Origins in any of the original peoples of Hawaii, Guam, Samoa, or other Pacific Islands
Some Other Race	Category included for respondents who were unable to identify with the preestablished categories

TABLE 2.2 *Population by Race and Hispanic Origin for the U.S.: 2000 (Based on information from the U.S. Census Bureau, Census, 2000b)*

Race and Hispanic or Latino	Percent of Total Population
White	75.1
Black or African American	12.3
American Indian and Alaska Native	0.9
Asian	3.6
Native Hawaiian and Other Pacific Islander	0.1
Some Other Race	5.5
Two or More Races	2.4
Hispanic or Latino, total population	*100.0*
Hispanic or Latino	12.5
Not Hispanic or Latino	87.5

Examining these questions can provide insights into communication patterns, discipline techniques, familial expectations, and beliefs surrounding children who are born with special needs.

In the space of this chapter, an in-depth examination of the diversity found within and between cultural groups is not possible. However, by highlighting values and beliefs cherished by each of these ethnic groups, a thumbnail sketch of the vast multicultural variations exhibited by America's families can be represented. It is critical that these factors receive consideration when engaging in any discussion pertaining to the nature of family dynamics. Although caution must always be taken when attempting to describe any group in a brief generalized exposé, by recognizing that differences exist, family patterns can be examined within the context of their ethnic and cultural roots.

Families with Anglo-European Roots

This group is comprised of individuals who have immigrated to the United States from several countries in Europe. Originally representing England, Germany, Ireland, and Italy, they brought their cultural beliefs and values with them when they entered this country. Their backgrounds, coupled with the experiences they encountered in a new land, contributed to the shaping of the major cultural values and practices reflected by the dominant culture found in America today.

Some of these values include a focus on independence, freedom, assertiveness, equality, self-help skills, and self-directness. From an early age, children are taught to be self-reliant and independent. Individualism and privacy are stressed and a high premium is placed on job success and materialism (Lynch & Hanson, 1998).

Communication is open and direct, with one expected to make eye contact when conversing. Anglo-European Americans believe that trustworthiness, sincerity, and directness are communicated through this acceptable form of eye contact (Asante & Davis, 1989). During communication exchanges, emotions may be expressed freely. However, personal topics are avoided unless the discussion occurs among family and close friends. The concept of family life typically refers to members of the immediate family and may include the grandparents, who may or may not be actively involved, as extended family members. Other family members are usually termed "relatives" (Lynch & Hanson, 1998).

Traditionally, nuclear households were characterized as male dominant, with the father employed outside of the home and the mother responsible for household duties including childcare. However, as of 2002, more than one of every two mothers with a child under the age of 5 was employed and more than two of every three with a child from 6 to 17 years of age were engaged in the workforce (Santrock, 2002). These women have continued to work while retaining their primary household and childcare responsibilities.

Disabilities are ascribed to a variety of causes, including genetic disorders, diseases, and perinatal trauma. Familial acceptance of the disability is dependent on several factors. These include, but are not limited to parental familiarity with the physical condition, expectations and attitudes projected by extended family members and friends, religious beliefs, and support from significant others.

Families with African American Origins

The people referred to as African Americans originated from many of the tribes located in central and West Africa. They arrived in this country representing individuals from highly varied backgrounds. Although some came as indentured servants, many more arrived as slaves against their will (Bennett, 1966; Holloway & Bass, 1993). Through the centuries, the majority of them have shared in their common experience of racism, prejudice, and economic oppression (Terrell & Jackson, 2002).

In contemporary America, blacks represent a diverse group. This is evidenced in their values, lifestyles, and cultural preferences. Today they represent individuals who are born in America, the Caribbean, and Africa, and thus reflect the traditions of of three ethnic groups, as well as distinct social classes (Davis, 1993; Hill, with Billingsley, 1993; McAdoo, 1997).

The terms "family, my folks, my kin, my people" are used to describe the family unit and the individuals who feel they belong to each other (Willis, 1998). Although family members may elect not to live together, the extended family, including distant relatives, is a tremendous source of social and/or financial support (Hill, 1993; Taylor, 1994). Key to the socialization process is instilling in children a sense of an African American consciousness. Through this process they become familiar with a common history, heritage, and an awareness of being a black person in a white dominant culture (Willis, 1998).

African Americans believe that children are the future and thus place a high premium on the attainment of one's potential through the acquisition of education and life skills. Furthermore, they value religion and view it as a confirmation of identity, of being God's children (Billingsley, 1974). Although they ascribe to a variety of denominations, children are taught from an early age that they must "believe in something."

When children are born with a disability it is often interpreted in one of two ways: as bad luck or misfortune, or occasionally because of the "sins of the father." Although blame may be initially assigned to one family member or another, this phase is usually of short duration. Then family members devote time to securing the necessary health, medical, and social services that are needed to assist in the development of their child (Willis, 1999).

Families with Asian Origins

One of the largest groups of immigrants entering the United States are people of Asian decent. This population represents approximately 30 distinct ethnic groups with very diverse national origins and histories (Chan, 1986). The initial group originated from three distinct regions on the Asian continent: East Asia, Southeast Asia, and South Asia. Each of these regions is characterized by a unique national heritage, language, beliefs, and customs. From the onset they have faced discrimination and have formed segregated communities to protect themselves.

The dominant groups residing in the United States today include Chinese, Filipinos, and Japanese. The Japanese American population constitutes the largest subgrouping of the Asian American population with numbers approaching one million, many of whom were born in this country (McAdoo, 1993). Profound intra- and interethnic differences can be noted among the various groups. These distinctions are reflected in subpopulation sizes, regional concentrations, preferred residential location, degree of acculturation, educational level, occupational skills, socioeconomic status, language, religion, ethnic identity, and cultural values and beliefs (Fong & Mokuau, 1994; Lee, 1996; Min, 1995; Uba, 1994).

In Asian culture hierarchical roles and status govern behavior, and subordination and interdepence are valued. Furthermore, in traditional Asian cultures, cooperation, obligation, and reciprocity are valued over Western values that place a high premium on competition, autonomy, and self-reliance. Rules and roles are considered of utmost importance when determining context and content of social interaction (Chan, 1986).

The family is viewed as the basic unit or backbone of society; it serves as the tie between the individual and society and is a model of society as a whole (Major, 1989; Te, 1989). Central to the individual's life is the focus on loyalty, mutual obligations, cooperation, interdependence, and reciprocity among family members. Furthermore, within the family unit efforts are ingrained to promote the welfare of the group, with little emphasis placed on individuality or on self-serving activities.

Children are viewed as gifts from God, and from the beginning their parents set very high expectations for them. A child's behavior is thought to reflect on the family, and therefore respect, obedience, and discipline are highly valued. Communication is unidirectional from parent to child, and children are not expected to express feelings, wants, likes, and dislikes (Cheng, 2002).

Children born with severe disabilities (developmental disabilities, physical/sensory impairments, and serious emotional disturbance) can be viewed with considerable stigma. This is created in part by traditional views that link specific disabilities to various causes (Lynch & Hanson, 1998, p. 310). Many of the Asian beliefs presume that a disability is caused by the mother's failure to follow prescribed dietary and other healthcare practices during pregnancy and/or during the postpartum period. The mother may also believe she is directly responsible because she violated certain cultural taboos. In essence, feelings of embarrassment and shame may arise, thus impacting child development.

Families with Native American Origins

Contemporary American Indian families emanated from a variety of tribal groupings spread throughout the United States. Each group has its own unique geographic distinctions, tribal histories, religious beliefs, and practices. Eight different language groupings categorize the Indian language, including Iroquoian, Muskogean, Caddoam, and Athapaskan (Joe & Malach, 1998). The uniqueness associated with each group is often rooted in a core value system that is shared collectively by most tribes of like or similar descent (Sipes, 1993). Values that some American tribes share include the extended nature of the family structure, and the ultimate value of the group rather than the individual (Joe & Malach, 1998). Although there is evidence of some shared values, it is critical to note that the diversity within their cultures is as great as in all of the European cultures.

Native Americans have been residing in every state and in most major cities of the United States since 1998. While approximately half of this cultural group lives on the 278 reservations and in the 200 Alaskan native villages, the other half live in urban areas (Westby & Vining, 2002). However, because they comprise less than one percent of the population, they frequently remain an "invisible" part of the population.

Many of the tribes share similar views on the importance of the tribe and child-rearing practices. Generally speaking, members feel a strong sense of pride in their heritage, tribal identity is important, and the clan and the family comes first before the individual. Elders hold a place of respect and are considered valued members of both the family and the tribal unit.

Children are taught by example rather than by direction, and in many tribes grandparents carry on parenting roles. Extended kinship structures are very common, and in some tribes the uncles rather than the parents provide most of the discipline

(Joe & Malach, 1998). At an early age children are taught to be self-reliant; they are exposed to tribal humor, religious beliefs, and cultural values.

The general tendency among Native Americans is to accept natural and sometimes unnatural events as they are. This is representative of the Indian belief that events occur as part of the natural order of life; therefore, they are taught to accept both the good and the bad (Coles, 1977). When children are born with a disability it may be attributed to supernatural or natural causes.

Upon hearing that their child has a disability due to a genetic disorder, parents may accept the medical professional's diagnosis, but will frequently turn to cultural resources in an attempt to discover why it occurred. Traditional ceremonies may be conducted to begin the healing process and to prevent the condition from weakening the individual. Many hesitate to receive assistance from public agencies, based on previous experiences with them that have resulted in a sense of distrust being established. Frequently subjected to racism, discrimination, and/or cultural insensitivity, they avoid the help offered by public agencies (Joe & Malach, 1998).

Families with Latino or Hispanic Origins

Latinos and Hispanics are the fastest growing ethnic group in the United States. They represent a variety of nationalities that have immigrated to this country from Cuba, Mexico, and Puerto Rico, as well as several Central and South American and Caribbean countries (Zuniga, 1998). Residing on the coasts and along the southern border, most are familiar with the Spanish language. Between the various groups there are considerable local, regional, and national variations in their dialects, colloquialisms, and speech patterns. However, in spite of these differences, the language serves as a unifying feature of this cultural group (Epanchin, Townsend, & Stoddard, 1994).

Within the literature there is evidence to suggest that in addition to a common language, persons of Latino and Hispanic descent are likely to share a worldview that is grounded in a religious ideology with widespread Christianity (Harry, 1992). The purpose of marriage is to bear children, and the role of the family is valued as the central operating principle in the life of this population (Bernal, 1982; Garcia-Preto, 1982).

The majority of Latino families are two-parent families, with the extended family configuration providing support to the nuclear family. Parents exhibit strong nurturing tendencies toward their children and interdependence on other family members is encouraged. From the onset male and female roles are established among the children. While daughters are instructed to develop positive attitudes and suppress emotions such as anger and aggression, sons are taught how to be dominant and independent (Kluckhohn & Stodtbeck, 1961). Parents encourage their children to develop close emotional ties with their siblings and fighting among brothers and sisters is discouraged (Goodman & Beman, 1971).

Families view children first as members of the extended family unit, and second as individuals. All adults and extended family members, as well as godparents, may be involved in child rearing and decision making (Ortiz, 1998). Furthermore, all are expected to discipline the children (Vega, 1990). Within this family setting, children are assigned responsibilities around the home that often relate to childcare or to working with other family members.

Oftentimes, the perception held by those outside of this group is that Hispanic and Latino families do not value education. However, this is often a fallacy, fueled by erratic school attendance and lack of parental involvement. However, upon closer inspection, it becomes apparent that older children may be required to stay at home when the need arises to care for their younger siblings. This is frequently the case among migrant families due to their poor economic conditions. At other times this occurs due to the lack of knowledge parents posses regarding school policy. It is important to bear in mind that one of the driving forces behind them moving to this country is to secure a quality education for their children.

When a child is born with a disability, it may be interpreted as happening because of one's belief in a punishing God. Furthermore, it may be attributed to "evil in one's environment" or to a "curse" placed on the child (Zuniga, 1998, p. 234). Because folk beliefs may play a role in the explanation of causation, children may be the recipients of folk remedies or the services of spiritual healers (Delgado, 1988). Social class, degree of acculturation, and educational background all contribute to the family's acceptance of the child's disability. As previously emphasized, diversity occurs within every ethnic group and caution must be taken to insure that global generalizations are not made.

Table 2.3 provides a summary of these characteristics, as well as the beliefs, values, and practices described in previous sections.

Families with Biracial/Bicultural Origins

A discussion of families representing various ethnic groups would not be complete without mentioning individuals of biracial/bicultural origins. Information gleaned from the Childcare Health Program in Oakland, California, indicates that between 1970 and 1990, birthrates for children with one black and one white parent escalated. As early as 1968, 8,758 births were recorded, compared with 26,968 in 1981, and 52,232 in 1991. From 1970 to 1995, the number of black-white couples more than quintupled, reflecting an influx from 65,000 to 328,000. Furthermore, the number of interracial marriages (marriages between people of different races) increased from 321,000 in 1970 to more than 1.4 million in 1990. Additionally, this agency indicates that almost one-third of the children adopted from the foster care system are placed with families of a different race, and that Americans adopt nearly 16,000 children from other countries.

These family units illustrate another unique segment of American society that merit consideration when discussing the dynamics of psychosocial development. Although space does not warrant an in-depth discussion of the dynamics that ensue when biracial children interface with the larger society, it is critical that this part of the population be recognized when family units are discussed.

TABLE 2.3 *Cultural Diversity: Contrasting Beliefs, Values and Practices (Based on information in Lynch & Hanson, 1998)*

Anglo-European Roots	Native American Roots	African American Roots	Latino Roots	Asian Roots
Communication				
• Low-context communication. • Expression is direct, explicit, informal, spontaneous, emotionally expressive, egocentric.	• Some Native American people are brought up to show respect for those in authority by not asking direct questions and not giving eye contact.	• High-context communication that includes not just the actual words offered to convey a message, but also relies heavily on personal delivery that resonates the affective as well as the factual (Harry, 1992, p. 238).	• High-context communication that includes not just the actual words offered to convey a message, but also relies heavily on personal delivery that resonates the affective as well as the factual (Harry, 1992, p. 238).	• Expression is indirect, implicit, nonverbal, formal, emotionally controlled, self-effacing, modest.
Significance of Family				
• Nuclear and immediate family bonds. • Less respect for the elderly in the family. • Tendency for more democratic family structure.	• Group life is primary. • Respect for elders. • Family is defined as extended family members and fictive kin.	• Kinship and extended family bonds valued. • Respect for elderly and their role in the family.	• Tendency for more patriarchal family structure. • Overt respect for elderly. • Extended family system promoted.	• Family as primary unit or backbone of society. • Each individual views self as an integral part of the totality of the family. • The larger social structure encourages a social/psychological dependence on others. • Respect for elders.

Child-Rearing Practices

- Males and females may share equally in child-rearing practices.
- Children may spend extended periods of time with caregivers outside the home.
- Frequently children are involved in the decision-making process from an early age.

- Grandparents, not parents, may hold primary responsibility for the care of the children.

- More authoritative child-rearing practices.
- All responsible adults take part in the education and discipline of the child.

- More relaxed with child development.
- Parent/child relationship has more importance than marital relationship.
- Class, region, and acculturation stage may contribute to more or less traditional format for child rearing.

- Parent provides authority and expects unquestioning obedience.
- Family makes decisions for child.
- Older children are responsible for the sibling's actions.
- The strongest family ties are between parent and child rather than between spouses.

Perceptions on Disabilities

- No single causation is ascribed to disabilities.
- Sometimes the care the mother takes during pregnancy is blamed for the disability.
- View individuals as masters of their own fate.
- Feel adverse nature of the condition can be overcome through resources, work, and ingenuity.

- Most attribute disabilities to illness, misfortunes, or to supernatural or natural causes.
- Within the natural category, disability may be attributed to breaking a cultural taboo.
- Parents may accept medical diagnoses, but turn to tribal healers to prevent the condition from worsening.

- Disabilities may be interpreted in one of two ways: as bad luck or misfortune, or occasionally as the result of "sins of the fathers."
- The attitudes of causation have no real effect on how parents interact with the person with the disability.

- Can interpret the birth of a child with a disability as due to a curse.
- Amulets may be worn to ward off evil spirits.
- Folk beliefs may be used to explain disabilities.
- Those from middle and upper class may have a more educated view of causation.

- Varies within the different Asian cultures.
- Some view deafness as a curse, ostracizing individuals from society.
- May be viewed as a personal embarrassment.
- May view the person as mute and incompetent to learn oral language.

Economic Variability and the Family Unit

Structural variation, ethnic diversity, and socioeconomic status are key components frequently discussed when describing the family unit. All have a direct bearing on the home environment and the quality and quantity of interaction that occurs between family members. While structural differences and ethnicity influence value formation, economic variability determines the amount of resources each family has available to them.

Children raised in poor socioeconomic conditions are faced with challenges unfamiliar to those who are nurtured in middle- and upper-class settings. As parents struggle to provide for their children, their energies may be consumed in basic needs, leaving little if any time to nurture those around them.

According to the U.S. Census Bureau (2000), 16.2 percent of children, residing in the United States live in poverty. Furthermore, the poverty rate for children is higher than for those who are age 18 and older. Although children comprise 37 percent of the poor, they only account for 26 percent of the total population. When individuals are subjected to poor economic environments, daily survival is of paramount importance. Parents may find that their primary foci revolve around protecting their children from violence, locating affordable housing, keeping food on the table, and finding the means to purchase prescribed medications (Lynch & Hanson, 1998). Poverty strikes at the heart of family dynamics. Oftentimes it reduces the parent's ability to provide a structured and stimulating environment. Furthermore, it robs them of planning for the future while leaving family members vulnerable to the stressors that are frequently associated with lower-income groups.

These three factors of family structure, ethnic background, and socioeconomic status are all intact when infants enter the world. The environment that surrounds their arrival, the unique personal characteristics all babies bring with them, and the interactions that follow characterize each family unit. By recognizing that these variables exist, one can gain a broader perspective of the dynamics that occur when a deaf child is born into a hearing family. In these instances, all of the above variables must be considered, with deafness adding another unique dimension. As this new individual begins to find his or her place in the family, members will begin to form their perceptions of what deafness is and how it relates to them.

Hearing Parents/Deaf Children: Cultural Conflicts

Most hearing adults are raised from infancy in homes where spoken communication is taken for granted. Through a lifetime of verbal exchanges, ideas are shared, values are formed, and social expectations are instilled. From the onset "we are socialized to look at ourselves, the world, and our role in certain ways" (Gonzalez-Mena, 1997). This socialization process originates at birth and continues through adulthood. It influences the way individuals view themselves in relation to those around them and eventually influences how they interrelate to those residing in the larger community. In turn, it affects the way parents will eventually socialize their children.

Hearing culture places a high premium on spoken communication, a communication system that requires both hearing and speech. Members of the group assume that their offspring will hear and give little if any thought to the possibility of producing a child with a hearing loss. Therefore, when the diagnosis of deafness is confirmed and becomes a reality for the parents, they are frequently flooded with a plethora of emotions. Alternating between feelings of pain and disbelief, parents struggle to decipher medical jargon in an attempt to discover what to do for their child. Caught between feelings of anger, guilt, and self-doubt, they begin their journey to determine what they can do to ensure that their child will develop into an independent adult with an identity reflecting the underpinnings of self-esteem and self-confidence.

Volumes have been written about the grief hearing parents experience when they discover their child is deaf. However, much of this grief is a result of the way society views deaf people. According to Thomas (1994), "The severe stigma of deafness, its low incidence, and early medical intervention in deaf children's education all collaborate to intensify this grief and make it very difficult for parents to see that their child is first and foremost a child who can't hear."

Oftentimes when the diagnosis is made, parents turn to their own parents for support and understanding, only to find that they too are struggling with the same set of emotions. Caught in a web of preconceived perceptions of deafness, the grandparents may view the child as an "afflicted human being" rather than as a child who cannot hear. Unable to offer advice, they may turn back to their children for support and information. Cognizant of the fact that the child's grandparents are grieving, feelings that would normally be shared with them are instead turned inward, thus fostering feelings of psychological loneliness and/or resentment.

According to Luterman and Ross (1991), the pain of deafness and the sense of loss never totally disappear. Although these feelings may lose some of their initial intensity, they resurface as the child progresses through various life events. Even as the child reaches adulthood, parents are frequently brought to tears when they question what their child would have been like had he or she not been deaf (Luterman & Ross, 1991).

Throughout the developmental process parents of deaf children may fluctuate between periods of overprotection and bouts of withdrawal. In an attempt to become "perfect parents" and compensate for their child's deafness, they may focus all of their energies on this one particular child, oftentimes to the total exclusion of other family members. While some become overwhelmed with the socialization process, others attempt to raise their child as a hearing member of the family. Drawing from their personal experiences, they respond to the child as an individual with imperfect hearing rather than as a deaf child with special communication needs. When this occurs, deaf children are frequently left in limbo, struggling to decipher the verbal exchanges that surround them.

Communication: Providing Inroads into Psychosocial Development

Communication relies on a shared language base for understanding to occur. It becomes one with our identity, allowing us the freedom to express and interact with others. The language a group uses becomes central to its identity. Furthermore, it provides one of the primary threads in the fabric of a culture. Therefore, when we change a basic fiber, such as a belief or a language, it creates a change in the overall design (Battle, 1998). Such is the case when a deaf child is born into a hearing family. Unable to access language through auditory means, he or she must rely on other senses to gain inroads into the communication system.

Language and communication are crucial factors in creating a healthy home environment for children (Ogden & Lipsett, 1982). Regardless of family structure, ethnic background, or socioeconomic status, all children have a need to feel they are part of the family unit. It is critical that this is communicated through a language that they can comprehend.

Hearing children are fortunate in that they are born into an environment that is "an exquisite system of dynamic, interdependent, and interactive processes" that occur within the child and also between the child's environment (Luterman et al., 1999). Because they are equipped with auditory, cognitive, and motor skills, they are able to receive and transmit spoken exchanges. Furthermore, this motivates them to become competent language users (Luterman et al., 1999). From the onset, as babies babble and caregivers speak in "motherese," the foundation is established for the eventual development of the complex communication system that will follow.

This system is far greater than the sum of all of its parts. It is not limited to spoken exchanges but rather expands to include the social context where these interactions occur. By examining the message that is being transmitted, both spoken and implied; the developmental stage of the child; the intent of the speaker; and the responsiveness of the individual receiving the message, one can gain a greater understanding of the total function of the communication system. In essence, the language the child is exposed to, how and when the communication occurs, and the social framework where the communication transpires are all variables that play a critical role in language development (Luterman et al., 1999).

How adults mediate communication allows babies access into the language system whereby they can express their needs. Furthermore, when caregivers respond to a child's expression of communication, they provide the opportunity for linguistic mapping to occur (Dapretto, 1999). Later, as these exchanges become more sophisticated, the child learns how to model appropriate communication behaviors and responses.

Deafness affects the entire family unit, including the communication system. From the onset, it influences the critical bond that needs to be established between the primary caregiver and the child. As parents are faced with the initial diagnosis of deafness, they are forced to rapidly determine methods whereby they will communicate with their child. As families recover from their initial feelings of shock, members are required to return to a "state of equilibrium." Here they can focus on their strengths and discover what works best for their child as well as their family unit (Bodner-Johnson & Sass Lehrer, 1996). This is a pivotal point, for the method of communication they select and the success or failure of their choice will have a significant impact on their child's overall development. By establishing the appropriate language scaffolding, deaf children are provided with the necessary tools to assist them as they engage in conversations, establish relationships, and acquire a sense of belonging. When this does not ensue, feelings of insecurity and isolation may take root. All children, including those who are deaf, have mutual communication needs that are associated with the desire for affiliation, affection, and control (Luterman & Ross, 1991).

Affiliation

Affiliation originates with a bond between the mother and the child wherein the foundation for psychosocial development is anchored. In turn, this sense of belonging expands to include other family members and individuals within the home neighborhood environment. Later, it broadens even further as children enter school and become involved in various clubs and activities.

Deaf children may encounter difficulties when attempting to establish these bonds of affiliation. This is due in part to the difficulty that parents and other family members have in adjusting their verbal communication to the visual attentiveness of the child. Although deaf children are exposed to the same amount of speech as hearing children, it is unlikely that they receive comparable amounts of language. As both Harris (1995) and Gallaway and Woll (1994) have indicated, even though the child may be raised in a language-rich environment, what he or she assimilates becomes the yardstick for measuring language manipulation and flexibility.

Research conducted by Lederberg and Everhart (1998) indicates that although hearing parents may opt to sign to their deaf children, communication delays still exist. When conducting a longitudinal study comparing 20 hearing and deaf children between the ages of 22 months and 3 years, their findings revealed that both groups of children increased the amount of communication they had with their mothers from 22 months to 3 years of age. However, upon further comparing the two groups, it was noted that those who could hear experienced a significant increase in the amount they communicated with their mothers compared with those who were deaf.

The study further revealed that at 3 years of age the deaf children still relied primarily on nonlinguistic communication; only 38 percent of utterances of the deaf 3-year-olds contained language (either signs or speech) compared with 76 percent of the hearing children whose utterances contained language. Furthermore, the language development displayed by the deaf 3-year-olds was equivalent to that displayed by hearing 22-month-olds (Lederberg & Everhart, 1998).

This study also examined the mode of communication employed by the mothers. Thirteen of the 20 mothers who had deaf children indicated they had received some training in sign language. However, when their children were 22 months of age they only averaged 1.6 sign utterances per minute. Furthermore, when their children reached 3 years of age, the amount of sign communication only increased to 4.6 sign utterances per minute. In essence, these 3-year-olds were only receiving 30 percent of their mother's messages in both a spoken and a signed format (Lederberg & Everhart, 1998).

Limited messages affect the quality of both the content and the process that is inherent in effective communication exchanges. In addition, these early interactions provide the child with the tools to participate in conversations both at home and at school. Those who develop a successful repertoire of communication skills are able to enter social situations where they can actively participate with their peers and thus develop a sense of affiliation. They become part of the "feedback loop" where they receive reinforcement for their involvement in the group (Kluwin, Moores, & Gaustad, 1992).

As infants grow into childhood and transcend into adolescence it is critical that they stay abreast of the communication skills that are accepted as the norm by their various peer groups. They must possess the sophistication that will allow them to enter the group and speak to the issues that are relevant to group members. To accomplish this they must possess communication clarity and connectedness, knowledge of appropriate play activities, the ability to exchange information, and knowledge of conflict resolution skills (Parker, 1986, as cited in Kluwin, Moores, & Gustad, 1992).

Deaf children raised in hearing families may struggle at various times in their development as they attempt to establish a sense of affiliation. As they begin to recognize that they are the only family member who wears a hearing aid, struggles with communication, and experiences difficulties academically, their self-esteem may be affected, thus prompting them to search for a group where they can develop a sense of affiliation.

Affection

Self-esteem can be viewed as a reflection of the individual's self-worth or self-image. From early parent-child interactions, children begin to form their perceptions of who they are. Coopersmith (1967) conducted an extensive study of parent-male child relationships and self-esteem. He noted that expression of affection, concern about the child's problems, harmony in the home, participation in family activities, availability to give help when it was needed, and the establishment of clear and fair rules were all attributes that were associated with high self-esteem (as cited in Santrock, 1999).

Luterman and Ross (1991) stress that it is fundamental to one's self-esteem to recognize that the individual is loved for himself or herself. When children are accepted for who they are and are praised for what they are capable of doing, their self-esteem is enhanced. However, when children do not receive the emotional support and social approval they need, their self-image can remain low.

Frequently parents of deaf children apply the same communication standards to their deaf children that they expect from their hearing children. When this occurs, those who are deaf are faced with the overwhelming task of mastering speech and language. When they attempt to develop these skills and are successful, they may be showered with affection. However, if they experience failure, they may perceive that their parents are withdrawing their love. Therefore, from an early age, they may begin to equate deafness with a negative connotation, and view it as something that must be overcome.

Control

Communication affords parents the opportunity to transmit expressions of freedom and control. By discovering a healthy balance between these two, they are able to promote independence and foster critical thinking skills. Through a process of trial and error parents determine how much responsibility their children can handle and what they are capable of doing. When parents expose their children to situations that are reflective of their maturity level, they create learning environments for them whereby ultimate growth can occur. Consequently, if they routinely subject them to experiences that they are ill equipped to handle, they set the stage for failure. When this ensues, early feelings of worthlessness begin to take root, that later manifest into feelings of low self-esteem.

Speech and language are the primary instruments of control. As children respond to various situations, their behaviors are accepted or reprimanded. In turn, they form the association between their behaviors and the consequences that follow, and thus assume responsibility for their actions. When children are provided with growth-producing experiences they can claim ownership for their actions, thus enhancing their feelings of self-worth.

Frequently deaf children are denied access to these growth-producing experiences. Raised in homes with overprotective parents, they may have things done for them, decisions made that affect them, and responses made on their behalf that are contrary to their beliefs. When this occurs, deaf children may develop a sense of "learned helplessness." In essence, they exhibit a lack of social competence and are reluctant to accept responsibility for their actions.

Based on the assumption that deafness affects the child's ability to understand and therefore learn, some parents lower their expectations for their child. Fearing that communication is not clear, they may devise mechanisms for protecting their children from society. However, when parents come to terms with the concept of deafness and allow their children to have ownership of it, they are able to relinquish their power of control over them. When this occurs, deaf children are provided with the opportunity to make decisions, face the challenges of communication, and ultimately mature into independent adults.

Fostering Independence within the Family Unit

When family units allow children their deafness and create strategies that will enhance healthy psychosocial development, they are promoting independence. If this is not accomplished, the task of parenting has not been successful. As Luterman and Ross

(1991) have so aptly stated, "Parenting is a painful process because in order to succeed we must do ourselves out of a job" (p. 16).

The task of parenting deaf children in healthy home environments entails preparing them to function in the outside world. This includes providing the child with a firm social base whereby he or she can navigate the challenges imposed by the larger hearing community. By discovering the fine line that exists between developing feelings of closeness versus fostering a sense of dependence, parents are capable of conveying love without stifling their children's needs for independence.

Deaf and hearing children alike are capable of developing into well-adjusted and psychologically healthy young adults. Through a lifetime of interactions, where mistakes become the springboard for learning, and expectations for social behaviors are clearly defined, children learn that they can attempt familiar as well as unfamiliar tasks, succeed, or fail, and still be accepted by the family unit. Furthermore, when their social behaviors fall short of parental expectations and they are disciplined with consistency and love, they are afforded the opportunity to grow and develop. When parents employ effective discipline techniques, children learn to separate their negative behaviors from their personal self-worth. They garner a sense of parental acceptance, even when they recognize that their behavior deviates from the anticipated norm.

Discipline Techniques: Working with Deaf Children

The term "discipline" has several definitions. It can denote forms of punishment or actions that are employed for the purpose of shaping or modifying behavior. Parents incorporate disciplinary measures as a teaching device, and when they feel the need to prevent, suppress, or redirect behavior. Generally speaking, discipline is only administered if the child exhibits behaviors that are considered inappropriate in the existing setting or situation.

Social scientists have described five types of misbehaviors that may warrant punishment. Listed in descending order of seriousness, they are aggression, immorality, defiance, disruptions, and "goofing off" (Charles, 1999). Parents select specific techniques to modify their children's behaviors. These methods are contingent upon their cultural backgrounds, the parenting techniques their parents employed, the nature of the child's personality, and the type and severity of the child's problematic behavior.

While some parents are proactive and expend energy in developing positive discipline strategies, others are reactive, often responding to their children's misbehavior with controlling, punitive actions. Termed "authoritarian parenting," these caregivers place firm limits on the child, and administer a form of punishment, either corporal and/or verbal to control their child's behavior. Authoritarian parenting is frequently employed when parents do not have a firm rule system in place, and when they want to remain in control of the situation. In these instances, children are directed to do as they are told with little if any opportunity for discussion. Their behavior may be controlled by threats, ridicule, or withdrawal of love (Marion, 1995).

In order for children to learn from their behavior and develop a sense of self-control, they must be nurtured in environments that foster independence within the confines of set behavioral limits. This is indicative of authoritative discipline. When parents adhere to this philosophy, children are taught to value themselves and others. Furthermore, they learn how to solve problems and develop a sense of social competence. Through a myriad of discussions, children are afforded to opportunity to gain insights into their behavior, learn acceptable ways to respond to social situations, and develop a sense of ownership for their actions. In turn, parents foster growth while allowing their children to take responsibility for their actions. By transferring parental control to their children, they provide them with the opportunity to develop an internal locus of control, thus setting the stage for self-control to flourish.

Although various techniques may be applied, the underlying goal of all discipline is to reduce the need for adult intervention. This is accomplished by helping children develop effective strategies that, when implemented, will assist them in independently controlling their behavior (Charles, 1999). Children do not master self-control after one or two encounters with punishment. It is a learned process that occurs gradually over time. It entails the ability to form associations between punishment and cause, and the capacity to form and apply generalizations from one situation to another. Furthermore, it relies on clear communication to ensure that the child comprehends not only the form of the punishment, but also the intent of the disciplinary measure.

When discipline is administered under the auspices of clear communication, both the nature of the punishment and the intent of the message can potentially be conveyed. However, when clear communication does not exist, children are left on their own to determine what specific behavior warranted the reprimand. While hearing children can depend on subtle communication cues and incidental learning experiences to aid them in forming cause-and-effect relationships, oftentimes deaf and hard-of-hearing children cannot. Frequently punished by removal or physical discipline rather than by verbal admonishment or denial of a privilege related to the misdemeanor, they may not comprehend the "precise dimensions of their misconduct" (Higgins & Nash, 1996). Furthermore, when parents remove their children from situations without affording them an explanation, they demonstrate that avoidance and physical action are acceptable techniques to incorporate when attempting to resolve problems.

In these instances, children may sense that they have done something wrong. However, because they have had few opportunities to learn from their past difficulties, they may not make the appropriate associations that are required to ensure that a change in behavior will be forthcoming (Greenberg, Calderone, & Kusche, 1984). Instead, based on parental role modeling, they learn to approach problems in one of two ways. They may respond by avoiding unpleasant situations entirely, or they may react with displays of inappropriate "acting out" behavior. Later, when problems arise and children model these learned behaviors, adults may question why their responses reflect a lack of impulse control, and a level of maturity that is indicative of a much younger child. They may fail to recognize that learned social behaviors are implicit in hearing children's daily exposure to spoken communication, but must be explicitly taught to deaf and hard-of-hearing children. If this instruction does not occur, deaf children are left with voids in the socialization process. Lacking the information they need to develop cause-and-effect relationships and effective problem-solving strategies, they struggle to develop an internal locus of control.

The method of discipline incorporated in the home impacts the overall development of the child. It influences the child's feelings of self-worth and productivity. Furthermore, it plays an integral role in assisting the child in his or her pursuit of emotional, social, moral, and psychological development.

These interactions are learning experiences that can potentially foster emotional security. When discipline is administered in a constructive and caring manner, the stage is set for children to develop a sense of who they are and what they are capable of achieving. However, if this does not happen and the foundation remains shaky, children are frequently faced with the challenge of overcoming obstacles as they strive to develop into emotionally healthy young adults.

Stanley Greenspan (1995), in his text *The Challenging Child*, outlines eight developmental stages that children pass through on their way to becoming healthy, mature individuals. Referred to as "emotional milestones," he describes the challenges that children are confronted with as they progress from preschool though the elementary school years. Although his book does not pertain specifically to deafness, his treatment of the family unit in regard to communication, forming relationships, and emotional thinking applies to all children.

Greenspan's Emotional Milestones and Their Relationship to Deafness

Fundamental to Greenspan's philosophy of child development is the premise that children learn basic abilities at different stages in their lives. From the onset, mastery of these skills provides them with the building blocks upon which future skills are added. Furthermore, once mastered, these skills remain with individuals indefinitely, allowing them the opportunity to develop a sense for who they are and what they are capable of doing.

From the onset, infants must feel secure and develop the ability to focus on individuals, sights, and sounds in their environment. Once accomplished, children and later adolescents are equipped to engage in interactions with their parents, peers, and other adults. These exchanges provide them with the opportunity to develop a sense of trust and closeness with those around them. Evidence that children have mastered this developmental task can be observed in infants, when they mirror their parent's facial expressions. It can also be seen in young children when they exchange pleasantries with adults, and in adolescents when they join a group of their friends and freely and effortlessly engage in their banter (Greenspan, 1995).

When children struggle with decoding spoken communication, as is often the case with deaf and hard-of-hearing children, they are confronted with challenges as they attempt to establish and enjoy relationships. Faced with the possibility of misunderstanding and ultimately feeling humiliated, some withdraw and isolate themselves from the larger group. Greenspan states that if children experience difficulties developing one-on-one relationships with other children or with adults, they will struggle with subsequent developmental tasks:

> This is because in the early years of life not only intimacy and self-esteem but also most learning—insights, intuition, and principles—come from what we learn from relationships . . . All abstract, intellectual concepts that children will master at later ages are based on concepts they learn in their early relationships. If children haven't the fundamental ability to relate, much of their learning is in danger of being undermined and sabotaged (Greenspan, 1995, p. 17).

The ability to look, listen, and remain calm and the ability to feel close to others is followed by intentional two-way communication. Dependent on the previous two abilities, this form of communication involves two stages. The first requires that children learn how to read body language and facial expressions; the second stage involves communicating through nonverbal patterns. As children progress from pointing and gesturing to spoken exchanges, they develop an understanding of communication patterns. In essence, they learn to recognize basic emotional themes such as approval, anger, love, or danger. Later, as words are added, they exchange ideas through spoken language.

When children experience difficulties comprehending the facial expressions of others, or are denied access to changes in their vocal tone and modulation, they may fail to recognize the patterns exhibited in nonverbal communication. Hence, their ability to develop a sense of intuition is hampered. Based on the ability to recognize patterns or clues, intuition is used when children need to decipher the context of the message that is being delivered. For some, this becomes an easy task; for others, like those who experience difficulty hearing, it becomes an ultimate challenge, thus inhibiting the effectiveness of two-way communication exchanges (Greenspan, 1995).

With intuition in place, children progress through the stage of developing emotional ideas. At this juncture, emotional feelings are represented by thoughts or ideas, rather than by outbursts of physical expressions. In essence, children learn how to integrate their wants into vocal expressions while representing how they feel. This ability opens up a whole new world for the child.

> Children can begin to exercise their minds, bodies, and emotions as one. In the school years, emotional ideas and symbols become the basis for understanding not only relationships and playground games but also the story the teacher is reading, principles in math, and the basic logic involved in arguing one's own point of view (Greenspan, 1995, p. 19).

As children go beyond labeling their emotional feelings, they enter the stage referred to as emotional thinking. At this time they develop the sophisticated ability to distinguish the differences between their viewpoint and the viewpoints of others. Furthermore, they begin to establish the mindset that one event can cause another to happen. When this connection is made, associations are formed between external experiences and internal feelings. In turn, children begin to realize that their external behaviors impact others, creating feelings of happiness, hurt, or anger. In addition, they learn quickly that when they behave inappropriately, punishment may follow. Thus, as children come to the realization that their actions merit consequences, the foundation for logic and cause-and-effect relationships is established. When children fail to make these associations their comprehension of cause-and-effect relationships may be lacking.

Throughout Greenspan's remaining stages he examines "the age of fantasy and omnipotence," "the age of peers and politics," and the development of "an inner sense of self." He outlines the process involved as children emerge from family-centered relationships to the world of peers and group dynamics. Furthermore, he examines how these experiences help children define their roles in the group, and to some extent, what their relationship is to the larger community.

Each family determines the most effective way to support their children as they navigate through these emotional milestones. For some the task is manageable; for others it becomes an awesome responsibility. Drawing from their cultural backgrounds, childhood experiences, and parenting models, caregivers fashion strategies that will promote the growth and development of psychologically healthy, well-adjusted children.

Summary

Contemporary U.S. families can be characterized as unique, diverse, and multifaceted. Shaped by family structure, cultural and ethnic diversity, socioeconomic status, and parenting techniques, they comprise a fascinating segment of society. Each family unit relies on a shared communication system to convey values and beliefs to their offspring. Furthermore, through daily interactions they model child-rearing practices that will be reflected in future generations.

Deaf and hard-of-hearing children add yet another dimension to the hearing family unit. Although these infants enter the world equipped with the same strengths and weaknesses as their hearing siblings, their inability to hear impacts the overall communication system. Challenging their parents to interact with them, they begin their journey toward independence.

Their innate personalities, coupled with early childhood experiences, will ultimately influence their overall development. While some will come to terms with their deafness and view it as an added dimension of their persona, others will perceive it as a debilitating feature that becomes the focal point of their existence.

Deafness by itself does not characterize the child or the family unit. It becomes an added variable to be recognized, understood, and accepted. Furthermore, it provides an additional layer that must be examined when family dynamics are explored. Sharing the playing field with ethnicity, cultural background, and socioeconomic status, it becomes another facet in the total composite. Thus, when it is placed in perspective, it becomes a contributing factor, rather than the sole identifying feature of the family unit.

3

Sociolinguistics and Deafness

The socialization process begins at birth as significant others engage in communication with newborns. Through these early interactions, emotions and basic needs are conveyed, and a sense of interconnectedness is formed. These initial exchanges establish the underpinnings for language formation, thus providing infants with inroads into the rich vernacular that surrounds them. Once established, this language base becomes the link between children's minds and the outside world, affording them a mechanism through which to partake in the exchange of information, while according them a venue for self-expression. Furthermore, the child's language base serves an integral role in psychosocial development.

What is language, and how is it defined? What role does language play in communication? How do individuals from different language domains converse with one another? What bearing does hearing loss have on language development? What is the relationship between language and psychosocial development?

Linguistics: A Study of the Nature and Structure of Language

Linguistic theory has been defined as "the study of the psychological system of unconscious knowledge that underlies our ability to produce and interpret utterances in our native language" (Parker & Riley, 2000). It entails the examination of pragmatics, semantics, syntax, morphology, and phonology. It also encompasses the realm of language acquisition, language processing, and the expression of thoughts through a written format.

Language has been defined as a socially shared code that represents ideas through a system of arbitrary symbols governed by an agreed upon set of rules. These rules govern sounds, words, sentences, meaning, and use (Bernstein & Tiegerman-Farber, 1997). Embedded in the structure of language is meaning and purpose that is conveyed through semantics, syntax, and pragmatics. Language users manipulate these symbolic forms as they engage in social discourse. Furthermore, through this complex system, they are provided with a medium whereby they gather information, form attachments, and interact with their social environment.

According to Bloom and Lahey (1978), language can be divided into three areas: form, content, and use. Form refers to the surface structure of the language and is represented in phonology, morphology, and syntax. In essence, it reflects the grammatical features of the language. Content refers to the semantics of the language, describing the meaning of words. Through semantics languages have the capacity to refer to content and expand upon the implied meanings of words. The third area, use, refers to pragmatics, the communicative function or intent of the words. It describes how words are used to deliver information, make requests, and convey ideas within various situational contexts.

Phonology

Phonology refers to the system of rules that govern sound production in a language. Each language can be characterized by the specific phonemes, or speech sounds, that distinguish it as a language.

A phoneme can be defined as the smallest linguistic unit of speech that signals a difference in meaning. Phonemes consist of vowels and consonants and when one or both of these components are altered, the meaning of the word changes. Words such as "pig" and "dig" differ in initial sound only, "dig" and "dog," in medial sounds, and "dog" and "dot" in final sounds.

There are two rules that govern phonemic use. The first is the distributional rule, which describes how sounds can be placed in various word positions. The second is the sequencing rule, which dictates which sounds can be used together within the same syllable (Bernstein & Tiegerman-Farber, 1997).

Morphology

Morphology studies the structure of words and word formation. It examines the smallest linguistic units that have meaning and those that represent a grammatical function. While some words can be viewed as a single unit, others can be broken down into smaller units. The smallest unit of a word is called a morpheme (Valli & Lucas, 2000).

Morphemes that can stand alone as words are described as free morphemes. Words such as *cat, serve, give*, and *house* are examples of words that cannot be broken down into smaller parts. However, morphemes can be added to words to reflect plurality or tense. When this occurs they are referred to as bound or inflectional morphemes. For instance, the "s" or the "ed" as in dog(s) or attend (ed) perform a grammatical function, thus altering the meaning of the word. Although the "s" and "ed" are the smallest units of the word, they have no meaning by themselves and therefore cannot function as free morphemes.

Bound morphemes function as affixes. When added to the beginning of words they are referred to as prefixes, as in unstable. Likewise, when they occur at the end of the word, they are identified as suffixes, as in strongest. Furthermore, they can be used to change one word into another, thus reflecting a different part of speech. In these instances they are called derivational morphemes because they are used to derive new words (Bernstein & Tiegerman-Farber, 1997).

Syntax

Syntax focuses on the structure of a language and thus becomes the rule system that describes how words must be arranged and organized within sentences. It studies phrases, clauses, and sentence types. Moreover, it allows language users the flexibility to combine words into phrases, phrases into sentences, and transform one sentence type into another sentence. In essence, it provides a mechanism for generating an almost infinite number of sentences from a finite set of words. It assists in the orchestration of sentences by establishing parameters for appropriate word order (correct use of the parts of speech) and phraseology.

Syntactic rules alert us to the fact that sentences have different structure and/or meanings as illustrated in the sentences below:

The dog bit Manual and Katie.	Manual and Katie were bitten by the dog.
Did the dog bite Manual and Katie?	Manual bit the dog and Katie.
The dog was bitten by Manual and Katie.	

These rules also assist in the recognition of those sentences that are not grammatically correct, such as:

Dog the and bit Manual Katie.	Were bitten Manual Katie dog the by and.

Syntax allows for the development of simple and complex sentences. It provides the structure for word use and the flexibility to convey a multitude of thoughts and ideas.

Semantics

Semantics focuses on the meaning of words (lexicon), phrases, and sentences. It directs its attention to how words are used to describe objects, people, and situations, and how they can further be used to refer to animate as well as inanimate objects. Semantics relies on the mental word dictionaries of language users. It recognizes the fact that children's comprehension of words varies appreciably from that of adults, and that breakdowns in the transmission of messages can lie in the connotation as well as the denotation of the word choice.

Pragmatics

Pragmatics addresses how language is used to communicate in social contexts. It examines the rules that govern the exchange of language, and focuses on the reasons why individuals converse with each other. It delves into the realm of discourse and analyzes how speakers organize their thoughts into coherent conversations. Furthermore, it takes into consideration the speaker's word choice, the recipient's knowledge base, and the choice of words that are selected to convey the message. Pragmatics differs from semantics. Although semantics examines what words mean, pragmatics reflect on the intent of the content. In addition, it observes the rules speakers must follow as they enter and exit conversations, how they initiate and maintain a dialogue, and how they learn how to make appropriate comments once they begin conversing with someone.

Stages of Language Development

The foundation for language learning originates in infancy. From the first weeks of life babies begin to attend to and imitate facial expressions. Furthermore, they quickly become adept at distinguishing emotions such as happiness, sadness, and surprise (Meltzoff & Moore, 1977). By the third month of life, they have all the major emotional expressions in place and begin to make judgments about how to respond when placed in a variety of situations (Walden, 1993).

From these early interactions, infants develop attending behaviors. Then between 3 to 6 months of age they begin to show an interest in sounds and respond to voices. Throughout the next three- to six-month period, babies engage in babbling, and at approximately 6 to 9 months of age they begin to develop their receptive vocabularies. Their understanding of spoken language increases dramatically between the first two years of life. Although they may only comprehend approximately 12 words at their first birthday, by the time they reach their second birthday their receptive vocabularies have increased to 300 or more words (Santrock, 1999).

Between 10 and 15 months of age babies generally express their first spoken words, and by 18 to 24 months of age, they are expressing themselves in two-word statements. During this time they quickly grasp the importance of expressing concepts and the role that language plays in communication with others (Slobin, 1972). By the time they arrive at two years of age, their expressive vocabularies consist of an average of 200 to 275 words.

Furthermore, as they continue through the early developmental years their ability to express themselves by using more than one morpheme in a sentence increases. Roger Brown (1973) has proposed that children's language development can be examined in light of the number of utterances they make in one sentence. Referred to as the mean length of utterance (MLU), Brown has identified five stages that he contends are reflective of children's language maturity levels. An explanation of Brown's stages is presented in Table 3.1.

TABLE 3.1 *An Explanation of Roger Brown's Five Stages of Language Development (Based on information found in Santrock, 1999).*

Stage	Mean Length of Utterance	Sample Sentence
Stage 1: 12–26 months	1.00–2.00	Sentences primarily consist of nouns and verbs: "Daddy, bye-bye" "Soft kitty"
Stage 2: 27–30 months	2.00–2.50	Incorporation of plurals, past tense, articles (the, a, an): "Cookie all gone"
Stage 3: 31–34 months	2.50–3.00	Incorporation of yes/no and wh- questions, negatives (including no, not, none) and imperatives (commands and requests): "Mommy go store?" "Missi no want juice"
Stage 4: 35–40 months	3.00–3.75	One sentence may be embedded in another: "I think it's blue."
Stage 5: 41–46 months	3.75–4.50	Simple sentences may be coordinated with propositional relationships: "I like hamsters 'cause they're soft."

During these early years children learn to talk and how to interact socially with others. Initially they use language to express their basic needs, gain control over their environment, and establish a sense of connectivity with others. While some infants actively seek opportunities to interact with those around them, others do not. According to Thomas and Chess (1977), babies enter the world with their own personalities or temperaments. While some possess an easy or flexible temperament, others are slow to warm up or are fearful. Still others reflect a personality that is feisty or difficult. The nature of the infant's temperament is a major contributing factor in language development, influencing the extent to which he or she actively becomes involved in social exchanges. This, coupled with the child's motivation to master the language, plays an integral role in how quickly and efficiently proficiency is accomplished.

Initially, children use language to sustain and maintain emotional attachments. As they continue to grow and their life experiences are expanded, they intentionally begin to search for words to express their feelings. Prompted by a desire to share these new experiences with others, they look to language as a vehicle for sharing their experiences, thoughts, and feelings (Bates et al., 1982).

From the onset their thoughts are directed inward, focusing on self-expression. This introspection gradually turns outward as they begin to realize that other people experience emotions too, and that they have experiences that they want to share. This recognition marks a pivotal point in establishing social conversational interactions, because at this juncture children begin to develop the ability to predict the behaviors of others, and thus can effectively participate in social conversations (Bretherton, 1991; Bruner, 1986; Hewitt, 1994). From these early interactions basic communication skills emerge that, when refined, provide the child with the tools he or she needs to become an effective communication partner.

During the preschool years children learn to talk and thus to express themselves. However, as they enter school the focus changes and children talk to learn (Westby, 1998). Throughout the elementary years they become skilled at employing syntactical rules to construct lengthy and complex sentences (Singer, 1991). Their knowledge of word meanings expands dramatically, while their expressive vocabulary increases significantly. According to Carey (1977), the speaking vocabulary of a 6-year-old child ranges from 8,000 to 14,000 words.

As children enroll in school they rely on this word base to gather knowledge, perform academic tasks, and engage in social discourse. As they enter classrooms it is generally assumed that they are "language ready." Spending the majority of their day in language-rich settings, they are required to draw upon these skills to comprehend the academic aspects of what is being taught. Within a very short period of time it becomes apparent to them that their command of both spoken and later written language is critical if they want to be successful. Furthermore, they realize that they are also expected to be familiar with the rules for social interaction so they can participate in classroom exchanges.

Throughout these early school years important linguistic growth occurs. Perhaps the most significant advances are made in the area of language use, or pragmatics. During this time children learn how to become good communication partners, how to make indirect requests, and how to process language that is exchanged in the classroom (Bernstein & Tiegerman-Farber, 1997). Development of pragmatics involves more than the mastery of syntactic structures. It entails developing a familiarity with sociolinguistic rules that are related to language use within a variety of communication settings. These rules involve the act of speech; however, they also govern the discourse structures in which speech acts are embedded (Hayes & Shulman, 1998).

From an early age children become adept at incorporating different registers as they address their friends, parents, siblings, and authority figures. They quickly learn that speech can be used to administer directives as well as to elicit responses. Furthermore, they become aware of the fact that what precedes a statement can oftentimes be as critical as the message that is delivered. During this time they enhance their skills in conversational discourse. Children learn how to initiate a conversation, how to sustain a dialogue once it has begun, and how to terminate or change topics (Hayes & Shulman, 1998).

Throughout this time period children develop the ability to make use of indirect requests. This involves administering a directive in an indirect manner, such as "It's very cold in here," which is an indirect request for increasing the heat. The incorporation of this aspect of pragmatics is noteworthy, signifying that the child is growing in his or her awareness of what is considered a socially appropriate request within a designated communication context (Hulit & Howard, 1993).

As children progress from kindergarten through third grade their metalinguistic skills begin to develop. During this time they begin to think and talk about language. According to VanKleek (1984), as this evolves children begin to recognize that language is an arbitrary and conventional code, that it is a system of units and rules, and that this system can be used for communication. Throughout middle and late childhood, children use these skills to analyze how words are used. This provides them with insights into the world of abstractions and affords them the opportunity to understand that words can represent inanimate objects and thus have no direct bearing on their personal experiences.

The transition from childhood to adolescence can be observed in classrooms where students are expected to translate their "word knowledge" into "world knowledge" (Wiig & Secord, 1992). At this juncture new words and concepts are added to the lexicon, and old words assume new and subtle meanings. Double-functioning words such as "cold" and "bright" assume a psychological meaning as well as a physical meaning, thus reflecting the development of advanced language skills (Asch & Nerlove, 1960).

Throughout high school, students are exposed to technical terms, abstract concepts, and words that have multiple meanings, as well as words that serve multiple functions. Thus, at the time of graduation, these individuals have been exposed to, and have learned the meaning of, at least 80,000 different words (Nippold, 1998b). This period is further marked by adolescents who are capable of producing complex sentences, use communication for purposes such as persuasion and negotiation, and engaging in some metalinguistic discussions (Nippold, 1994; Whitmore, 2000).

Subtle changes can be observed in the adolescent's ability to comprehend spoken communication. Furthermore, during this time their understanding of figurative language, metaphors, and idioms increases (Reed, 1994, Galda, 1981; Nippold, 1998c). Changes can also be observed in the maturity level that is expressed during conversations. Research conducted by Wiig (1982) has revealed that by age 13, youths are able to make the transition between informal register, used with peers, to a more formal register when they encounter adults.

Throughout this developmental period, adolescents master more sophisticated communication strategies. They are able to take the perspective of the other listener, and are capable of recognizing and correcting inept communication acts. Inept communication acts occur when inappropriate responses are made to statements (Ritter, 1979).

Adolescence is further characterized by socialization, whereby "talk" becomes the major medium of social interaction, thus representing a new aspect of the young person's relationship to the social world. In addition, the shared activities upon which friendships were formed during childhood are replaced by friendships that revolve around "just talking." In these instances intimacies are shared and experiences are communicated for the sake of communication alone (Rafaelli & Duckett, 1989). These conversations are interspersed with idioms, puns, and sarcasm, as well as slang and "in-group language." The ability of adolescents to discern the appropriate uses of this slang is a contributing factor in group membership and peer acceptance (Nippold, 1998a).

Language learning spans one's lifetime. From early word recognition to complex sentence structures, individuals interconnect with others as they exchange thoughts and ideas and acquire a wealth of information. Language development is fostered through direct and indirect learning experiences. It is based on the premise that children can hear, and that they have early caregivers that can be described as language role models.

What impact does deafness have on language development? How does it affect spoken word acquisition and later complex written forms of expression and recognition? Furthermore, how does hearing loss impact both social and academic experiences, and what, if any, are the implications of these experiences on psychosocial development?

Language Development and Deafness

Extensive research has been conducted in the area of language development as it relates to deafness. Studies reveal that the majority of deaf babies are born to hearing parents and that their language-learning situation differs considerably from deaf infants who are born to deaf parents (Spencer & Lederberg, 1997). Furthermore, as a group, deaf children with hearing parents display significant language delays as evidenced in school-aged children who possess limited vocabularies while struggling with English syntactic structures (Meadow, 1980; Moores, 2001).

Factors that impact language development include age of onset of deafness, degree of hearing loss, hearing status and communication mode utilized by the primary caregiver, language environment where the child resides (rich or deprived), the presence of any cognitive deficits, and opportunities for mediated learning experiences to occur. These variables not only contribute to word development, but also play a crucial role in the ongoing evolvement of pragmatics. For words, by themselves, mean nothing if they cannot be used to communicate with others.

Deaf children acquire their language through three domains: the conversational domain, the literate domain, and the metalinguistic domain (Hoffmeister et al., 1998). The conversational domain encompasses those skills required to engage in discourse with peers and adults. Those who have a command of conversational language are knowledgeable in the rules of turn taking and initiating and ending conversations, and can relate to peers and adults on a wide variety of topics. Furthermore, they are skilled at manipulating their words to insure that their message will be understood by a variety of conversation partners.

The literate domain of language refers to the individual's ability to "decode and encode either a representation of language in another form, or understand how the rituals of stories or narratives are established" (Hoffmeister et al., 1998). Furthermore, it entails comprehending or decoding printed text by being familiar with both the language and the rules of the culture to which the language belongs (Lane, Hoffmeister, & Bahan, 1996).

The third domain, metalinguistic, involves learning how to identify and manipulate the parts of the language to capitalize on using words to their fullest potential. At this level, one is able to distinguish between exposés that are well written and those that are poorly constructed. Additionally, this is where children learn how to use language appropriately, and why certain words are chosen to ensure clarity of expression. As they become familiar with the grammar and semantics of the language, they are granted passage into the world of academia. Here they rely on their metalinguistic skills to complete written classroom activities.

What affect does deafness have on these three domains? Do deaf children develop conversational strategies that are similar to their hearing peers? Do they develop comparable literate and metalinguistic skills? If differences exist, what impact, if any, do they have on psychosocial development?

The Conversational Domain and Deafness

Communication that transpires within the conversational domain is instrumental in shaping one's thoughts, beliefs, values, and behaviors. Through this venue feelings are expressed, relationships are developed, and identity is projected. Conversational exchanges originate in the home and later expand into educational and social settings. Within this domain expressive and receptive language skills flourish as children mature into competent interpersonal communicators. Such is the case when deaf children are born to deaf parents. However, when deaf children are born to hearing parents the process of instilling language and engaging in spoken exchanges becomes challenging. While some parents opt to communicate with their children through sign language, others elect to rely on an aural/oral method.

Numerous studies have been cited in the literature regarding early aural/oral communication that occurs between mother and child. These studies reveal that mothers of deaf children between the ages of one and two relate to their children using the same simplified, concrete, grammatical register that is similar to that used by mothers of hearing children (Cheskin, 1982). However, frequently their deaf children appear to be unresponsive, passive participants who, by the very nature of their disability, react to nonverbal stimuli rather than verbal stimuli. As a result, these mothers tend to dominate and control the conversation (Cheskin, 1982; Schlesinger & Meadow, 1972; Wedell-Moonig & Westerman, 1977). When this occurs opportunities for communication exchanges are limited.

Research conducted by Griffith, Johnson, and Dastoli (1985) indicates that the frequency of parent/child interactions differs significantly when deaf rather than hearing children are involved. During their study, they observed the interaction between mothers and their children during 20-minute sessions. Their results revealed that hearing mothers of deaf or hard-of-hearing children who relied on oral/aural communication initiated interactions on an average of 21.8 times per session, whereas the deaf or hard-of-hearing children initiated interactions approximately 2.3 times throughout the same time period. By comparison, initiations by hearing mothers and their hearing children were more equitable, with these mothers initiating conversation on an average 12.7 of times per session and their children initiating conversations approximately 9.6 times per session. Furthermore, additional research conducted by Wedell-Monnig and Lumley (1980) indicates that although hearing mothers initially make frequent attempts to converse with their deaf children, the number of these spoken interactions decreases over time.

Interactions between hearing mothers and their deaf children who rely on simultaneous communication have also been cited in the literature. These findings reveal that these mothers, who utilize a form of manual communication, are able to engage in more sustained conversations with their children than when speech is used alone. Greenberg (1980) examined the social interaction of 14 aural/oral and 14 simultaneous communication mother-child dyads. The children involved in this study were between 3 and 5 years of age. Although mothers and children in both groups were able to initiate interactions on an equitable basis, those who engaged in conversations utilizing simultaneous communication were able to maintain their interactions over a longer period of time. Furthermore, these conversational exchanges were more complex than those expressed by the aural/oral group.

Pragmatics lies at the heart of interpersonal exchanges. Research indicates that hearing children acquire these needed skills within the first eight years of life due to their active, early involvement in meaningful conversational interactions (Owens, 1996; Romaine, 1984). Much less is known about the effects of hearing loss on the development of pragmatic skills.

Because deafness is a low-incidence disability, there are fewer opportunities for deaf children to have meaningful conversational interactions in naturalistic settings with those who can communicate freely with them (Clark, 1989; Gallaway & Woll, 1994; Ling, 1989). As a result, they are less likely to develop the full range of conversational pragmatic skills.

Research indicates that deaf children's conversations have many similarities when compared to normal hearing children with regard to range of communicative intent and in their ability to give feedback to conversational partners (Day, 1986; Greenberg, 1980; Mohay, 1990; Skarakis & Prutting, 1977). However, limitations have been cited in deaf children's use of informative or heuristic communicative functions and in the strategies they employ to enter conversations (Day, 1986; Pien, 1985).

In addition, studies conducted by Nicholas and Geers (1997) and Yoshinaga-Itano (1992) reveal that children with hearing losses ask very few questions at young ages. At 36 months of age, children with normal hearing spend the majority of their time in conversations making statements, asking questions, and providing answers. However, 36-month-old deaf or hard-of-hearing children who are learning spoken language spend the majority of their time making directives and performing imitations (Nicholas & Geers, 1997).

In part, this reflects the language role modeling children are exposed to at very young ages. From the onset, mothers of both hearing and deaf children ask questions, supply answers, and maintain an ongoing dialogue for their children. Thus at an early age hearing children become accustomed to this pattern of discourse that they later model as they develop their expressive skills. Relying on their command of the language, hearing children manipulate it to make statements and ask questions.

Deaf babies of hearing mothers are often raised in language environments where emphasis is placed on establishing word/meaning associations. In these instances mothers engage in early direct instruction as they attempt to foster vocabulary growth. Even when this occurs, delays in both expressive and receptive vocabulary may be evident.

Although the rate of vocabulary growth is similar to that documented in children with normal hearing, differences are still apparent. Hearing children's expressive vocabulary increases steadily with age. At 18 months they are able to produce an average of 110 words; at 24 months, 300 words; and at 30 months, 540 words (Fenson et al., 1994). Studies conducted with deaf children demonstrate overall deficits in their expressive abilities when compared with their hearing peers.

Studies reflect that even when a philosophy of sign-supported speech is embraced in the home, language delays occur. In a cross-sectional study conducted by Yoshinaga-Itano (1994), deaf children, using a variety of communication methodologies, demonstrated mean inventories of 300 signed or spoken words between 3 and 4 years of age and 514 words between 5 and 6 years of age. This research is further supported by the findings of Calderon, Bargones, and Sidman (1998), who noted average delays in 3-year-old deaf children enrolled in a total communication program. Their investigation revealed that at age 3 their language scores reflected average delays of 11 months for expressive language and 8 months for receptive language. Further research conducted by Fenson and colleagues (1993) using the MacArthur Communication Development Inventory (CDI) indicates that the average expressive vocabulary size of 30-month-old hearing children is 530 words, compared to 396.5 words for 32- to 37-month-old deaf children.

Based on these expressive delays, hearing mothers of deaf children frequently assume that their children do not have the word knowledge base to respond to questions. As a result, the language pattern frequently modeled by these mothers is a monologue rather than a dialogue. When this occurs, deaf children are denied early access to language models whereby the art of asking questions is initiated and later developed.

Research conducted by Nicholas (2000) examined vocabulary development in deaf children. Within this study he compared hearing children to those with severe to profound hearing losses between the ages of 12 and 54 months of age. His findings revealed significant differences between the two groups. While the hearing children involved in the study made large gains in vocabulary between 18 and 24 months of age, the deaf children's largest acquisition occurred just before 36 months of age. Although both groups reflected an increase in number of words/utterances between 18 and 36 months of age, those with normal hearing represented a gain of 2.1 words in average sentence length, while those with hearing losses reflected a gain of only 1.3 words over the same period of time. Results from this study also revealed that children with normal hearing, at 36 months of age, engaged in twice as many informative/heuristic statements, questions, and responses than deaf children at 48 months of age. (Nicholas, 2000).

The ability to ask questions, request clarification, respond appropriately when requests are made, and employ appropriate strategies when communication breakdowns occur are all key components mastered within the conversational domain. For without these skills, effective face-to-face interactions cannot occur (Jeanes, Nienhuys, & Rickards, 2000).

Research conducted in the area of pragmatic skill development reveals that hearing children develop these skills throughout early childhood. By 2 years of age, they can respond to neutral requests (Fey, Warr-Lepper, Webber, & Disher, 1988), and by 3 years of age children can respond to clarification requests (Brinton, Fujiki, Loeh, & Winkler, 1986). Between 4 and 5 years of age, they begin to improve and revise their original message as they respond to listener feedback (Patterson & Kister, 1981). By 5 years of age children begin to appraise the quality of the speaker's message (Asher, 1976), and by 7 years of age they begin to develop the skills needed to abstract information from ambiguous messages (Bearison & Levey, 1977, as cited in Jeanes, Nienhuys & Rickards, 2000).

Although numerous studies have been conducted with hearing children that focus on the acquisition of spoken language, it has not been determined if pragmatic skill development is related to a child's age or more closely dependent on the child's communication experience. Jeanes, Ninhuys, and Rickards (2000) investigated the pragmatic skill development of one group of hearing students and two groups of profoundly deaf students, one using oral and one using signed communication. Within each group of participants there were three pairs of 8-year-olds, three pairs of 11-year-olds, two pairs of 14-year-olds, and two pairs of 17-year-olds.

Students in each of the groups were placed in dyads and presented with communication tasks. Their responses were analyzed to determine the degree of specificity in their requests for clarification, the types of responses made to these requests, and the appropriateness of the responses.

Results revealed the following. Regarding requests for clarification, 86 percent of the hearing group made specific requests for clarification, compared with 65 percent of the oral deaf and 52 percent of the signing group. Fourteen percent of the hearing group, 35 percent of the oral deaf, and 48 percent of the signing group expressed nonspecific requests. These results indicate that the oral group recognized communication breakdowns and made an attempt to clarify requests more often than their hearing or signing counterparts. Furthermore, the greater number of specific requests for clarification exhibited by the hearing group suggests a more mature communicative competence reflected by this group.

Results also revealed that each of the three groups of speakers provided a high percentage of appropriate responses to their listeners' requests for clarification. Those in the hearing group responded appropriately 99 percent of the time, the oral deaf responded 90 percent of the time, and those in the signing group answered 87 percent of the time. Although the signing group responded appropriately, the quality of their responses differed significantly from the other two groups. Whereas the hearing and the oral group responded to breakdowns in communication by engaging in confirmatory responses and major modifications when necessary; the signing participants frequently limited their responses to simply repeating their original misunderstood utterance. It is critical to note that this strategy was rarely used by the other groups, and is reflective of a lack of skill development.

In order for effective communication to transpire, those involved in the discourse must be capable of discerning when communication breakdowns occur. Furthermore, they must possess strategies to assist them in making conversational repairs, if and when they are required. These pragmatic skills are developed throughout childhood as children interact with a variety of communication partners.

Deafness can pose a communication barrier, impeding conversations between deaf and hearing individuals. It affects peer/peer relationships, teacher/student interactions, and those involving parents and siblings. It equalizes the playing field, frequently creating mutual barriers and thus fostering a less than optimum communication environment.

Regardless of the mode of communication selected (oral or sign) by the deaf individual, difficulties can and often do arise. When children are raised in environments that promote the use of oral language, communication difficulties with family members and peers may occur because of the "mutual unintelligibility of the speech code" (Antia & Kreimeyer, 1997).

Even when parents, siblings, and hearing peers sign, their command of the language may be inferior to the fluency of the deaf individual, therefore reducing "the cognitive and linguistic complexity of their communication" (Greenberg & Kusché, 1993). Furthermore, even when the immediate family embraces the philosophy of conversing through sign communication, it rarely extends beyond the immediate family. Thus, it is rare among those who are deaf to have experienced extended or expanded conversations with their grandparents, aunts, uncles, or cousins (Foster, 1989b). This has a significant impact on deaf children and adolescents, restricting their opportunities to develop social communication skills.

Several researchers have explored the interaction between deaf students and their hearing counterparts in mainstreamed and integrated settings. Results reveal that young deaf children interact less frequently with their peers, both deaf/hard-of-hearing and hearing, than do their hearing classmates (Antia, 1982; Levy-Shiff &

Hoffman, 1985; McCauley & Bruininks, 1976). This reduced pattern of interaction frequently originates in childhood and continues through adolescence, impacting deaf students' opportunities to develop friendships with hearing peers.

They often miss the informal "joking and messing around" that is a prerequisite for the formation of friendships. As a result, conversations with hearing peers are often limited to a casual "hi and bye" (Foster, 1989b). Deaf students are very cognizant of what they are missing, and express regret over their lack of establishing close friendships. They frequently sense their hearing peers' lack of motivation or patience to work through difficult communication situations. As a result, many perceive their experiences in mainstreamed programs through the lens of academic and social isolation (Foster, 1989b).

Libbey and Pronovost (1980) conducted a national survey of 557 deaf and hard-of-hearing adolescents between the ages of 11 and 16 in mainstreamed programs to determine what types of communication strategies they employed. Fifty percent of those responding had been attending mainstreamed programs for seven or more years. Respondents to the survey indicated that their mode of communication differed according to the situation and the individual(s) to whom they were speaking. The majority reported that they spoke to the majority of hearing people, used writing to communicate with hearing peers, and utilized signing with their deaf friends.

In a "self-perceptions" section of the survey, only 38 percent of the students indicated that they started conversations with others. Furthermore, they expressed their discomfort with talking to their hearing peers and teachers, and indicated that they experienced difficulty in being able to comprehend what was said during a conversation. In addition, they stated that they felt hearing individuals wanted to converse with them, but when they instigated these types of interactions they were often plagued by their inability to understand one another. They further revealed that they experienced a great deal of difficulty engaging in classroom discussions. Twenty-five percent of those responding reported that they never joined in.

Brackett and Donnelly (1982) have also studied the abilities of hearing and hard-of-hearing individuals to identify junctures in conversations whereby it is appropriate to insert comments. They surmise that both visual and paralinguistic cues are necessary for both groups to enter conversations successfully. Although many hard-of-hearing individuals can identify these cues in one-on-one exchanges, they find they have fewer linguistic cues available to them in groups where there are multiple speakers. Because adolescents rarely identify who is speaking before the discourse begins, deaf and hard-of-hearing youth struggle from the onset with locating the speaker. Once identified, critical information may be lost and the deaf/hard-of-hearing person is left to piece fragments together while trying to decipher the message. Forty-eight percent of those involved in Brackett and Donnelly's survey indicated that they felt left out of peer conversations and that they tended to limit their discourse to one-on-one dialogues.

As deaf and hard-of-hearing adolescents transition from high school and either continue their education or enter the workforce, they continue to be confronted with conversational challenges. Although some of these exchanges may be facilitated smoothly, others result in breakdowns in communication whereby one or both parties are left feeling frustrated, embarrassed, or inadequate.

Using ethnographic research, Foster (1998) has interviewed more than 350 deaf and hearing individuals to gain insights into the causes of communication breakdowns that can and frequently do occur. Termed "spoiled communication," Foster describes some of the major causes of problems evident when deaf and hearing individuals engage in face-to-face exchanges. Within the area of spoiled communication, she examines stalled communications, miscommunications, and social discomfort that may arise when hearing people engage deaf people in a conversation, only to discover that they cannot hear.

Stalled communication refers to the frustration both deaf and hearing individuals experience when spoken exchanges are not clearly understood by both parties. Causes of stalled communication stem from deaf individuals using their own voices that are not clear enough to be understood by the listener, or when hearing people attempt to speak louder or more clearly, only to realize that their message is not generating the response they anticipated. Although writing, mime, or gestures can be used to alleviate these misunderstandings, these tactics may not always be successful, leaving both parties feeling embarrassed, disappointed, or even angry. Furthermore, hearing people, upon being asked to repeat or clarify, oftentimes interpret this to mean that the person is not paying attention or doesn't understand the idea that is being conveyed. When this occurs, those who can hear frequently characterize the deaf person as being socially inept or incompetent. Because deaf people are aware of these possible perceptions, they may refrain from asking for repetition even when they sense they have misunderstood.

Foster defines miscommunication within the context of exchanges whereby both parties feel communication has been successful, only to realize later that they were mistaken. Examples where miscommunications frequently occur include information shared in casual conversation, gossip and banter at the workplace, informal directives, and the general sharing of information. Deaf and hard-of-hearing consumers who wear hearing aids and/or are excellent speechreaders may be particularly vulnerable to this type of communication breakdown. Frequently those who can hear perceive hearing aids as rectifying one's hearing loss or assume that if the individual has any speechreading skills, that he or she is are fully capable of understanding the full intent of the message, thus they do not modify their spoken delivery of the message and they do not check for comprehension.

Additionally, individuals who rely on speechreading to engage in conversations are required to "watch" conversations closely, not only for information but also to alert them to appropriate junctures whereby they can interject comments or ask questions. Hearing individuals, unfamiliar with this need to remain visually attentive, may misconstrue the observer's intent and label the individual as rude or nosy.

Deaf individuals who elect to use sign language as their preferred mode of communication also adhere to the social norms ascribed by Deaf culture. As a result, they may rely on touching someone's shoulder, waving, or stomping the floor to get someone's attention. Hearing individuals, unfamiliar with this protocol, may find these behaviors intimate or rude. Conversely, when hearing people engage in discourse they frequently break visual contact with the speaker, in order to maintain a comfort level with the individual. Those steeped in Deaf culture view this as rude and as monopolizing the conversation, and thus consider it unacceptable behavior.

When any of these breakdowns in communication occur, both parties can be left feeling inadequate and uncertain of how to rectify the situation. Although spoiled communications impact both deaf and hearing individuals like, the long-term effects on those who are deaf/hard-of-hearing are generally more negative. From an early age, young deaf children may be subjected to teasing and ridicule as their playmates struggle to understand their speech. Later, as they mature into adulthood, deafness may form an invisible barrier that prevents them from engaging in social situations where those who can hear form a sense of belonging.

Throughout Foster's interviews many deaf persons described their feelings of loss and isolation from hearing colleagues, schoolmates, and family members. Several expressed that they had experienced social rejection, due in their opinion to spoiled communication. Anecdotes were shared by teenagers who felt that "guys wouldn't accept me because I couldn't hear on the phone" and adults commented that they felt they were not accepted by their colleagues because of their hearing loss. Others expressed sentiments that they knew they couldn't "force" hearing people to be their friends (Foster, 1989a).

Hearing people who responded to the interview questions indicated that when they entered conversations with deaf people, their exchanges were frequently difficult and time consuming. As a result, some admitted that they occasionally avoided having contact with deaf persons. They further related that communication in the workplace was consumed by work-related issues and that time did not permit the exchange of casual comments. In this setting, employees and employers reiterated that they frequently felt awkward because they did not believe they could communicate effectively with their deaf employees. As a result, information that could enhance a working relationship and foster promotion was withheld.

Foster emphasizes that one of the most profound long-term implications of spoiled communications between deaf and hearing persons is the development of social networks and communities of deaf persons. Through a lifetime of sensing isolation from family members, hearing peers, and later colleagues, deaf individuals seek the company of those with whom they can communicate as equal partners. Through these interactions they can share in the banter of informal comments, engage in discussions involving complex topics, and establish social bonds with those around them.

The Literate Domain and Deafness

The literate domain relies heavily on metalinguistic knowledge. It entails having an understanding of how words can be manipulated to express information clearly, succinctly, and accurately. At the rudimentary level, it involves identifying and differentiating the basic parts of speech. At a more advanced level it allows the reader to know when sentences are well constructed and when corrections need to be made. This knowledge base provides children with insights into the grammatical features of the language. Furthermore, it furnishes them with inroads into the mastery of academic tasks that are required for them to become competent readers and writers.

Literacy is based on developing fluency in one's language whereby words can be manipulated freely and easily without giving thought to the process that is involved. Termed "automaticity," it reflects how thoroughly individuals have acquired the flexibility of the language, thus allowing them time to process information that is conveyed through either conversations or printed texts (Hoffmeister, Philip, Costello, & Grass, 1997).

According to deVilliers, deVilliers, Hoffmeister, and Schick (1996), fluent language users are characterized by their proficiency in making inferences, abstracting meaning from complex sentences, and their ability to incorporate new vocabulary into their written exposés. Furthermore, they are capable of recalling, recognizing, and utilizing an extensive vocabulary as they read, write, and tell stories. All of these are skills that are related to academic success.

Currently, the majority of students who are deaf and hard of hearing attend public schools and receive at least part of their education in included settings (U.S. Department of Education, 1989). They compete with their hearing peers in most if not all of their academic subjects, where they rely on their ability to read to comprehend and master the subject matter. While some are very successful, many more struggle with the complexities of the English language as they endeavor to comprehend the multiplicity of texts set before them.

There is a plethora of information within the field of deaf education that addresses the reading abilities of deaf children. According to a literature review by Luetke-Stahlman, Griffiths, and Montgomery (1999), extensive research has been conducted describing how deaf students access phonological processing, utilize short-term memory, and process English. This body of research indicates that several factors pose potential comprehension problems for deaf and hard-of-hearing readers. These include vocabulary, multiple-meaning words, indefinite pronouns, subordinate structures, figurative language, and inferencing (Luetke-Stahlman, Griffiths, & Montgomery, 1999). All of these factors have a direct impact on the overall reading ability of deaf and hard-of-hearing children.

This is evidenced in the depressed scores depicted on standardized tests that reflect only 10 percent of the deaf school-aged population exceeding the fourth grade in reading achievement upon their completion of high school (Allen, 1994; Trybus & Buchanan, 1973). Studies also reveal that deaf students tend to reach a plateau around 12 years of age and demonstrate very little semantic or syntactic language or reading development after this age. Furthermore, "it appears that more than 30 percent of deaf students now leave school functionally illiterate, compared to fewer than 1 percent of their hearing peers (Allen, 1986).

How do these language delays affect the psychosocial development of deaf and hard-of-hearing students as they compete with their peers on a daily basis? What effect do these shortcomings have on these individuals, if they experience routine failure with English-based tasks? Can any strategies be implemented to promote academic success?

From the time children arrive at school they are bombarded with an achievement-oriented environment characterized by standards that tell them that success is important (Eccles, Wigfield, & Schiefele, 1998). Some become quickly attuned to the external rewards that can be earned and this compensation motivates them to achieve. For others, their internal desire to be competent in the tasks at hand prompts them to work diligently. When motivation is intrinsic children learn to attribute their successes and failures to themselves, and in particular to the amount of effort they expend (Ryan, 1998). Intrinsic motivation coupled with classroom expectations, or extrinsic motivation, influence children in their quest for success, and both components play an integral role in motivating achievement.

Achievement in the literate domain encompasses the ability to read and respond in a written format. In order to determine if students have met these standards, they are frequently tested on their ability to recognize and recall printed text. From the elementary grades forward, hearing, deaf, and hard-of-hearing students are evaluated in terms of reading comprehension, vocabulary identification, and later their ability to abstract information and draw inferences from printed materials. When students possess word attack skills and strategies and can incorporate contextual clues to assist them as they decipher unfamiliar passages, the task at hand can become a challenging but enjoyable exercise. However, when students lack these fundamental skills, they are frequently met with failure and the exercise becomes one of dread.

Although there is a plenitude of research that describes the deficiencies of deaf students' reading abilities, there is very little if any that explores how these deficiencies, especially when exacerbated within the realm of peer comparisons, affect psychosocial development. Studies conducted with hearing students enrolled in public school settings reveal the negative effects of social comparison when it is utilized as the sole motivator to encourage achievement. Results from these studies indicate that when students' accomplishments, or lack thereof, are compared with their peers, their energies can become focused on ego-involved, threatening, self-focused states, rather than on task-involved, effortful, strategy-focused states (Nicholls, 1984). One can surmise that the social comparisons students frequently engage in among themselves can be equally detrimental.

Children want to succeed and receive recognition for their accomplishments. They want to be considered part of their peer group and compete with their classmates on an equal basis. When their assignments are less than satisfactory they begin to question their abilities and their self-worth. Although some deaf and hard-of-hearing students flourish in included settings, others find the experience overwhelming. At the same time they are struggling to master the English language they are also attempting to use it to compete academically with their peers, as they seek recognition for their accomplishments both inside and outside of classroom settings.

The Metalinguistic Domain and Deafness

During the preschool years children begin expressing themselves through language. It becomes a communication tool allowing for inquiry and self-expression. Then, as they enter elementary school, they begin to reflect on language as a "decontextualized object." At this juncture they begin to develop their metalinguistic skills as they start to think and talk about language while using these skills to analyze language. Based upon emergent literacy skills that are formed throughout the preschool years, these abilities continue to develop during the elementary years, and are most noticeable during middle childhood between the ages of 5 and 8 (Bernstein & Tiegerman-Farber, 1997).

As these skills develop children begin to recognize that language is an arbitrary conventional code. Furthermore, they become familiar with multiple-meaning words, figurative language, and how they can vary their sentences to convey the same meaning. They begin to recognize grammatical errors while becoming familiar with register and how to use it appropriately with different listeners (Berstein & Tiegerman-Farber, 1997).

Research studies that have examined the written language of deaf and hard-of-hearing children highlight their lack of syntactic and semantic knowledge. Writing samples of those with severe or profound losses reflect a lack of complexity, and are marked with frequent grammatical errors including additions, substitutions, and deviant word order. Furthermore, their writing is characterized by shorter sentence and clause length, and demonstrates a lesser degree of abstraction when compared to the writing of normal-hearing children (Yoshinagra-Itano, 1986).

Grammatical acquisition in deaf and hard-of-hearing children follows the same general order as it does in hearing children. In addition, there is evidence of significant delays that impact all modalities including written communication (Quigley, Power, & Steinkamp, 1977). When deaf children write they frequently omit words and use fewer adverbs, conjunctions, and auxiliary verbs when compared with their hearing classmates. However, their incorporation of nouns and verbs is comparable to their hearing peers (Quigley & Paul, 1984).

Findings further indicate that deaf children tend to have smaller and more concrete vocabularies than their hearing peers and that their writing is more literal (Blackwell et al., 1978; Everhart & Marschark, 1988). Numerous studies lead to the general conclusion that the average deaf 18-year-old writes on a level comparable to that of a hearing 8-year-old (Kretschmer & Kretschmer, 1978).

Writing is the most widely used response mode in academic settings. Furthermore, it provides an essential link to social interaction. When children struggle with expressing themselves through this domain it impacts all areas of their psychosocial development. From the early mastery of the alphabet to later expressions of complex thoughts, writers are able to convey their mastery of content knowledge, as well as their views and insights on contemporary issues.

Written communication provides deaf individuals an avenue whereby they can relate to those who can hear. It frequently serves as a resource when breakdowns in spoken communication occur. However, if the written exchanges that follow confuse rather than clarify the situation, both parties may leave feeling frustrated and confused.

Research indicates that mediated learning experiences may help rectify this problem. Studies conducted by Dickinson and Smith (1994), Andrews (1984), and Andrews and Mason (1991) document that these mediated reading experiences provide a 'bridge between the familiar, contextualized (spoken, spoken and signed, signed) language and the decontextualized, analytical language of written texts" (Luetke-Stahlman, Griffiths & Montgomery, 1999, p. 144). Thus, by engaging deaf students in these types of interactive experiences the stage is set to enhance semantic and syntactic language development.

Summary

Language emerges in infancy and has the potential to flourish throughout one's lifetime. It provides the building blocks for spoken and written expression, and grants one passage into the world of literature. Through language, individuals connect with others, gather information, form beliefs, share ideas, and establish a sense of identity.

Language originates in the home and is influenced by the cultural and ethnic backgrounds of the family unit. As children enter school, they bring this rich diversity into the classroom, where it is molded, shaped, and used to access academic subjects. Within the educational domain, students also use language to form friendships, develop social skills, and transition into adulthood. It becomes a valuable tool, fostering academic success and social acceptance.

Deaf children born to hearing parents begin life in a linguistically altered environment. Unlike hearing infants, who share a mutual language base with their caregivers, deaf babies are not privy to the auditory channel taken for granted by those who can hear. From the onset they are faced with the challenge of developing language through their visual domain, filling in the gaps when words are not understood. As they enter school they are faced with the challenge of developing a language base that is auditory in nature, while simultaneously mastering the information placed before them. While some excel in their endeavors, others struggle as they attempt to access class materials. Through these experiences, deaf individuals, like their hearing counterparts, begin the process of forming their identity and establishing their feelings of self-worth.

4

The Educational Domain: Promoting Social/Emotional Growth and Development

Contemporary classrooms reflect a microcosm of the larger communities that they serve. Characterized by diversity, those embarking on their educational journey epitomize contrastive segments of society. Representing numerous socioeconomic levels, a variety of family structures, a multiplicity of ethnic groups, and special needs populations, young learners arrive at classroom doors with their own thoughts, fears, and expectations. While some enter their academic domains mirroring childlike innocence and enthusiasm, others arrive already jaded with a wisdom that far exceeds their chronological ages. Commencing with prekindergarten and concluding with their high school years, their experiences paint a portrait that characterizes the nation's educational system.

Although some students progress through the system with relative ease and minor frustrations, others encounter countless obstacles and drop out of school prior to receiving their diplomas. According to the United States Department of Education, over the last decade, between 347,000 and 544,000 tenth- through twelfth-grade students left school each year without successfully completing a high school program. Statistics further reveal that in October 1997, 3.8 million young adults were not enrolled in a high school program and had not completed high school. These youths accounted for 11.2 percent of the 34.2 million 16- to 24-year-olds residing in the United States. Of those who elect to leave school, 28.6 percent are Hispanic, 12.6 percent are African American, 7.3 percent are white, and 4.3 percent are Asian/Pacific Islander (U.S. Department of Education, 1999).

What factors contribute to these statistics? Why do some students make the decision to remain in school while others feel compelled to leave? What types of learning environments actively promote programs that support the total growth of the student? How are students with special needs included in these programs and what effect do these experiences have on their total growth and development? And, more specifically, how do deaf and hard-of-hearing students fare as they enter the mainstream and begin competing with their hearing peers?

Characteristics of the School-Aged Population

Before discussing what transpires within the classroom, it is important to briefly examine the family structure and the social environment where the child resides. For these two elements, coupled with the student's peer group, are instrumental in fostering emotional growth and development, as well as influencing academic success. In order to design learning environments that will enhance this type of growth, educators must be familiar with the experiences and the amounts of stress that their students confront on a daily basis.

Family Structure and Economic Status

Today, children are growing up in a greater variety of family structures than those experienced by their predecessors. Many of them find themselves in the care of siblings, extended family members, and afterschool programs since their mothers spend the greatest part of their day employed outside the home. More than two of every three mothers with a child between the ages of 6 and 17 is in the labor force, leaving less time for them to spend with their children (Santrock, 1999). These women enter the world of work for a variety of reasons. For some it is in pursuit of a career, for others it becomes a prerequisite for survival. This is particularly true when divorce becomes inevitable. Taking its toll on the economic stability of the family unit, divorce thrusts these mothers into the employment sector as they search for means to support themselves and their children.

According to Armstrong, Henson, and Savage (1997), poverty has become very commonplace among today's school children: "almost half of the nation's white children (45.4 percent), over four-fifths of all African American children (81.8 percent) and 43.8 percent of all Hispanic children live in poverty" (Armstrong, Henson, & Savage, 1997, p. 213). Furthermore, in homes where extreme poverty is evident, the parents usually do not have the educational background or the time to provide proper support for their children's education.

In a country where divorce rates are staggering, approximately 23 percent of the children under the age of 18 grow up in single-parent families. The age and gender of the child; the amount of conflict experienced in the home prior, during, and after the divorce; the arrangements in custody and visitation rights; and the overall impact of the socioeconomic status will all contribute to the child's social/emotional development.

Although some individuals remain single after divorce, others opt to remarry, thus creating step- and blended-family units. In recent years, the number of children involved in remarriage has increased significantly. Stepfather families, in which the mother has custody, occur 70 percent of the time, while those involving a stepmother comprise approximately 20 percent of these newly formed relationships. Additionally, both partners may bring children into the marriage, creating blended families (Santrock, 1999).

Characteristics of Families Who Have Deaf and Hard-of-Hearing Children

Deaf and hard-of-hearing children are not strangers to these familial and socioeconomic structures. While a significant number of them experience the ramifications of divorce, others are raised in homes where conflict seems inevitable. These daily conflicts are further exacerbated by frequent breakdowns in conversations. Because approximately 90 percent of deaf and hard-of-hearing children have hearing parents, the lines of communication may repeatedly become tangled if not altogether broken.

As a result, when these children arrive at school, they may bring with them all the emotional baggage that is typical of children from low-income and/or divorced or single-parent families. Furthermore, many of them also exhibit characteristics typical of those who have been denied the benefit of access to spoken communication. Their lack of clear incidental learning bases, coupled with limited opportunities to engage in informal language promoting activities, render them disadvantaged. Therefore, as they are introduced into formal learning environments, their teachers may quickly discover that they are missing some of the fundamental tools that they will need to compete.

Whether the child enrolls in a residential school, a day class specifically designed to meet the needs of the deaf or hard-of-hearing, or is included in his or her neighborhood public school, the elements that are critical to foster academic success remain the same. For students to succeed academically they must be placed in environments where they sense that the benefits of being there outweigh the lure of dropping out.

Today, approximately 70 percent of deaf and hard-of-hearing students are enrolled in general education settings (Schildroth & Hotto, 1995). While some receive the majority of their education sitting along side their hearing peers, others remain in resource rooms for the larger part of their days and only interface with their hearing counterparts during selected times. For those who attend residential school settings, their education is conducted exclusively among deaf and hard-of-hearing peers. Although the majority of these students reside on campus, some live within the community and commute on a daily basis.

What types of learning environments promote the optimum amount of social and emotional growth? What kind of programs set the stage for students to succeed and remain in school? What types of classroom management techniques encourage student involvement and independent learning? Can all students from diverse backgrounds benefit from these strategies? What elements must be in place for deaf and hard-of-hearing students to take advantage of these techniques?

Classrooms That Promote Social Competence

Creating safe learning environments for today's students has become increasingly challenging for administrators, teachers, and related school personnel. Recognizing that the structure of the American family has changed, educators are often faced with the daunting task of instilling a sense of self-discipline into children who emerge from chaotic and often fragmented family environments. As these students enter the classroom, they are met with expectations and standards that have previously been determined by the teacher. The atmosphere that he or she sets, and the rapport that is established between the teacher and the individual students, play a significant role in orchestrating the degree of learning that transpires throughout the academic year. In classrooms where feelings of respect, acceptance, and self-worth are felt, a sense of security exists, and one's freedom of expression is enhanced. Likewise, in classrooms where students feel pressured to succeed and failure seems inevitable, feelings of worthlessness, inadequacy, and inferiority flourish.

In order to construct optimum learning environments, several theorists have recommended that strategies involving communication, interaction, and intervention be implemented. Based on the philosophy that feelings of respect, thoughtfulness, emotional integrity, and authenticity must exist for learning to occur, they have developed models for effective classroom and behavior management. Three of these paradigms promote collaborative decision making between instructors and their students. Engineered by William Glasser, Rudolph Dreikurs, and Haim Ginott, these theories have provided the foundation for subsequent classroom management approaches (Larrivee, 1999).

Glasser's Philosophy of Classroom Management

Glasser has authored several texts relating to student needs and techniques for classroom management. Based on his early work in reality therapy, he maintains that all individuals strive to fulfill two basic needs: the need to establish a sense of belonging, and the need to cultivate a sense of worth to self and to others. From his early writings he has maintained that students must develop a sense of responsibility for their behavior. Cognizant of individual differences, Glasser contends that a student's background and/or socioeconomic status does not exempt him or her from behaving appropriately (Glasser, 1969). He ascribes to the belief that appropriate classroom behavior can be elicited from students if their learning environments are structured to meet the four fundamental needs that are inherent in all students: the need to belong, to have power, to experience a sense of freedom, and to have fun (Glasser, 1969).

Glasser upholds that when we are young, most of our motivation for our actions comes from the love and attention we receive from our parents when we follow their directives. In turn, these interactions create positive pictures in our minds of our basic needs being satisfied. Furthermore, they provide us with an early sense of having "power" or "control" over our lives.

When children enter school their mental pictures begin to change. For those who are prepared and encounter success, their basic needs are met, and they are motivated to excel. However, for those who lack the maturity and/or the knowledge base to conform to the rigors of formalized education, they may find they are confronted with tasks that end in failure. After experiencing a series of these events, their mental picture of school begins to change and they develop a sense of feeling "powerless" or "void of control." In turn, they may begin to question their role within the larger group.

In order to reestablish their place in the class, they frequently resort to disruptive behavior. Attention derived from these antics may provide the child with the recognition he or she needs and help instill a sense of power that was previously perceived as missing. Although the child's immediate needs may be met, he or she is completely oblivious to the long-term negative consequences that can follow.

Glasser asserts that if we want our schools to be effective we must insure that students' early classes are satisfying. When this occurs, those enrolled will maintain positive mental images and be motivated to learn. Furthermore, from the onset, classrooms must be structured in such a fashion that provides students with the opportunity to engage in meaningful dialogues and make choices. By affording them this right, they develop a sense of ownership for their behavior and feel they have some control within their environment (Glasser, 1986).

Dreikurs' Approach to Classroom Discipline

Like Glasser, Rudolf Dreikurs' background stems from psychiatry. After a long association with Alfred Adler, Dreikurs immigrated to the United States, where he eventually became the administrator for the Alfred Adler Institute. Throughout his career he focused on family-child counseling while authoring several texts on classroom behavior.

Dreikurs based his theory of classroom management on the premise that a student's underlying motives influence his or her classroom behavior. He determined that students develop defense mechanisms when they experience negative feelings or their self-esteem is threatened. Based on the belief that all students seek recognition, he postulated that misbehavior usually occurs when an attempt to be acknowledged is thwarted. In order to reduce or eliminate misbehavior, Dreikurs devised an approach to classroom discipline based on three key ideas:

1. Students are social beings and as such their actions reflect their attempts to be important and gain acceptance.
2. Students are capable of controlling their behavior and choose either to behave or to misbehave.
3. Thus, students choose to misbehave because they are under the mistaken belief that it will get them the recognition they want. Dreikurs refers to such beliefs as "mistaken goals" (Larrivee, 1999, p. 163).

Because all students want to belong they will resort to all types of behavior if it will get them the recognition they are seeking. When behaving in an appropriate manner does not generate the response they desire, students may feel that the only way to receive credit for their actions is through inappropriate behaviors. This, in Dreikurs's terms, is what he delineates as mistaken goals.

Grouped into four categories, these mistaken goals are: attention getting, power seeking, revenge seeking, and displaying inadequacy (Larrivee, 1999). He views these behaviors as occurring in sequential order and recommends strategies that teachers can follow to help students confront and examine their mistaken goals. By asking students specific questions pertaining to their motives (to get attention, to seek power, to get revenge, to display inadequacy) teachers can begin to implement actions that will defeat the students' purposes while initiating more constructive behaviors.

Dreikurs further advocates that teachers develop a comfortable dialogue with their students, and that they promote a sense of team spirit and cooperation. He encourages instructors to establish clear directives for student behavior while allowing them input into the prescribed classroom rules and outcomes. He further believes in teaching students to impose limits on themselves so that they in turn become responsible for their own discipline.

The ultimate goal of Dreikurs's approach is to bring about "genuine attitudinal change among students, so that they eventually behave more appropriately because they choose to do what they think is the right thing to do." In order for this endeavor to be successful, teachers must be willing to spend considerable time talking with their students about their actions. By confronting mistaken goals and encouraging appropriate behaviors, personal growth can be fostered and an inner sense of responsibility and respect for others can be cultivated (Larrivee, 1999).

Ginott's Theory of Communication in the Classroom

Haim Ginott has written extensively on the topic of communication between parents and children and teachers and students. In an attempt to get adults to incorporate communication styles that humanize rather than dehumanize children, he has been given credit for being the first to emphasize the importance of how teachers talk to their students, and how what is communicated is linked to their behavior.

Ginott is a firm believer that "adult messages are a direct line to a child's self-esteem" (Larrivee, 1999, p. 176). Therefore, based on what they say and how they say it, teachers can be either instrumental or detrimental in influencing the development of a child's self-concept. He further contends that if instructors want to create positive learning environments, they must first master self-discipline. Based on the premise that all individuals need to feel respected and understood, he portends that it is critical for teachers to convey feelings of warmth, respect, and empathy to their students. When this occurs, those under their direction will be provided with the ideal classroom setting where growth can and will occur.

Ginott has established six key principles for teachers to follow. The first one emphasizes the need to distinguish between the worth of the student and the worth of his or her accomplishments. He emphasizes the need for teachers to acknowledge students even when they perform poorly. When students are led to believe they will be accepted even when they fail, they remain open to learning and are willing to attempt new tasks. Conversely, when teachers limit their praise to those who accomplish the task, those who fail will develop feelings of inferiority, and may become defensive about participating (Cangelosi, 1997).

The second principle focuses on establishing a healthy emotional climate in the classroom. He advocates treating students with respect and encourages teachers to deal openly with their feelings. When classroom conflicts occur he maintains that teachers should remain in control and address the issues rather than verbally attacking the students.

This requires self-discipline, the third of Ginott's principles. He ascertains that when teachers model appropriate behaviors students will be presented with a window of opportunity to observe alternative methods for resolving conflicts.

The fourth principle focuses on sending "sane messages." Ginott emphasizes the need for teachers to consistently distinguish between the "deed and the doer." When communicating sane messages the teacher addresses the situation causing the difficulty rather than the student. This affords the students the opportunity to explore their feelings and learn appropriate ways to deal with them.

Praise is the focus of the fifth principle. While Ginott supports appreciative praise, giving recognition for what a student has done while acknowledging his or her effort, he is cautious about administering evaluative praise. This, he believes, can be as detrimental as negative comments. He warns teachers to be cautious, indicating that when students fall short of the standard, they cannot reap the benefits that are derived from evaluative praise. Rather, as they hear others praised, they become cognizant of the fact that the quality of their work is substandard. Thus, this form of praise can be internalized negatively.

The last principle focuses on why teachers should avoid asking the "why" question. Ginott believes that questions prefaced with "why" automatically signal criticism or disapproval. Thus, the student may feel threatened or judged. By rephrasing questions, teachers help compel students to respond openly without the fear of being judged (Larrivee, 1999).

Ginott suggests that adherence to these principles establishes classrooms that will foster optimum learning environments. When teachers show empathy, respect, and warmth for their students and evaluate their behavior rather than their self-worth, students feel more compelled to engage in the learning process.

Glasser, Dreikurs, and Ginott all embrace the philosophy that classrooms need to foster a democratic learning environment. Founded on the belief that schools should be structured to meet students' basic needs, these approaches encourage teachers to elicit appropriate behavior through open communication, empathy, recognition, and the development of the students' abilities to develop an internal sense of behavior control. With these elements in place, they ascertain that classroom disruptions are minimized, and the stage is set for optimum learning to occur. Others, like Skinner and Canter, feel a more structured approach is needed for effective classroom management to transpire.

Incorporating Skinner's Principles of Behavior Modification into the Classroom

Although democratic classroom environments can be very conducive to learning, there are times when teachers must rely on consequences to control, suppress, or redirect behavior. When students become aggressive or abusive, teachers may need to employ a form of behavior modification to repress these negative actions. Implementing rewards and punishments can help students become extrinsically motivated to comply with the rules and the expectations established by the teacher.

Noted for his work with behavior modification, B.F. Skinner's theory can be applied to situations that occur both inside and outside of the formal classroom setting. Based on the premise that one's voluntary behavior is largely determined by the events or consequences that immediately follow it, it is critical to insure that the reinforcement the student receives will serve to strengthen the behavior that the teacher wants modified, since over time behaviors that are reinforced will be strengthened, while those that are punished will be weakened. There are four basic reinforcement principles; each of them has a different effect on behavior.

The first involves the implementation of positive reinforcement. This is employed when individuals respond in a desired way and are rewarded for their behavior. These rewards may be given in the form of tangible and/or social reinforcers. While some situations require food, tokens, or toys, other events are rewarded with recognition, special responsibilities, or free time.

A second type of reinforcement focuses on weakening behaviors. When this principle is applied, punishment follows a behavior in the form of a negative consequence. When this occurs, the behavior is weakened. This type of punishment is frequently used by schools in an attempt to change and control behavior. Even though this method is popular in some settings, its effectiveness is usually short term in duration and it is ineffective in promoting long-term changes in behavior. Furthermore, it can generate feelings of resentment and hostility on the part of the student and lead to the expression of other inappropriate behaviors.

A third type of punishment relies on the removal of a positive reinforcer. By incorporating time outs (removing the child from the source of positive reinforcement) and response costs (removing a specific reinforcement from the child, such as tokens), the behavior is weakened. This type of punishment is generally more effective than the previous type where negative consequences are applied.

The fourth principle operates by applying negative reinforcement. When employed, a desired behavior is strengthened when the negative reinforcer is removed. Teachers who incorporate this approach will frequently reduce the amount of work that is required if students can demonstrate comprehension of a concept by producing accurate work. In these situations, students who do not want to complete the task at hand will apply themselves, thus demonstrating that they have mastered the assignment. Therefore, they can fulfill the requirement by doing less.

Other reinforcement principles that may be applied include extinction (no reinforcement is given) and shaping (reinforcing behaviors as they begin to approximate the desired outcomes). While extinction can become a powerful tool for eliminating unwanted behaviors, it can also be used inadvertently to extinguish appropriate behaviors. Students want to receive recognition when they are adhering to classroom standards. When teachers fail to acknowledge that their students are behaving appropriately, they will frequently revert to negative behaviors until they receive the attention they are searching for. Reinforcing appropriate behavior, even in small increments, and applying the principle of extinction can form new behaviors.

Those who advocate using behavior modification strategies in the classroom caution instructors to be especially careful when punishment is used. Keeping in mind that the student will perceive it as hurtful, it should be used discriminately rather than routinely and should be combined with positive procedures. Furthermore, it must be administered immediately after the behavior, emphasizing to the child that it is the behavior rather than the individual that is being rejected. While punishment may need to be employed as part of a short-term immediate solution, other strategies such as time out and positive reinforcement are more effective in the long-term shaping of desired behaviors.

Applying the Canters' Assertive Discipline to the Classroom

Assertive discipline can be applied within the confines of the classroom and within the mainstream of society. Popularized in the educational setting by the Canters (1976, 1992), assertive discipline is based on the premise that teachers as well as students are entitled to some fundamental basic rights. Teachers have the right to establish environments that maximize student learning, and the right to expect that students will behave in a manner that is conducive to learning taking place. Likewise, students have the right to expect that teachers will establish and maintain a safe learning environment, will communicate clear expectations for student behavior and performance, and will hold students accountable for their behavior (Larrivee, 1999).

The Canters believe that students have the right to make choices. When they choose to behave appropriately they are rewarded. However, if they choose to misbehave, they pay the consequences. Before students are given the opportunity to make choices it is essential that they have a full understanding of the teacher's expectations and the consequences that will follow. Furthermore, for this type of discipline to work, the teacher must consistently adhere to his or her expectations. When students misbehave, they must be confronted and the consequences must be enforced.

When assertive discipline is implemented in the classroom, teachers are enabled to deal directly with their own as well as their students' feelings without experiencing anger or guilt. It also provides them with an avenue to comfortably place demands on others without yelling or resorting to threats. In this type of learning environment, excuses for misbehavior are not condoned and students realize from the onset that they do not have the right to interfere with the rights of others as they pursue their education.

Before introducing this type of discipline into the classroom, teachers must have an action plan in place. Their plan should include expectations, routines, rules, and intervention approaches that will be used when students misbehave. Although assertive discipline can be instrumental in assisting teachers in clarifying their expectations for classroom behavior, it cannot be used as a formula for a comprehensive classroom management plan.

Adapting Classroom Management Approaches for Deaf and Hard-of-Hearing Students: Fostering Social and Emotional Growth and Development

Deaf and hard-of-hearing students find themselves enrolled in a variety of school settings where any one of these classroom management approaches may be employed. While some are exposed to a democratic learning environment, others find themselves placed in settings that are rooted in the philosophy of behaviorism. The approach that is selected reflects the teacher's philosophy of education and sets the tone for how interactions will be handled in the classroom. However, it is only one of the dynamics that contributes to a successful learning environment. Other variables that influence academic success include teachers' perceptions of deaf and hard-of-hearing students, their ability to communicate with them, and their expectations for them both academically and socially. These factors, coupled with the attributes, needs, and communication requirements that deaf and hard-of-hearing students bring to the classroom, are instrumental in contributing to the learning process.

Deaf children enter school with the same basic needs as those expressed by their hearing contemporaries. They have a fundamental need to belong, a desire to experience a sense of accomplishment, and a need to cultivate a sense of self-worth. Emerging from home environments where many have had a restricted range of interpersonal interactions, they arrive at school exhibiting behaviors that may differ substantially from children who share effective communication with their parents (Marschark, 1993). As a result, the educational setting becomes a mecca for the acquisition and development of mature social skills that can only be accomplished through communication. In this arena, children must have the opportunity to engage in discourse, both with peers and with teachers, in order to gain insights into an understanding of how their own emotions interface with the emotions of others (Kluwin & Stinson, 1993).

Where the child attends school—residential, day, or mainstreamed setting—how the child communicates—orally, manually, or a combination of both—and how the classroom teacher receives the student will all contribute to the enhancement or destruction of the child's self-esteem. Recognizing that educational settings provide fertile soil for young minds to develop and grow, attitudes and information conveyed both inside and outside the classroom will ultimately shape deaf children's perceptions of who they are, where they belong, and what they can accomplish. By examining the various school settings one can gain insights into the factors that contribute to the psychosocial development of deaf children and adolescents.

Deaf and Hard-of-Hearing Students in Mainstream and Included Settings

Prior to the 1970s the majority of deaf students received their education in residential or special day schools designed specifically to meet their needs. Then with the advent of two pieces of legislation—the Rehabilitation Act of 1973, in particular Section 504, and the Education for All Handicapped Children Act (PL 94-142) passed in 1975 and later renamed the Individuals with Disabilities Education Act (IDEA)—the face of deaf education began to change.

This mandate was prompted by the early desire to provide a free appropriate education for all handicapped children in the least restrictive environment. The law stipulated that handicapped children should be educated with nonhandicapped children to the greatest appropriate degree (Harvey & Siantz, 1979). With this legislation in place, residential placements began to decline, with enrollment decreasing almost 11 percent in a 12-year period (Craig & Craig, 1987). This pattern has continued into the twenty-first century, leaving approximately 30 percent of the deaf school-aged population receiving their education in the residential setting.

The original intent of the law was to insure that students with disabilities could receive their education in their neighborhood schools alongside those who are nondisabled. For some, this mandate opened pathways to opportunities that were previously out of reach. For others, it opened doors to classrooms where they would experience social isolation, language barriers, and academic challenges that they were unprepared to meet. Although the focus of this legislation was to provide equal academic access to all students, it overlooked the potential negative ramifications that could affect social and emotional development.

It has been well established in the literature that students have a strong need to interact socially both inside and outside of the classroom. This requires that students possess a communication base that will enable them to engage freely in conversations with their peers. Furthermore, it provides them with the vehicle to participate in classroom discussions, thus gaining them peer recognition and approval.

This "interaction creates avenues for mediating activities. That is, through social intercourse maturing children harness cultural tools, their language acquisition unfolds, and their knowledge of the world is accumulated and interpreted" (Ramsey, 1997, p. 4). Language provides them with a symbol system that, when manipulated, grants them entry into their social group, as well as the larger membership group who rely on this shared system to exchange information. In this respect, it becomes an integral tool for participation in academic activities.

Research supports the fact that academic success can be correlated with self-concept and perceived social acceptance by one's peers, both factors that rely on communication skills (Coyner, 1993). Bearing this in mind, this mandate failed to consider what could happen when students from a low-incidence disability group (deafness), who rely on a form of sign language to communicate, were placed alongside their hearing peers. What affect has mainstreaming had on deaf and hard-of-hearing students' psychosocial development?

Effects of Mainstreaming on Psychosocial Development

The terms "mainstreaming" and "inclusion" bring to mind images of classrooms where deaf and hard-of-hearing students sit among their hearing peers, interacting with them and their teachers on a daily basis. One further may assume that these students have a deaf peer group at the school with whom they can identify as well as hearing friends who will want to spend time with them. However, upon close examination of these settings one may find that in reality this is not the case.

Throughout the United States there are approximately 50,000 deaf and hard-of-hearing students enrolled in public school programs (Schildroth, 1988). Of the schools surveyed, 52 percent indicated that their program served only one hearing impaired student and 16 percent reported that they served only two students (Ramsey, 1997). This is striking in that it suggests that a portion of the deaf and hard-of-hearing school aged population either does not know any other deaf children or potentially has contact with only one other deaf or hard-of-hearing child (Ramsey, 1997).

Holt (1990) has also collected data on deaf and hard-of-hearing students attending school in mainstreamed settings. Table 4.1 summarizes these findings.

Holt's findings correspond with the Annual Survey of Deaf and Hard-of-Hearing Children and Youth conducted by the Center for Assessment and Demographic Studies that further indicated that the majority of 12- to 17-year-olds attend special schools for the deaf, and those students with profound losses are the most likely to receive no academic integration (CADS, 1992–1993).

These statistics reveal that mainstreaming can have far-reaching linguistic and academic implications for deaf and hard-of-hearing students. Furthermore, within this domain, limited time spent in the regular classroom combined with decreased

TABLE 4.1 *Characteristics of Deaf and Hard-of-Hearing Students Attending Mainstreamed Programs (Based on Holt, 1990)*

- 64 percent of elementary-aged deaf students (ages 8–12) attended local public school programs; however, only about a third of them were integrated for six or more hours per week. This equates with barely an hour per day.
- More than half of the students with less than severe losses, who used speech as their primary mode of communication, were integrated six or more hours a week; most of them attended class without an interpreter.
- Among all white deaf and hard-of-hearing students, 58 percent were mainstreamed for more than six hours per week.
- Only 30 percent of those from minority groups were placed in mainstreamed settings for more than six hours per week.

opportunities to engage in typical peer exchanges can significantly impact social and cultural development (Ramsey, 1997). It is generally conceded that the foundation for all interactions is communication. Educators are attuned to the fact that classroom instruction must be accessible to those who cannot hear. However, they frequently overlook the fact that a mutually understood language base must be in place for acquaintances and friends to interact with each other. Unfortunately, these communication needs may remain transparent; the students may not receive the support they require to develop appropriate social skills; therefore, there is an increased possibility that they will be denied access to group membership and social activities.

The link between language and social identity is a strong one, and one that has not received the pedagogical attention that it deserves. In order for children to mature into social beings who reflect desirable behaviors, they must be provided with opportunities to actively participate in those group events that will encourage peer interactions. This requires learning, and like other educational tasks, it demands practice for mastery to occur. As Vygotsky (1978) states, this type of learning "awakens a variety of internal developmental processes that are able to operate only when the child is interacting with people in his environment and in cooperation with his peers" (Vygotsky, 1978, p. 90). When children are lacking the conversational skills needed to engage in these social activities, their development is truncated and their overall social development is stymied. Although they may share the same physical space with their hearing counterparts, they remain on the outside of the mainstream, going through the motions as they try to discover where and how to "fit in."

Those experiences that lead to social and personality development cannot be ignored. Having the opportunity to share intimate secrets with their friends, feel part of a group and be privy to the gossip that is shared, tell and hear dirty jokes, and flirt on the playground all hold significant implications for the child. For it is through these encounters that children are able to acquire an internal locus of control, and begin to formulate an accurate self-image. These characteristics, coupled with positive self-esteem, play an instrumental role in children's desire for achievement and eventual success in academic and social settings (Janos & Robinson, 1985).

In reality, inclusion does not exist for the deaf child. For all children, "being truly integrated means having access to one's peers and to one's teachers. This is manifestly not the case with Deaf children who are placed in hearing classrooms" (Lane, Hoffmeister, & Bahan, 1996). How do deaf and hard-of-hearing children participate in classroom discussions? How do teachers understand their questions and comments? How do these students fare in classrooms that are designed for spoken language users?

Effects of Classroom Environments on Psychosocial Development

Upon entering mainstreamed programs, young deaf and hard-of-hearing students find themselves encased in auditory environments. Oftentimes they function as members of a minority group, as they struggle to communicate with those around them. Placed in resource rooms for part of their day, they are frequently faced with professionals who exhibit rudimentary sign language skills. Although these teachers are trained in the field of deafness and are attuned to the academic needs of their students, they have rarely acquired the sign proficiency needed to engage in complex conversations. As a result, some teachers find they are unable to comprehend the nuances of the language. Therefore, they limit communication exchanges and present classroom material in a didactic manner.

Even though many contemporary teacher preparation programs require that their students complete between one and four classes in sign communication, time constraints frequently limit these courses to the mastery of signed vocabulary. This leaves only a minimal amount of time to devote to the complexities found within the grammar and syntax of American Sign Language.

Many of these professionals only understand a third to a half of the signs their students use. However, not wanting to admit what they do not comprehend, they subsequently refrain from asking for clarification. Consequently, they attempt to respond with coherent responses without fully understanding the questions. Unfortunately, their answers frequently do not match what the students want to know. Furthermore, the sign choices they use to express themselves are either inaccurate or close approximations for the intended sign meaning, and the message becomes muddled in the process.

Through a series of guesses deaf students try to construct meaning from the piecemeal information they are given. Instead of focusing on the content of the lesson, they spend their time developing strategies to decipher signs used by the teacher. If the child becomes frustrated or repeatedly asks that information be repeated, he or she may be perceived as having an intellectual or an emotional disorder (Lane, Hoffmeister, & Bahan, 1996).

Communication within the classroom can be problematic for both the teacher and the student. It is the avenue through which information is imparted and students demonstrate what they have learned. By utilizing a shared language system, students reveal what they have mastered, receive praise for their accomplishments, and develop feelings of self-esteem.

The time that is spent in resource rooms varies from student to student, and is dependent on each of their individual needs. However, the majority of these students are integrated into classes with regular teachers for a portion of their day. Here they rely on the skills of a sign language interpreter to facilitate communication between their instructor and the other members of the class.

Educational Interpreters: Providing the Communication Link

Although the skills of the interpreter vary, with some possessing outstanding credentials, the fact remains that the students, both hearing and deaf, must communicate through an adult to converse with their peers. Although this may not be problematic at the elementary level, by the time the adolescent reaches middle or high school it can become cumbersome and at times awkward.

There is currently no body of research that explores the role of the interpreter from the student's social and emotional perspective. Do deaf students feel self-conscious with an interpreter sitting next to them? Do interpreters impede interactions with other class members because students are uncomfortable discussing certain subjects when the interpreter is within such close proximity (Stedt, 1992)? Or, due to the relative ease of interacting with interpreters, do these professionals become surrogate peers, party to the discussions typically generated between friends rather than with adults? In turn, does this become a contributing factor in social stagnation, creating a conversational comfort zone for those who are either uncomfortable with or intimidated by their hearing peers?

Upon arriving at school, many deaf students have not mastered the language skills that are required to fully access the services of an interpreter. Their English language bases may be weak, and most do not possess a fluent sign vocabulary. These two factors render them ill equipped to receive instruction through a visual language. From the onset, they must learn to recognize the signs and associate them with the appropriate English words. Only then will they be able to comprehend the signed message.

"For a Deaf child to function with an interpreter requires that the child have great language facility, high intelligence, and a strong background in school-related tasks, as well as a skilled interpreter" (Lane, Hoffmeister, & Bahan, 1996, p. 249). Recognizing that many of these students enter the mainstream with an impoverished English language base and that the schools require that they be "language ready," it stands to reason that they will quickly fall behind their peers academically, often entering middle school reading at only a third-grade level (Scheetz, 2001). The linguistic pressures placed on them are significant as they struggle to communicate, compete, and form successful social relationships.

Classroom Participation and Emotional Security in Mainstream Settings

One of the goals of education is to promote social competence in all students. By providing them with opportunities to actively participate in class, school, and social activities, a sense of emotional security is formed and their social identity is shaped (Stinson and Whitmore, 1992). Deaf and hearing students alike value the camaraderie of their peers. Through these interactions they develop a sense of self-worth and a feeling of belonging.

Deaf and hard-of-hearing students may find this aspect of their academic life lacking. Although the majority of their classmates are hearing, their daily interactions with them may be limited to greetings in the hall or upon entering a class. Rarely are they included in discussions surrounding dating issues, current music groups, or fads. Research indicates that the interplay between the two constituencies is minimal and close friendships are usually not established. Only on rare occasions are they invited to participate in parties, afterschool activities, or special events (Foster, 1988).

In these programs where there are very few deaf students, there is almost inevitably a severe lack of social interaction. Those who are deaf may form friendships with other deaf or hard-of-hearing students, but oftentimes these associations find their roots in a shared disability rather than in the mutual enjoyment of the other person's company (Lane, Hoffmeister, & Bahan, 1996).

In a public school program study conducted by Stinson, Chase, and Kluwin (1990), results indicated that there was no evidence that the increased mainstreaming of deaf and hard-of-hearing students promoted identification with their hearing classmates. Furthermore, it was reported that when emotional security was examined:

- Mean ratings of emotional security with hearing-impaired peers were higher for students who were mainstreamed less (0–2 to 3–4 classes).
- Ratings of emotional security with hearing-impaired peers by students who were mainstreamed more frequently were also significantly higher than their ratings of security with hearing peers.
- The ratings with hearing peers were relatively constant across the levels of mainstreaming that were examined.
- Students who were most frequently mainstreamed reflected a discrepancy between ratings of participation and emotional security. While participating in class and school was more frequent with hearing than with hearing-impaired peers, emotional security was greater with hearing-impaired peers. The implication is that some students may have unmet needs for more social contact with hearing-impaired classmates (Stinson, Chase, & Kluwin, 1990).

This study highlights a discrepancy between class participation and emotional security. It also illustrates that although deaf and hard-of-hearing students have ongoing contact with their hearing peers, the depth of these relationships can be characterized in terms of "acquaintanceships" that are casual in nature and of relatively short duration rather than being viewed as deep friendships (Foster & Brown, 1989).

When students actively participate in school and out-of-class activities, the stage is set for them to cultivate feelings of emotional security. This in turn contributes to a sense of perceived social competence. It is desirable for students to nurture both within the confines of the academic setting. Even though mainstreamed programs frequently provide outstanding educational offerings and lend themselves to activities that foster group interaction, those who are deaf and hard-of-hearing may find they are confined to superficial relationships that are dependent on classroom interpreters for the majority of their social interaction. How do students fare who attend residential school programs?

Psychosocial Development in the Residential School Setting

The history of residential schools can be traced to the early 1800s, when the first school for the deaf was established, in Hartford, Connecticut. Designed specifically to meet the academic and social needs of the deaf student population, these facilities became the cornerstone for future educational endeavors. Prior to the 1970s they served the majority of these school-aged children, providing them with a place to live while they attended classes.

Since their inception, residential schools have provided a fertile ground for social interactions with peers and with deaf adults to take place (Marschark, 1993). In these settings, where communication flows freely, students can compete on an equal basis. They can participate in a multiplicity of extracurricular activities, including student government, sports, and dramatic performances. Furthermore, they have the opportunity to interact with deaf students of all ages.

Residential schools are one of the largest employers of deaf adults. Although only 7 percent of the teaching staff is deaf and most of them teach at the middle or high school level, others are employed as counselors, cooks, and groundskeepers. These adults, coupled with the older deaf students, provide excellent role models for young deaf children. These professionals generally have high expectations for their students and view their deafness as an integral part of their individualism, rather than perceiving it as an impediment to their academic success.

In these settings, young deaf children are likely to have more playmates and more opportunities for collaborative play than would typically occur in public school settings. Furthermore, by having contact with older deaf students and adults, younger children can gain insights into how to function in the larger hearing world. For this environment is one of the few where Deaf perspectives are shared readily with younger group members (Lane, Hoffmeister, & Bahan, 1996).

From the time deaf children enter residential schools they have opportunities to interact socially with peers and deaf adults that go beyond what is available in most homes and public school settings. They are among others with whom they share a sense of identity and belonging. As a result, most of these students graduate from school exhibiting an enhanced sense of self-identity and a healthy self-esteem (Lane, Hoffmeister, & Bahan, 1996; Marschark, 1993).

Although there are many positives to sending deaf children to residential schools, they, like the public school arena, have negative drawbacks. One of the most striking of these is the removal of children from their home environments. Once removed, they do not have daily contact with family members that includes routine outings, family gatherings, and everyday living experiences. Additionally, they are not privy to the values that are instilled through role modeling, ongoing interactions that occur between parents, siblings, or related incidental learning experiences.

Furthermore, the academic offerings provided in residential school settings may be limited due to the small enrollments. This is particularly true at the high school level, where students need to explore career options prior to graduation. Traditionally, many students attending residential schools are placed on vocational tracks and many fail to enroll in college preparation courses. Some of these vocational tracks may be outdated, and upon graduation, students may find themselves ill prepared to enter the world of work.

Although these students may have the luxury of communicating easily with their instructors and their peers, they may be faced with teachers who have not left the residential setting for a number of years. Thus, there is a risk that the academic standards set by these individuals might not be on par with the public school setting.

Enhancing Self-Esteem: Promoting Social Competence

Regardless of the school setting, it is essential that each student has the chance to feel important and that each feels that they are a valued member of the learning community. If and when they feel inferior, rejected, or alienated from their peers, problems will develop. Ziezula and Harris (1998) conducted a nationwide survey of directors of counseling in educational programs serving deaf students to determine the problems and issues they encountered. The information they obtained was reflective of a one-semester time period. The results of their survey, indicating these problems and concerns, are listed below in the order of frequency that they were reported:

1. Strained relationship with peers
2. Inability to make decisions
3. Problems with self-esteem
4. Inappropriate relationships with others
5. Aggressive behaviors
6. Teaching
7. Parental relations
8. Communication
9. Interaction with hearing individuals
10. Career decisions (Ziezula & Harris, 1998, p. 43)

These findings mirror an earlier study conducted by Marie Curtis in 1976. In this respect, both studies reflect similar problems and issues that are brought to counselors by deaf students. The issues counselors face today are similar to those encountered by this same body of professionals two decades ago. Problems surrounding family and peer relationships, ineffective communication, difficulties experienced when interacting with hearing peers, lack of decision-making skills, feelings of social isolation, and feelings of low self-esteem still exist today. However, when the two studies are compared, there are five primary differences between them. In the more recent study the students expressed additional areas of concern. These included topics surrounding aggressive behavior, sexual concerns, sexual acting out, histories of sexual abuse, and suicidal behavior (Ziezula & Harris, 1998).

Deaf students are no different from hearing students with respect to their social and emotional needs. They experience the same problems, frustrations, and insecurities, and have the same basic desire to feel a sense of acceptance, belonging, and self-worth. In order for students to become contributing members of learning environments rather than disruptive classroom agents, these basic needs must be met. Challenged by students who arrive from homes where social skills and language may be deficient, teaching skills must be implemented to assist in filling these voids.

Recognizing that many of these students enter classrooms lacking the social competencies required to compete both inside and outside of the classroom, a concerted effort must be made to insure that these skills are imparted. Only then will students be empowered with the skills they need to become responsible and independent individuals (Sorenson, 1992). By incorporating a social skills curriculum into the framework of the classroom, teachers have the opportunity to foster responsibility and independence on the part of their students. In these instances, when programs are structured in a fashion to render cooperative learning environments, then both teachers and their students work together as a team. This provides opportunities for discussion to occur within decision-making and problem-solving areas. Furthermore, it sets the stage for students to become responsible for their decisions.

When teachers invite students to become active members in the decision making process, they encourage them to care about themselves, care about others, and care about the world they live in (Pendergrass, 1982). In turn, these fundamental principles form the basis for the development of self-esteem and interpersonal relationships.

Additionally, when students are empowered by their school experiences they develop the ability, confidence, and motivation to succeed academically. Not only do they participate competently in academic areas, but through these experiences they develop appropriate types of attitudes toward school and life (Sorenson, 1992). This motivation to succeed usually stems from the individual's desire to "match some internalized standard of excellence, a standard usually derived from significant others." Through encounters with family members, peers, teachers, and perceived role modes, they attempt to mimic those behaviors that will gain them approval and recognition (Marschark, 1993).

Teachers have the opportunity to create positive learning environments and serve as change agents. By creating classrooms where language differences are recognized, cultural diversity is acknowledged, and individual needs are considered, optimal learning experiences can be structured. Although deaf students have been labeled as being "relatively impulsive and egocentric," it is now thought that these characteristics can be attributed only partially to linguistic or sociocultural sources. Professionals have begun to acknowledge that these children and adolescents frequently have significant deficits in the knowledge and skills that are required for them to become independent members in both social and academic settings (Greenburg & Kusche, 1987). Recognizing this, it is imperative that curriculums are designed that include information that promote the development of positive social skills.

Summary

Children arriving at school embody the language, values, and patterns of social interaction that have been laid down in the home. All of these factors, in turn, will influence the social interchanges that will transpire once the child enters the classroom. Furthermore, the success or failure of these interactions will be dependent on the child's flexibility, the individuals that he or she encounters and interacts with, and the contexts in which these social interchanges occur.

Schools provide a vital link in the socialization process. In this arena, students are exposed to a multiplicity of views, social experiences, and academic expectations. For some, it becomes a very enjoyable experience, for others it becomes a drudgery, as they attempt to master the skills that are required to compete both academically and socially.

In order for deaf students to succeed, teachers must implement and integrate curriculums that will enhance each child's self-esteem and motivate them to compete in the classroom. It is imperative that students be provided with opportunities to develop appropriate social skills so they can successfully interact with both their hearing and their deaf and hard-of-hearing peers. Furthermore, it is essential that they be included as team players so they too will feel they have a shared responsibility for their behavior and for their eventual academic successes and failures. By empowering students with the responsibility to control their behavior, the teacher is free to focus on providing academic instruction.

By providing students with the educational background they need and the opportunity to participate in structured social activities, the stage is ultimately set for productive socialization patterns to be established. Academic experiences provide only a fraction of what students need to grow socially and emotionally. Other integral components are encompassed in out-of-class activities. Thus, it is critical that all students have the benefit of participating in both.

5

Sexuality and the Deaf Community

Sexual attitudes and behaviors have changed significantly since the early 1900s. From the early lectures and writings of Sigmund Freud to the highly publicized studies of Alfred Kinsey and Masters and Johnson, the United States has experienced an influx of articles that pertain to topics dealing with human sexuality. Highlights of this decade include the instigation of school-based sexuality education programs, the development of the contraceptive pill, the creation of the Sex Information and Education Council of the United States (SIECUS), the legalization of abortion, and the removal of homosexuality from the list of mental illnesses by the American Psychiatric Association.

Throughout this era Americans experienced the "pinup girls" of the 1940s, the creation of *Playboy* magazine in the 1950s, the identification of the first AIDS cases in the 1980s, and the abundance of sexual information via the Internet in the 1990s. The endless onslaught of articles has heightened our awareness of the issues, problems, and concerns that will continue to shape the sexual landscape of the twenty-first century (Czuczka, 1999).

Contemporary Explanations of Sexual Behavior

The media bombards us daily with reports containing health-related hazards due to contemporary sexual practices. Statistics are shared and warnings are given to those who engage in unsafe sexual activities. Is the information contained in these reports enough to alter the behavior and attitudes of those who are sexually active? Or, are other factors instrumental in influencing these behaviors?

Throughout the decades professionals have developed a variety of theories aimed toward explaining the function of sexuality in our lives. These theories all attempt to build a model or a picture of what we do and why we do it. All theories have strengths and weaknesses, and they continue to be refined as they are tested. Four of them merit discussion. Termed "approaches," they all endeavor to explain the reasons and motives that are instrumental in influencing our sexual behavior.

The Evolutionary Approach

The oldest of all the approaches is the evolutionary approach. Its origins can be traced to the early work of Charles Darwin, who proposed that organisms evolve through a process of natural selection. As genes are transmitted from one generation to another, characteristics such as the skill to attract mates increase the likelihood that the offspring of one generation will continue to produce children of their own. Therefore, "adaptive characteristics are 'selected' for continuation, producing reproductive success, a critical concept in the theory of natural selection" (Allgeier & Allgeier, 2000).

Contemporary evolutionists believe that previous generations exist because of their "fitness" regarding reproductive success. Therefore, these theorists focus their course of study on the inherited psychological mechanisms underlying behavior. They explore the origins of behaviors, as well as the proximate and the ultimate cause of a behavior. They examine the genetic, biological, and psychological causes in their attempt to explain a variety of sexual behaviors (Allgeier & Allegier, 2000). In essence, their concern lies with the early history of a species, and how and why certain characteristics of sexual behavior are transmitted. This perspective is biological in nature and provides us with a panoramic view of sexuality and reproduction.

The Psychoanalytic Approach

Considered the "father of psychoanalysis," Sigmund Freud was one of the most influential thinkers of the twentieth century. His views of sexual development continue to fascinate and shock those who study his theory. A medical doctor by training, he developed his ideas from his work with psychiatric patients.

Freud was a firm believer in the power of the unconscious mind. He envisioned our lives in terms of tension and conflict, convinced that these turmoils were stored in our unconscious. Therefore, in order to understand an individual's behavior, it was essential that one probe those repressed subliminal thoughts. Freud's views on sexuality and sexual behaviors are intertwined with his posture on personality development. Key to his theory are three structures: the id, ego, and the superego.

The id is the Freudian structure of the personality that deals with instincts such as hunger and sex. Present at birth, it is not controlled by any knowledge of reality or morality. It works strictly according to the pleasure principle, always seeking pleasure and avoiding pain.

As reality begins to place constraints on young children, the ego begins to develop. Termed the executive branch of the personality, it makes decisions based on rationality. In essence it attempts to "bring the individual pleasure within the norms of society" (Santrock, 1997, p. 402). Although the ego differs from the id in that it is partially conscious while the id is completely unconscious, neither makes the distinction between right and wrong; they have no morality.

The moral branch of the personality is found within the superego. This entity serves as the individual's conscious. Its primary function is to determine if the id's sexual and aggressive impulses can be satisfied in moral terms.

Freud is also noted for his psychosexual stages of development: oral, anal, phallic, latency, puberty, and genital. He believed that early in life, libido is channeled into certain body zones; these zones then become the center of eroticism (Allgeier & Allgeier, 2000). His views, while primarily masculine in nature, focused on complexes, fears, and jealousy relationships children have with their parents.

Freud's theory has received a great deal of attention and has undergone significant revisions by several psychoanalytic theorists. Contemporary practitioners from this school of thought place less emphasis on sexual instincts and more emphasis on cultural experiences. Although unconscious thought remains a key tenet of this theory, conscious thought is given more credence for its role in the development of the personality.

Learning Approaches

Unlike the evolutionary and the psychoanalytic approaches that emphasize a biological explanation of sexual behavior, the learning approach examines the learning processes and how it impacts sexual activities and behaviors. Learning theory stems from a school of psychology known as behaviorism. Fundamental to this doctrine is the belief that human behavior can only be studied by observing overt behaviors. Thus, mental events such as thoughts, attitudes, and ideas are disregarded, while attention is placed on studying what we do, with whom we engage in activities, and how these interactions transpire.

John Watson was one of the first behaviorists to study sexual response. He was instrumental in initiating a school of research that has provided the foundation for most contemporary theories of learning (Allgeier & Allgeier, 2000). Classical conditioning and operant conditioning are two of the key principles that provide the foundation for learning theory. (See Chapter 4 for a discussion of B.F. Skinner's theory of operant conditioning).

Classical conditioning has been employed to study sexual arousal in both men and women. Nonsexual stimuli are paired with sexual stimuli to determine if sexual arousal can be conditioned. Research indicates that while men can be conditioned to become aroused, the same has not been documented with women (Letourneau & O'Donahue, 1997).

Operant conditioning principles can be applied to sexual behaviors when studying both physical and psychological responses. Sexual activities that generate pleasurable responses are far more likely to be repeated than those that create adverse reactions. Furthermore, we are more likely to become attracted to and involved with people who praise and compliment us and display attitudes similar to ours, and whom we perceive as physically attractive (Byrne & Schulte, 1990).

Because most learning does not occur in a vacuum, a group of behaviorists have expanded their perspectives and now view the development of behaviors within the context of social interactions. One of the most influential of these social learning theorists is Albert Bandura. His belief that sexual behaviors can be learned without the individual receiving any direct reinforcement has prompted researchers to examine the concept of modeling.

Modeling refers to the process of observing someone being rewarded or punished for a behavior. According to Bandura, when one observes someone receiving a reward, he or she is more likely to engage in a similar activity. Likewise, if someone's behavior were punished, those in observance would be less likely to instigate similar behaviors (Bandura, 1986). This hypothesis has been expanded to examine the role of peer pressure and sexual activity. Research indicates that perceived peer sexual behavior is a strong predictor of early sexual involvement (Christopher, Johnson, & Roosa, 1993).

In an attempt to explain contemporary sexual attitudes and behaviors, social learning theorists are applying cognitive and learning principles to the social arena. By observing the transmission and reception of sexual messages, and conversely how this affects subsequent sexual behavior, these theorists are mirroring an approach similar to the approach that is reflected by sex researchers trained in the area of sociology.

Sociological Approaches

Social learning theorists and sociologists share similar beliefs. However, while learning theorists focus primarily on the individual, sociologists view the world through a broader lens. Sociologists examine the relationship between beliefs and norms that are shared by members of a specific society. Although they recognize the value of individual learning experiences, their goal is to gain a broader societal perspective of why people in one society differ in their philosophical beliefs from members of another society.

They study cultural expectations and societal differences. They acknowledge the fact that cultures differ in their philosophies of sexual beliefs and search for explanations for this diversity. They ascertain that each society dictates male and female gender roles, and that members of each specific group must learn a complicated sequence of behaviors before sexual or nonsexual interactions can take place. Embedded in these expected behaviors are the scripts or societal guidelines that members establish to outline proper behavior in social situations.

As individuals explore their sexual identities they often follow male and female scripts. Male and female scripts exist as well as the traditional religious script and the romantic script. The male script emphasizes sexual conquest whereas the female script intertwines love and sex and is frequently limited to partners whom they consider marrying (Santrock, 1997).

Those adhering to the traditional religious script believe that sex is accepted only within marriage. They view extramarital sex as taboo, especially for women. Sex is equated with reproduction and occasionally affection. However, those who adhere to a romantic script equate sex with love and believe that if one develops a relationship and falls in love it is acceptable to have sex with the person whether they are married or not.

How do deaf individuals acquire their sexual knowledge and behaviors? Is their knowledge base comparable to their hearing peers? Do they adhere to the same scripts that are touted by the larger hearing community, or do they follow their own cultural guidelines? What role does their deafness play in their overall psychosocial and sexual development?

Acquiring Sexual Knowledge: Sources of Information

According to Allgeier and Allgeier (2000), children learn about sex from the onset of their lives. However, the accuracy of their sexual knowledge varies according to the source of the information. Most hearing children hear about sexual intercourse and its connection to pregnancy by the age of eight or nine. In the event that information is not provided children devise their own explanations.

Research indicates that 50 percent of all hearing 11-year-olds and 79 percent of all 13-year-olds can provide accurate descriptions of conception and pregnancy (Goldman & Goldman, 1982). Studies further suggest that the majority surveyed revealed that they preferred to receive sexual information from their parents. However, only 10 percent of the males and 16 percent of the females listed "parent" as their primary source of information about sexuality (Ansuinic, Fiddler-Woite, & Woite, 1996). Furthermore, when parents engage their children in discussions about sexuality, it appears that attitudes and values rather than factual information are conveyed (Fisher, 1986).

Deaf Children and the Acquisition of Sexual Information and Knowledge

It is well documented that the majority of deaf children are born to parents who can hear. It has also been well established that in the majority of these homes, communication between those who are deaf and those who can hear is marginal, and in some cases virtually nonexistent. As a result, familial information that is shared is frequently not received, thus creating gaps in the deaf child's knowledge base. This affects factual information that is presented, as well as any incidental learning that occurs as a result of these discussions. In a nonsigning family, the deaf child will not hear his or her sibling's sexual questions. Furthermore, they are often not privy to their brothers' and sisters' expressions of curiosity. The deaf child may have several questions relating to sexual topics but may lack the communication skills to express them (Shaul, 1981).

Even in homes that embrace a form of manual communication, conversations revolving around sexual issues do not necessarily take place. This can be attributed to several factors: the parents discomfort with the topic, their assumption that the material is being covered in school, or their lack of familiarity with sexual signs. Prior to the late 1970s, there were no texts depicting sexual signs. Although James Woodward's book *The Signs of Sexual Behavior* was published in 1979, it has not found its way into the hands of most parents. As a result, many of them lack the sign terminology that is required to engage in such a conversation with their children.

The communication concerns that plague the family unit also filter into the educational arena. Regardless of the type of learning environment—mainstream programs, day or residential schools—communication barriers can and do exist. As a result, health and sex education information that is accessed easily by hearing children may be restricted from those who cannot hear.

Understanding vocabulary is a prerequisite to engaging in conversational exchanges, because without a working knowledge of the terminology, one cannot identify, describe, or formulate questions that pertain to the topic being discussed. This is true in all areas, including subject matter that addresses sexuality. Without the fundamental vocabulary in place, parts of the body cannot be described, and more complex issues that relate to both health and sex education cannot be discussed.

Recognizing that a fundamental understanding of anatomy is a prerequisite to comprehending maturational changes in one's body, Jones and Badger (1991) designed a study to investigate deaf children's knowledge of internal human anatomy. Eighty deaf children and 190 hearing children between the ages of 5 and 15 were involved in the study. They were grouped according to age (5–7 years, 8–11 years, and 12–15 years). The study focused on two specific research questions. First, what knowledge do deaf children have about internal anatomy at different ages, and second, how do deaf children compare with their hearing counterparts at these same ages? Results revealed the following:

- Deaf children in successively older age groups had more information about internal anatomy than did the younger subjects.
- Deaf children in all three age groups knew far less than the nondeaf children involved in the study.
- Deaf children seemed most familiar with the heart, bones, and brain; however, they did not demonstrate knowledge of internal organs in the respiratory, reproductive, or immune systems.
- Many of the 5- to 7-year-old deaf children included arms, leg bones, and hearts in their drawings, but eliminated internal organs and blood vessels.
- Deaf children in the 8- to 11-year-old group added more detail to the bones, some muscles and blood vessels.
- The oldest group of deaf children added some internal organs such as stomach, liver, and kidneys.
- The mean number of body parts named by deaf adolescents (12–15 years of age) was lower than the mean number of body parts named by nondeaf children in the youngest group (5–7 years of age) (Jones & Badger, 1991).

Additional research by Swartz (1993) has been conducted with hearing and deaf college students to determine if there are any disparities in sexual knowledge between college freshmen. Swartz administered the Sex Knowledge Inventory (SKI) and the Sex Knowledge and Attitude Test (SKAT) to hearing freshmen enrolled at the University of Maryland and Loyola College in Baltimore and deaf college freshmen enrolled at Gallaudet University. The results of this survey indicated:

- Deaf students are not receiving information regarding anatomy and physiology.
- Hearing freshmen demonstrated more sexual knowledge than deaf freshmen.
- Educational level of the subject's father correlated with the subject's score on both the SKI and the SKAT (increased education correlated with an increase in the scores).
- Race of the subject was also determined to be instrumental in affecting the performance on the SKAT.
- Although race and educational level of the father can be viewed as covariates in this study, the findings still revealed significant differences between the hearing and the deaf populations (Swartz, 1993).

The results of these studies mirror the findings of earlier research conducted by Tripp and Kahn (1986). This study was designed to compare sexual knowledge of deaf-and-hard of hearing adults with adult hearing subjects in the Chicago area.

Tripp designed an eight-part sexual knowledge survey that addressed physiology, slang, anatomy (male and female), contraception, pregnancy, and fetal development, as well as general questions. The survey was administered to the hearing subjects and was interpreted in American Sign Language (ASL) for the deaf subjects. Data was gathered on the number of items that were answered correctly on each part.

A significant difference was found between the two groups on each of the eight parts, with the hearing subjects performing significantly higher than the deaf and hard-of-hearing subjects. The researchers concluded that the adult deaf community is in need of sexual education programs within the schools' curriculum (Tripp & Kahn, 1986).

School-Based Health and Sex Education Programs

There are over 47,000 American deaf and hard-of-hearing youth enrolled in the public school system. Of these students, approximately 70 percent of them attend local schools, either as mainstreamed students or in self-contained classes. Of the remaining students, about 21 percent attend residential schools with another 8 percent attending day schools for the deaf (CADS, 1992–1993). Those attending mainstreamed programs are subjected to the same curriculum as their hearing peers.

Allgeier and Allgeier (2000) report that, as of 1999, only 20 states plus the District of Columbia had mandated school-based sexuality education programs. However, 35 states and the District of Columbia had mandated the provision of education on sexually transmitted diseases and the human immunodeficiency virus (STD/HIV) (Allgeier & Allgeier, 2000).

Those students mainstreamed into public school programs are therefore exposed to a wide variety of topics housed under the auspices of health and sexual education curriculums. While some programs focus on anatomy and physiology, others examine family life and other sexuality-related subjects. Although the topics vary, few programs provide comprehensive, kindergarten through twelfth-grade programming for their students. According to the Sex Information and Education Council of the United States, fewer than 10 percent of American children receive comprehensive courses in sexuality education (Sex Information and Education Council of the U.S., 1991). Even though data has not been generated delineating the specific type of information shared with deaf and hard-of-hearing students, it is unlikely that the programming afforded these students would be any more comprehensive than that provided to the hearing students (Joseph, Sawyer, & Desmond, 1995). Furthermore, follow-up studies as to the effects of these courses indicate that they improve the accuracy of the student's knowledge about sex; however, this information does not necessarily produce major changes in sexual attitudes and behaviors (Kirby, Barth, Leland, & Fetro, 1991). "Research consistently shows that by age 16, the majority of North American adolescents have engaged in coitus and a variety of other sexual activities" (Coley & Chase-Lansdale, 1998; Day, 1992; King et al., 1998; Laumann et al., 1994).

In response to these trends toward early onset of sexual activity, the past two decades have witnessed the development of hundreds of curricula that pertain to sexuality education. These programs have since been implemented in various schools throughout the United States (Kirby, et al., 1991). Although these curricula may vary, the majority of them can be clustered under the umbrella of two approaches: abstinence-only programs and postponement and protection programs.

Abstinence-Only Programs

Of the two programs, this approach has received the political backing and the majority of funding from the federal government. Based on the premise that abstinence should be adhered to prior to marriage, these programs do not provide youth with information regarding sex education and contraception. Initiated in the early 1980s, abstinence-only programs have received millions of dollars annually from the government to promote this philosophy (Goodheart, 1992).

Although there has been very little systematic evaluation of these programs, research indicates that they are ineffective in delaying sexual initiation, and that in fact they may be instrumental in contributing to earlier sexual initiation (Christopher & Roosa, 1990; Roosa & Christopher, 1990).

Postponement and Protection Programs

Students exposed to programs that foster a postponement and protection philosophy receive sexual education that includes instruction on contraception. One of the most widely known programs of this nature is the Reducing the Risk (RTR) program developed by Douglas Kirby and his colleagues (1997).

In this program, instructors discuss social pressures that can be attributed to youth becoming sexually active. Common "lines" that are used when one is attempting to obtain sexual access are discussed, and students are taught strategies and skills to respond to these pressures. Within this curriculum, students can practice talking with one another about abstinence and contraception. They are involved in a variety of role-play situations and are also given the opportunity to practice obtaining contraceptive information from stores and clinics.

Kirby and his colleagues have implemented their program with seventh and eighth graders in California. They have determined that when this program is delivered in five sessions (each lasting approximately 45–60 minutes), changes are made in the students' sexual attitudes and behaviors. Furthermore, they indicate that there is evidence of this change three months after the presentations have been completed (Kirby et al., 1997). Studies have revealed that programs such as this one, as well as other postponement and protection programs, have shown the ability to "delay sexual initiation, increase contraceptive use, and decrease pregnancy rates among adolescents" (Frost & Forrest, 1995).

Deaf and hard-of-hearing students in the mainstream may be exposed to varying degrees of either of these approaches. However, what they glean from classroom presentations and discussions may differ from what is received by their hearing peers. Three fundamental components are essential for learning to transpire: the student must have the capacity to receive the information, the instructor must possess the ability to impart the information, and a mutual channel of communication must exist to facilitate the exchange of content, questions, and answers.

When these students enroll in the mainstream, frequently they have not had the opportunity to engage in free-flowing conversations at home and in the neighborhood. Therefore, when they arrive at school they demonstrate a deficiency in the realm of language arts, the area that provides the foundation for all other learning experiences. And when the base is weak, the building blocks of information that follow cause it to crumble, creating holes in the storehouse of information. This applies to many of those who experience a hearing loss. For without the effortless exchange of information and incidental learning, facts can be misconstrued and the development of appropriate behaviors is stymied.

This can affect all areas of the maturational process, including psychological, social and sexual development. Therefore, these students may enter the classroom on a plane that is very different from their hearing peers. As Baugh (1984) has described the situation:

> Sensory-impaired students usually experience retarded psychosocial-sexual development and demonstrate behavior inappropriate for their age. The teacher must recognize that such behavior is not a reflection of any innate mental deficiency but an indication of having missed the external input available to most nonimpaired individuals. The sensory-handicapped student has similar basic emotional needs and innate drives as others. Being impaired only interferes with the ability

to gain the information and skills required to cope with these drives; it does not eliminate them (Baugh, 1984, p. 407).

In order for them to benefit from either of the sex education programs outlined above, instructors may find that they need to provide remedial sexuality information. It is essential that teachers recognize that their students' fundamental knowledge of anatomy, the ease of communication that transpires in the classroom, their comfort level with asking questions, and their ability to interact with their peers will all contribute to their overall comprehension of the materials and the information that is presented.

Mainstreamed students find themselves challenged to compete with their hearing peers on a daily basis. How do students fare who attend residential schools or day programs for deaf and hard-of-hearing students? Do these programs provide more comprehensive health and sexual education programs? Are the materials that are utilized designed specifically for them?

Residential School-Based Health and Sexuality Education Programs

Sexual education programs in residential schools have undergone a metamorphosis since the 1950s. From the early pioneering work of Stanford Blish, dubbed the "father of Sex Education of Deaf Youth" to the contemporary programs that focus on controversial and complex issues, the field has struggled with developing appropriate and timely curricula (Fitz-Gerald & Fitz-Gerald, 1998).

Through Blish's early articles, residential schools were encouraged to establish a sex education curricula that would foster developing parent cooperation, promote teacher competence, and provide health education. Almost 15 years after his initial articles appeared in print, three schools for the deaf (Illinois, Clark, and New Jersey) independently designed sex education programs for their students. Although this early instruction was based on the thinking of the 1940s and focused on the importance of health and social hygiene, they provided professionals with a printed model to follow (Fitz-Gerald & Fitz-Gerald, 1998).

Even though these three programs were instrumental in establishing the initial curricula, it was several years before any of the other residential schools would follow suit. Prompted by the research conducted by Rainer, Altshuler, Kallman, & Demenging (1963), professionals began to sense urgency for providing deaf youth with sex education. This body of research revealed that within the residential population, over half of the students had never dated, and only 7.7 percent reported having had the opportunity to engage in "one-on-one" dating. Furthermore, the research reflected a high number of deaf individuals being arraigned on sexual delinquency charges. The researchers attributed this to a lack of sex education within in the schools, as well as minimal family education, coupled with the reduced opportunity to date and develop social skills (Fitz-Gerald & Fitz-Gerald, 1998).

Throughout the 1960s and 1970s researchers continued to explore how deaf adults received their sexual knowledge base, what information they had obtained and retained, and what additional information was needed. During that time Scott and Adams (1974) surveyed the residential schools to ascertain if they had sex education and drug education programs in place. Although 66 percent of the schools reported these programs existed, they indicated that they were either short term in nature or focused on crisis intervention. Three years later, Fitz-Gerald and Fitz-Gerald (1976) conducted a follow-up study. With 96 percent of the residential schools responding, the findings were similar: 66 percent reported they had programs. However, written responses again indicated these were short term and/or crises oriented.

In 1980 the First National Conference on Sexuality and Deafness was held. This landmark event brought together professionals from the fields of deafness and human sexuality. Throughout these meetings sexual sign communication, sex role development, childhood and adolescent sexuality, and sexual abuse topics were discussed (Fitz-Gerald & Fitz-Gerald, 1998). This conference prompted research and the development of materials specifically for the deaf and hard-of-hearing populations. By the mid 1980s, sex education programs were occurring at Gallaudet College (now Gallaudet University), NTID (National Technical Institute for the Deaf), and Gallaudet's Pre-College Programs.

During this same time period, sex education programs continued to be offered at the residential schools. While they varied in nature, they could now be categorized based on their delivery system. While some programs followed informal dormitory chat sessions, others infused objectives into their programs, while still others offered comprehensive, team-centered programs. Although some focused their programming on seniors who were preparing to graduate, others still adhered to crises intervention strategies (Fitz-Gerald & Fitz-Gerald, 1983).

Following along these same lines, Getch, Young, and Denny (1998) conducted a survey of all of the schools for the deaf in the United States (state residential, private, and public schools who indicated they had specific programs for deaf students) to determine the type of sexual educational curriculum that had been implemented in their schools. Of the 92 questionnaires that were mailed, 76 responded, reflecting a response rate of 83 percent. Of those who responded, 13 percent stated they had no curricula and therefore could not respond to the questionnaire. One school declined to complete the survey, and one school returned seven questionnaires reflective of the teachers instructing students in this subject area.

The questionnaire elicited information pertaining to topics that were covered, materials that were used, mode of communication, and instructor satisfaction with the materials. In addition to this data, teacher and student characteristics were also noted. Results of their survey revealed the following:

- The typical teacher of the deaf was female (68 percent), between 40 and 49 years of age (51 percent), white (89 percent), hearing (69 percent), and held a master's degree (76 percent). Most of them had been teaching for 15 years or more (69 percent); however, only a few (16 percent) had been teaching sex education classes for more than ten years. Most of the teachers signed for themselves (75 percent) and rated their skills as excellent.

- The primary mode of communication was ASL (39 percent) while 32 percent used a combination of ASL, PSE, and SEE.
- Topics in the sex education curriculum included hygiene, anatomy, communication, self-esteem, birth control, sexually transmitted diseases (STDs), and AIDS/HIV.
- 71 percent of the teachers reported that their materials were appropriate for students if deafness was their only disability. However, the majority indicated that these materials were not appropriate if the student was also mentally retarded or exhibited multiple disabilities.
- 90 percent of the teachers used visually based materials, indicating that these same materials were "verbally loaded."
- 82 percent used written texts or workbooks, 50 percent used videotapes signed in ASL. In addition, over 80 percent utilized overheads, diagram/charts, handouts, and written materials.
- 75 percent of those surveyed stated the materials they used were adequate but needed some modification.
- Of those teachers who responded, 56 percent spent one to two hours per week modifying materials.
- Composition of sexuality education classes typically included eight deaf students and three students with additional disabilities.
- The students' modes of communication were reflective of what the instructors were using in the classrooms (Getch, Young & Denny, 1988).

This data addresses some timely issues. First, many of the materials that are currently being utilized in these programs are "verbally loaded" and must be modified for deaf consumers. Second, students who experience secondary disabilities may not be able to fully access the information even when modifications are made. Third, the majority of the instruction is provided by white, female teachers. These teachers may or may not be sensitive to the cultural differences frequently embodied in the values and beliefs of the various minority groups that their students represent. In addition, many of these students may be in search of a role model reflective of their gender and ethnicity, with whom they can feel comfortable discussing sexual issues. These concerns, coupled with the ramifications of deafness, make designing and delivering a comprehensive sexual education program both a complex and challenging endeavor.

Homosexual Behavior and Gay Identity

One of the topics frequently excluded from sex education programs is the discussion of homosexuality and the establishment of a gay identity. Because of its highly charged emotional, social, and value-ridden nature, it is oftentimes omitted as if it does not exist.

In the past decade, researchers have attempted to determine the percentage of the American people who identify themselves as homosexuals. Due to the difficulty in obtaining accurate information, only estimates are generally provided. Surveys conducted by Diamond (1993) and LeVay (1996) indicate that "about 4 percent to 6 percent of men and 2 percent to 4 percent of women are predominantly homosexual for a large part of their lives." Research further indicates that a "substantial number of people who engage in homosexual behavior do not become exclusively homosexual" (Alligier & Alligier, 2000, p. 326). Although males may engage in homosexual contact during preadolescence and during their teens, for the majority of them, this diminishes; they indulge in heterosexual relations and maintain a heterosexual identity for the remainder of their adulthood.

Those who describe themselves as homosexual indicate that they first sensed they were "different" during childhood and adolescence (Telljohann & Price, 1993). One study conducted by Bell and his colleagues (1981) of 1,000 gay people indicated that boys typically experienced "homosexual feelings" by age 14, while females experienced like feelings at approximately 16 years of age. Furthermore, both groups revealed that these feelings were evident at least two years prior to when they made genital contact with a person of the same gender (Bell et al., 1981).

Even though one might engage in homosexual activities the process involved in acquiring a gay identity is a gradual one. After adopting the label "gay," one generally begins to associate with other gay individuals. This in turn is followed by the person's first homosexual love relationship (Harry, 1993; Rust, 1993).

Establishing a gay identity is a complex process. One must decide whether to stay "in the closet," keeping sexual orientation as private as possible, or whether to acknowledge sexual identity to others and in essence "come out." If a person chooses to "come out," he or she must determine how public to be with the declaration. Should disclosure be limited only to family and friends, or do they want to share it with their employers and their casual acquaintances? These are decisions that each individual must contemplate.

Do deaf individuals establish a sense of their sexual identity in the same manner as their hearing peers? Do they have a clear understanding of what it means to be a homosexual? Is homosexuality accepted within the Deaf community or are these individuals ostracized?

Deafness and Homosexuality

Research conducted by Swartz (1993) has shed light on how deaf homosexual males regard their sexual identity and how this compares with males who are hard of hearing and those who have normal hearing. In a comparative study, Swartz mailed the Homosexual Perceptions and Attitudes Questionnaire (Swartz, 1989) to the following four groups of male homosexuals:

1. Normal-hearing gay males with normal-hearing parents (HHP)
2. Deaf gay males with normal-hearing parents (DHP)

3. Deaf gay males with hearing-impaired parents (DDP)
4. Hard-of-hearing gay males with normal-hearing parents (HHHP)

Although his sample size was small and the subjects were nonrandomly selected, this pilot study has provided some insights into the cultural implications of deafness on homosexuality. Characteristics of his subjects and highlights of his research are listed below:

- The median age for all deaf and hard-of-hearing subjects was 25 years of age; the median age for all hearing subjects was 32.
- 57 percent of the hard-of-hearing subjects (HHHP) reported homosexuality within their nuclear family.
- 71 percent of the deaf gay males with hearing-impaired parents had homosexual relatives in their extended family (DDP).
- 52 percent of the normal-hearing gay males had no homosexuals in their family (HHP).
- The median age that DDP *first suspected* they were gay was 10 years of age; the median age for the other three groups (*HHP, DHP, HHP*) was 10–13 years of age.
- The median age that the subjects *knew* they were gay was 14–17 years of age, with the exception of the HHHP subjects (median age 18–21).
- The median age that the subjects *accepted* their homosexuality was 22–25 years for HHP and 18–21 for DDP, DHP, and HHHP.
- The age of first homosexual experience for both DDP and DHP was 10–13 and for HHP and HHHP was 14–17. Also noted were the high percentage of HHHP who had their first homosexual experience between the ages of 10 and 13.
- 70 percent of HHP reported that when they engaged in their first homosexual experience their partner was about the same age; however, 58 percent of DHP and 71 percent of HHHP reported that their partner was much older.
- All the subjects reported that they willingly participated in their first homosexual act, but 29 percent DDP reported that they were forced and 33 percent indicated they wanted it to stop once it had started. None of the other three groups reflected this sentiment (Swartz, 1995).

Additional information from this survey revealed that 67 percent of the DDP responded with negative emotions during their first homosexual experience, unlike the pleasure that was expressed by the other three groups. When asked whether they felt their first sexual experience determined their sexual orientation, 67 percent of the DHP supported this belief while 73 percent believed their early sexual experiences had significantly influenced the way they viewed themselves.

Further information revealed that while only 9 percent of the hearing subjects wished they were straight, 43 percent of the DDP wished they were straight and 31 percent of those who were hard of hearing reflected this sentiment (Swartz, 1995). Other insights gleaned from this study indicated that hard-of-hearing gays experienced the lowest amount of acceptance and the highest level of rejection and yet they still displayed the most positive attitude. On the other hand, hearing gays reported that they were lonely, depressed, and sensitive to criticism and did not feel a sense of camaraderie with other gays. It was also noted that although deaf gays had a more positive self-image when compared with those who could hear, the majority who had deaf parents felt distant from their families due to their sexual orientation (Swartz, 1995).

Swartz's research reflects earlier studies conducted by Grossman (1972), Zakarwesky (1979), and Lewis (1982). Grossman conducted extensive interviews with students at Gallaudet University and discovered that they had extremely limited knowledge of factual information regarding human sexuality and that they were involved in a greater variety of sexual experiences than was typical of that age group (Grossman, 1972).

Zakarewsky (1979) was one of the first to interview deaf homosexuals and report his findings. His early interviews reflected the degree of distress evidenced in deaf parents when they were confronted with the realization that their deaf child was gay. He further noted that being deaf and homosexual places the individual in double jeopardy of discrimination (Phaneuf, 1987).

Studies on sexuality conducted by Lewis (1982) indicate that deaf teenagers are lacking the vocabulary and the avenues of communication to discuss sexuality topics, both with their parents and with educators. He notes that this has frequently resulted in confusion, with deaf adolescents clinging to myths and misinformation. In no other area is this more tragic than in their lack of information surrounding the HIV virus and AIDS.

HIV and AIDS

In the past two decades world populations have witnessed the rapid spread of the human immunodeficiency virus (HIV), the virus that can lead to acquired immunodeficiency syndrome (AIDS). Although several cases began to be identified in the early 1980s, the first case was actually diagnosed in the United States in 1952 (Alligier & Alligier, 2000, p. 385). Prior to 1981, only 92 people in the United States were diagnosed as having the symptoms; however, from 1981 through December 1998, health departments reported more than 600,000 cases. Those infected were men, women, and children of all ages. Throughout the same time period more than 400,000 AIDS-related deaths were noted (CDC, 1998).

According to the Centers for Disease Control, AIDS is most prevalent in large urban centers; however, an increasing number of cases are being reported from smaller cities and rural areas. The rates of AIDS cases among men who have sex with other men has been decreasing and now accounts for fewer than half the cases. Although minority group members continue to be disproportionately represented, this can be attributed in part to their lack of education rather than their sexual practices. Reports indicate that intravenous (IV) drug use rather than homosexual activity appears to be the cause of most HIV infections among minorities (CDC, 1997).

What do we know about HIV/AIDS and the Deaf community? Are members of this cultural group at risk for developing the virus? What do deaf individuals know about this virus, and how do members view their peers who eventually contract the disease?

HIV/AIDS and the Deaf Community

It is difficult to compile accurate statistics on the number of deaf and hard-of-hearing persons who have contracted the HIV virus or who have full-blown AIDS. This is in part because the Centers for Disease Control does not include deafness on their forms. Estimates that have been reported indicate that the number of deaf people range from 7,000 to 25,000. Statistics further reveal that between 300 and 500 deaths have been attributed to the virus (Kennedy & Buchholz, 1995; Gannon, 1998a).

Anecdotal reports have suggested that the statistics at the higher end of this range are perhaps more accurate, based on the suggestion that there is a higher incidence of HIV/AIDS among deaf people than in the general population. There are several possible explanations for why this might be true:

- Early in the 1980s deaf people had limited access to information on the subject.
- Community/cultural factors and language have created barriers to accessing general community education programs.
- Lack of sex education information.
- Residential schools and other organizations serving deaf people have not always been sensitive to gay people; most of the organizations that have developed information for those who are deaf come from within the gay community (Langholtz & Ruth, 1999).

Although the AIDS epidemic hit the Deaf community at the same time it began to take hold in the larger hearing community, it was not until the end of the 1980s that services for deaf patients were initiated (Kennedy & Buchholz, 1995). Even today, minimal services are available for this population, and some facets of the medical community still remain insensitive to the needs of their deaf consumers.

Studies as recent as 1992 have reflected that deaf youth appear to be approximately eight years behind in terms of their knowledge and awareness of HIV/AIDS (Barres, 1992). This lack of awareness frequently takes a tragic turn when a diagnosis of AIDS is made. Although this happens countless times a day, when the deaf person involved has no comprehension of what AIDS is, the ultimate diagnosis and prognosis can be even more devastating.

Such was the case with James, a young deaf man who finally consulted with a physician after experiencing the symptoms typical of AIDS patients. When the diagnosis was made, James revealed he did not know what AIDS was, he agreed to the treatments, and because he did not comprehend the diagnosis, he continued with his active and unprotected sex life. He assumed he would get better.

Frequently it takes countless conversations with therapists who are trained to work with the deaf before comprehension takes place. Often, the realization is not reached until the person is close to death. Unfortunately this story is not an isolated case. However, it is reflective of what happens when deaf individuals are not privy to the information they need (VanBienna, 1994).

Disclosures such as these have had a sobering effect on professionals working in the field of deafness. As a result, numerous articles have appeared in the literature. Professionals have begun to examine the knowledge base, attitudes, and sexual practices of deaf high school and college students. While Luckner and Gonzales (1993) have focused on high school students in the Rocky Mountain area, Doyle (1995) has examined AIDS knowledge, attitudes, and behaviors among deaf college students. Both of these studies have provided insights into the knowledge base and the sexual practices of these students.

Luckner and Gonzales focused on 204 students enrolled in residential and day programs throughout Colorado. They administered a three-part questionnaire designed to determine the students' knowledge of how AIDS is contracted and spread, as well as their opinions about issues related to AIDS (Gonzales & Luckner, 1993). Their results revealed that:

- 94 percent knew that people die from AIDS, and 88 percent knew that you can contract AIDS by sharing an intravenous needle.
- 93 percent knew that you can't get AIDS from shaking hands or hugging someone, and 86 percent knew you couldn't contract it by being in the same room with someone who had it.
- 70 percent did not realize that HIV and AIDS cannot be contracted by giving blood; 46 percent were unaware that people who are *not* gay can get AIDS, and 43 percent did *not* realize that all gay people do not have AIDS. Furthermore, 62 percent thought married people cannot get AIDS (Luckner & Gonzales, 1993).

Doyle's (1995) study, two years later, also gathered information from a questionnaire whereby AIDS knowledge, AIDS-related attitudes (including those related to safe sex and condom use), and actual sexual behaviors were surveyed. Five hundred undergraduate students attending Gallaudet University were selected to participate in the study. Of the 500 questionnaires that were distributed, only 84 were returned (18 percent). Of those responding, 61 percent were female and 39 percent were male. Seventy-seven percent of those who returned the surveys indicated that they were white, 16 percent indicated they were Asian, with only 1 percent of blacks and 1 percent of Hispanics being represented. This study revealed that:

- The respondents' general knowledge of AIDS was moderate to high.
- 60 percent of the respondents indicated that they had engaged in at least one risky behavior (defined as engaging in one or more of the listed sexual behaviors without a condom or a latex barrier).
- 67 percent reported they had discussed safe sex with a partner but less than 50 percent indicated they would use safe sex practices (Doyle, 1995).

When reviewing statistics such as these, one must bear in mind that they are reflective of a college-age population. As with all college programs, certain academic standards must be met prior to admission into the college. Gallaudet is no exception, thus students completing the questionnaire represent those possessing above average academic backgrounds. Therefore, these results might not be indicative of the general deaf population, those who dropped out of school, or those deaf individuals who have a secondary disability.

Regardless of the age group, academic background, or educational setting, the majority of professionals in the field today agree that more needs be done to insure that deaf individuals receive critical sex education information. Furthermore, it appears to be the consensus that students should be given the opportunity to discuss this information, thereby providing them with the tools and strategies to think critically and make wise decisions. Several professionals have outlined the components that should be included in comprehsvie health and sexual education courses.

Designing Comprehensive Sexual Education Programs for Deaf Students

According to Baugh (1984), the ultimate goal of any sexuality education program should be to enable students to develop into sexually responsible and informed individuals who have sufficient knowledge to make appropriate decisions regarding their own sexuality. Programs should encompass psychosocial as well as sexual development that occurs throughout one's lifetime. Furthermore, a parental component should be included within the program. Because parents provide the initial instruction to their children regarding topics surrounding sex education, it is vital that they become part of the program development team (Baugh, 1984).

Fitz-Gerald and Fitz-Gerald (1983) mirror Baugh's belief that parents play an integral role in any sex education program. They also believe that this type of instruction occurs continually, both formally and informally, in the home, the school, and in the community. They further address the three types of programs schools can implement. These include daily informal learning, whereby instructors take advantage of spontaneous opportunities to answer students' questions or concerns that arise concerning sexual issues; infused concept learning, where selected sex education objectives are included in existing classes; and comprehensive program learning, where separate classes are taught in sexuality for a semester or a year (Fitz-Gerald & Fitz-Gerald, 1983).

They also emphasize the importance of establishing a partnership between the home and the school, establishing a sex education advisory committee, and designing an appropriate program. They highlight that community members and parents as well as teachers must agree upon program goals and community advisors should be instrumental in selecting the curriculum and materials that will be presented.

Getch and Gabriel (1998) have emphasized the need for accessible, user-friendly sexuality materials that can be used with deaf and hard-of-hearing students.

They stress that these materials cannot be based on the assumption that deaf students have the same sexual knowledge as their hearing peers. Rather, materials need to be designed to provide them with fundamental information. They further reiterate the need to prepare materials that contain accurate and explanatory information that the students will be able to comprehend.

Gannon (1998b) reminds us that hearing children as young as 4 or 5 hear about AIDS on television and radio and that deaf children are not privy to this information. She accentuates that programs in the schools should include topics that are sensitive to ethnic groups and sexual orientation, and that Deaf role models should be incorporated whenever possible.

Gannon also delves into the embarrassment that many deaf teens, who struggle with spoken or written communication, encounter when they want to visit clinics to obtain information or contraceptive devices. Furthermore, she describes the frustration these individuals encounter as they struggle to communicate with medical personnel, often limiting their exchanges and leaving their appointments with misperceptions and erroneous information. She asserts that our sex education programs should extend beyond the classroom and into the public sector where Deaf-friendly resources (HIV and STI testing sites, clinics, physicians that provide interpreters, and TTY sexuality hotlines) are available to meet the needs of deaf consumers (Gannon, 1998b).

Preparing professionals to meet the needs of the Deaf community frequently seems like an awesome and overwhelming task. Flinn (1982) recognized this and has designed an in-service model to train teachers of the deaf to teach sex education. Her model is based on the premise that any communication mode that works successfully in the classroom is appropriate. They key to this model is multidirectional communication where administrators, parents, teachers, and students have the opportunity to engage freely and openly in conversations with one another.

Critical training components within this model include teacher preparation, sensitivity to the subject matter, and a willingness to participate. It is essential that teachers are knowledgeable in the subject matter they will be teaching. They need to be familiar with anatomy and physiology, as well as social attitudes and habits, family and peer relationships, and cultural socialization. It is important that they have acquired a comfort level with topics that pertain to sexuality, and that they are willing to participate in the total program. Furthermore, they must be committed to adapting or developing materials that are appropriate for the age level they will be teaching (Flinn, 1982).

Flinn encourages colleagues to add a sex education component in their teacher training programs, thus preparing their preservice teachers to enter the classroom. By cultivating classroom teachers who are better prepared, deaf and hard-of-hearing students will have the opportunity to receive the same information that is accessible to their hearing peers. This in turn will benefit them, as well as those who comprise the larger hearing society.

Summary

The new millennium marks the continuation of the era of scientific discovery and technology. By continuing to travel down this information superhighway, people of all ages continue to be both enlightened and bombarded with the values, beliefs, and opinions of others. While some have the sophistication to decipher what they encounter, others do not. This is particularly true within the area of human sexuality. For although there is a proliferation of materials, many of today's youth do not possess the psychosocial maturity to sort through the abundance of information.

This is particularly true of a number of our deaf and hard-of-hearing youth. Faced with the barriers related to spoken communication, they enter the super highway deprived of incidental learning experiences, and with a weakened English language base. This further compounds their ability to comprehend the materials they encounter.

In order to keep deaf and hard-of-hearing individuals abreast of current sexual information, it is essential that educational programs begin to take the helm in programming and the development of materials. Teamwork must be established between the homes, communities, and educational facilities to insure that accurate information is delivered and that services are provided. Only then will the Deaf community have equal access to the information that is so readily shared among their hearing peers.

6

Social Development and Deafness

Society provides the backdrop against which human lives unfold. Comprised of individuals, social networks, and institutions, it is instrumental in shaping our thoughts, feelings, and behaviors. Defined by culture, values, role expectations, and diversity, global societies interconnect with each other to form a composite that represents the world population. As infants enter the world and are initially shaped by their surrounding societies, foundations are established that provide the stage upon which the socialization process can build. From these early encounters, the child's social identity initially takes form and thereafter is continuously defined and developed throughout the course of the individual's lifetime.

How do sociologists define the socialization process? What are some of the contemporary theories that pertain to social and emotional development? What effect, if any, does deafness have on the socialization process? By examining these theories we can gain further insights into the socialization process.

Sociologists define socialization as a lifetime of social experience whereby individuals develop their human potential and learn culture. These social experiences provide the foundation for personality further described as a person's relatively consistent pattern of acting, thinking, and feeling (Macionis, 1998). Social experiences occur throughout one's lifetime, impacting behavior and fostering change both to the self and society.

Numerous social scientists have explored the complex process of socialization, approaching it from cognitive, moral, and psychoanalytic perspectives, as well as from the viewpoint of social behaviorism. Key to this philosophy is the theory that "environment shapes behavior and highlights the centrality of symbols to human thought and action" (Macionis, 1998, p. 63).

One of the key proponents of social behaviorism is George Herbert Mead. Throughout Mead's career he studied the self in relation to social experiences. He perceived the self as being inseparable from society and determined that this connection was made through a series of steps. First, he postulated that the self is absent

124

at birth and develops only with social experience. He further surmised that an infant could biologically grow into childhood, but if this growth process occurred in virtual isolation the development of the self would be void of internalizing a personality.

Second, Mead described social experience as symbolic interactions, or the exchange of symbols. These include facial expressions, gestures, and spoken communication. Although he recognized that the environment and the exchange of these symbols shape human behavior he also adhered to the belief that humans had the capacity to use these symbols for intentional actions and thoughts requiring intuition.

Third, he believed that individuals comprehend intention by learning to take the role of the other person. By developing the ability to perceive ourselves as others see us, we can anticipate the other person's point of view, and generate thoughts of how others will respond to us. In essence, we establish a perception of ourselves based on how others think of us. This concept was further conceptualized by Charles Cooley, one of Mead's colleagues, and has been termed developing a "looking-glass self." As others respond to us we begin to shape our personas. Thus, if others perceive and respond to us in a loving manner, then we generate a persona representative of loving individuals. However, Mead contends that we would not develop this perception in isolation—it is purely the result of interacting with others.

The fourth step of Mead's theory states that when we take the role of another individual, we become self-reflective. In this instance, the self serves a dual purpose. It functions as a subject self whereby it initiates action and responds spontaneously to those in the environment. Second, the self also responds in an objective manner as we imagine ourselves from the viewpoints of others. By combining these two functions, the self as the initiator of interactions and the self that views our actions from other's perspectives, our behaviors are refined as we develop the ability to see ourselves through another person's eyes.

According to Mead, they key to developing the self is gaining sophistication in taking the role of the other. Through multiple experiences individuals learn how to model appropriate behaviors while simultaneously taking on the roles of several others. Originating with imitation in infancy, toddlers begin to acquire language and the symbol system required for play. Through these play experiences they mimic behavior, frequently those displayed by significant others (mothers and fathers) and thus begin imagining the world and themselves from a parental perspective. Furthermore, as children grow and begin to see themselves through society's eyes they begin to incorporate norms and values into their personalities. They respond to themselves as they imagine how any other person would respond in the same situation. In this respect the individual has grown into referencing his or her behavior in terms of the "generalized other," defined by Mead as the widespread cultural norms and values used by a particular group as a reference point.

Mead believed that the socialization process does not culminate with the emergence of the self. He felt strongly that changes occur throughout one's lifetime and that these changes are largely the result of our social experiences. He further stressed that life is interactional. Just as members of society influence our behavior, our actions have a reciprocal affect on group members, prompting both transactions to be viewed as integral parts of the change process. In this respect, he concluded that we play a large and vital part in our own socialization.

Mead's theory of social development is reflected in the contemporary views of psychologists such as Albert Bandura and Walter Mischel. Recognized for their belief that cognitive processes are important mediators of environment-behavior connections, these two individuals have been instrumental in what is termed "social cognitive theory." Central to this theory, previously labeled cognitive social learning theory, is the belief that learning and development involves the behavior, the person, and the environment (Bandura, 1986, 1998).

Social Cognitive Theory: The Work of Albert Bandura

Bandura believes that imitation is one of the primary ways individuals learn about their world. Through observational learning, or modeling, a person observes and imitates someone's behavior. Through this form of learning, people are able to master new tasks without experiencing the tedious requirement for trial-and-error learning. According to Bandura, four main processes are involved in observational learning.

The first process is referred to as attention. In essence, before people can reproduce a model's actions they must initially attend to what the model is doing or saying. The second step involves retention. Prior to reproducing the actions of others, a person must store observed information in memory so it can be retrieved when needed. The third process involves motor reproduction. Individuals are capable of attending to a model and coding in memory what they have seen. However, limitations in motor development may prevent the person from reproducing the model's actions. The final process required in observational learning involves reinforcement or incentive conditions. This implies that although all other factors—attention, retention, and motor reproduction—may be in place, the individual may fail to repeat the behavior because of inadequate reinforcement (Bandura, 1965).

Bandura views observational learning as an information-processing activity. Individuals observe information about the world, transforming it into cognitive representations that serve as guides for action. These cognitive activities can influence the environment, the environment can change the person's cognition, and so forth (Bandura, 2000).

According to Bandura, children learn how to interact with their peers based in part on what they observe. In the event a child observes a parent acting in a hostile or aggressive manner, the child will model these same behaviors when he or she interacts with younger family members and peers. Social cognitive theorists, who support this view, believe that people acquire a wide range of behaviors throughout their lifetimes through observing the behaviors of others.

Closely related to Bandura's social cognitive theory is Urie Bronfenbrenner's belief in the ecological theory. Based on the premise that environmental factors are critical to social learning, Bronfenbrenner has developed a model for examining environmental systems that he feels are instrumental in influencing social development.

Bronfenbrenner's Ecological Theory

Bronfenbrenner's ecological theory consists of five environmental systems ranging from the direct interactions one has with others to the broad-based influences of one's culture. Included in his model are five systems that he labeled microsystem, mesosystem, exosystem, macrosystem, and chronosystem (Bronfenbrenner, 1986, 1995).

The microsystem is the setting where the individual lives. In this context one has contact with family, peers, school, and neighborhood. It is in this environment that most direct interactions with social agents occur, and the individual is viewed as an active rather than a passive participant.

The mesosystem focuses attention on the activities or relations that occur between microsystems or between contexts. In this system he examines the relationship of family experiences to school experiences, family experiences to peer experiences, and school experiences to church experiences. In this regard the individual is studied from a multiplicity of relationships. Behavior is examined in terms of how it is displayed in one situation in correlation with actions exhibited in another setting.

The term *exosystem* is applied to experiences incurred in social settings where the individual does not share an active role in the decision-making process. Examples of events that occur in the exosystem include decisions made by the government, as in the case of medical care, or decisions made by employers that directly affect a family member, such as increased travel imposed on a parent, which impacts marital and parent-child relationships.

The fourth system, the macrosystem, includes the culture where the individual resides. The fifth system, the chronosystem, involves the patterning of environmental events and transitions that occur throughout the course of a lifetime. This system operates under the auspices of a sociohistorical framework and analyzes events and experiences in relation to the time period in which they occur.

Bronfenbrenner's theory of social development places a strong emphasis on the environment. He purports that one can gain a fuller understanding of human development by examining individuals' behavior in multiple settings. He further believes that through a systematic examination of the micro- and macro- dimensions of the environmental systems, insights can be gained into social behaviors.

Encapsulated in Mead's, Bandura's, and Bronfenbrenner's theories are descriptions of how individuals relate to their environment, and how the environment in turn is instrumental in sculpting the individual's cognitive development. Through these interactions the social self develops and is displayed in an outward manifestation of social actions and behaviors. Underlying these behaviors are thought processes that become the monitoring agent for controlling thoughts, feelings, and actions.

An in-depth look at these thought processes has resulted in the study of social intelligence or practical intelligence. Within this domain, insight formation—gaining insights into both the self and others—is examined and the ability to understand one-self is explored. In recent years one aspect of social intelligence has come to the forefront. Termed "emotional intelligence," it investigates how individuals learn to monitor their feelings and emotions, discriminate among these feelings, and use this information to guide their thinking and action (Salovy & Mayer, 1990). The main interest in the study of emotional intelligence can be associated with the work of Daniel Goleman.

Emotional Intelligence and the Work of Daniel Goleman

Goleman believes that individuals are capable of developing an emotional intelli-gence just as they are able to develop competencies such as those assessed by standardized intelligence tests that yield an intelligence quotient (IQ). Furthermore, he purports that of the two forms of intelligence the one that subsumes the emo-tional domain is the most critical. According to Goleman, one's emotional intelli-gence involves four main areas. The first one focuses on developing emotional self-awareness whereby the individual is capable of separating feelings from actions. The second area examines managing emotions that entail learning strategies to con-trol negative emotions such as anger. The third area, identified as reading emotions, is described as being able to take the perspective of others. Goleman refers to the fourth area as handling relationships that he defines as the ability to solve problems (Goleman, 1995).

His philosophy is based on the premise that all children need to develop healthy emotional skills so that they are equipped to handle life in general. Based on this belief, he postulated that when individuals learn how to monitor their feelings and master the ability to take another person's perspective, they develop critical problem-solving skills that are essential if and when they engage in conflict resolutions.

Developing self-awareness and learning how to manage strong emotions are both valuable life skills that are essential to the socialization process. Furthermore, recognizing the importance of relationships and learning how to take responsibility for one's decisions and actions are key dimensions for social survival. These skills unfold over the course of a lifetime as individuals experience life by interacting with the various social agents within their environment.

Agents of Socialization

The socialization process begins in infancy with the family and continues through-out the school years, when peer groups become highly influential. Furthermore, this process extends into adulthood with the workplace, and with memberships in social, political, and professional organizations. Through all these interactions, individuals form a self-image based on their involvement with their various affiliations.

The family is the primary socializing agency from birth until the child enters school. From these early beginnings parents convey their values, religious beliefs, and social standing to their children. They inadvertently teach them to trust or fear the larger world based on how they react in various social settings. Furthermore, they are capable of unintentionally transmitting signals to them that reflect their perceptions of whether they consider their child to be strong or weak, smart or stupid, loved or merely tolerated. Through these early interactions, children begin to form a sense of self that accompanies them into the classroom.

Although some children are born into families where there are no siblings, others enter this world immediately surrounded by brothers and sisters. In these settings siblings provide the first peer group for children, thus affording them opportunities to experiment with conflict resolution, to determine how to make friends, and how to deal with authority. The process of vying for attention and finding their place and role in the family unit establishes the early underpinnings for future adult roles. As children reach school age, they carry with them the knowledge they have gleaned from interacting with their siblings as they come in contact with those outside their family unit (Luterman, 1987).

As children enter school their world is enlarged as they encounter people of more diverse social backgrounds. These experiences heighten their awareness of their own social identities as they begin to join groups and become involved in play activities. As they progress through the educational system their focus turns to academics that include reading, mathematics, and foundation courses that they will rely on later for advanced coursework. In addition to their academic training, children are exposed to the "hidden curriculum" whereby cultural messages are transmitted.

Within the school setting children have their first experiences with formalized instruction and the need to adhere to a schedule. For many, these experiences mark their first encounters with structured regimentation. Encouraged to follow a schedule in a timely manner, they develop the need to be punctual while honing their organizational skills. Thus, from these early beginnings children are socialized to develop those traits that will serve them later as they enter the workforce.

Schools also provide a mecca for peer interaction. Free of direct adult supervision, children gain valuable opportunities to form social relationships. Together with their peers they share common interests, and discuss topics that they may or may not discuss with their parents. Furthermore, they learn to anticipate how others will respond to their actions and therefore they become adept at adjusting their behavior to match these expectations. The importance of peer groups typically peaks in adolescence as young people begin to separate from their families and declare their independence as young adults.

According to Mead, Bandura, and Bronfenbrenner, these agents of socialization are instrumental in shaping the self, instilling culture and values, and providing the arena for individuals to form opinions and make decisions. Based on social scripts prescribed by society, individuals are afforded opportunities to interact with one another. Thus, within these social parameters they begin to develop a sense of uniqueness that distinguishes them from others, a distinction that is held in a positive light unless it deviates considerably from the social script. In these instances the individual has not mastered the required social protocol and does not conform to the traditional norm. When this occurs, the larger society equates uniqueness with a negative attribute rather than a positive feature, thus rendering the person unacceptable for group membership.

Deaf and hard-of-hearing individuals do not fit the prototype of those who move freely within the mainstream of society. Based on degree of hearing loss, age of onset when the loss occurred, cultural preference, and communication background these individuals may experience varying degrees of difficulty as they attempt to navigate within the social constructs designed by those who can hear. What impact does this have on their socialization process? What views do members of the larger hearing society hold regarding this disability group? How do these views affect those who are deaf and hard of hearing as they engage in developing the "looking-glass self"? Through this interactive process, how do deaf and hard-of-hearing individuals perceive the larger hearing society?

Views of Deafness: Society's Perceptions and Expectations

Congenital deafness is a low-incidence disability that affects a small percentage of the population. As a result, when deaf children enter the world the majority become part of hearing families and communities who know little if anything of the ramifications of deafness. From the onset, parents and hearing community members harbor preconceived ideas of a social image of deafness. These attitudes are conveyed to the deaf child and are instrumental in affecting his or her personality development. According to Oblowitz, Green, and Heyns (1991) and Stuart, Harrison, and Simpson (1991), "deafness per se does not determine the emotional and social development of the individual. Rather, it is the attitudes of hearing people that cause irreparable harm to the personality of the deaf person."

This view is shared by Martinez and Silvestre (1995), who contend that deaf individuals are affected by the consequences of deafness and the implied barriers that interfere with the acquisition of oral language skills. Furthermore, they hold that hearing society imposes a series of limitations that are rooted in the social image of deafness. Social images are formed based on previous experiences, observations, input from the media, perceptions of events, and hearsay.

Research conducted by Cambra (2000) has provided insights into the personality descriptors that are attributed to the deaf. Through a survey of 222 university students she determined that deaf people were specifically thought to be significantly more reserved, more solitary, slower, more dependent, and less confident than individuals without a sensory disability. Additionally, deaf individuals were perceived as being significantly less communicative, less kind and pleasant, possessing fewer friends, and less assertive than people without a sensory disability.

When the initial diagnosis of deafness is made parents experience a plethora of emotions. Furthermore, they react in part based on their preconceived ideas of what "deafness" means. As they seek advice regarding how to relate to their child, they frequently find themselves fraught with frustrations as they attempt to establish communication. Those in closest contact with the deaf child may find it difficult to adjust to the situation of having deafness in the family. Parents may experience feelings of guilt that they cannot explain. By outward appearances, their child has all of the external features of a hearing child. As a result many parents, either consciously or unconsciously, attempt to mold their child into the image of one who can hear. Initially relying on spoken language to convey their thoughts and feelings, they are unaware of what is not being heard, what is not understood, and what they are failing to convey.

As the child continues to grow, both parents and deaf children may find themselves caught in an ongoing struggle of attempting to make their needs understood. While some are successful, many more experience failure and eventually retreat to solitude, where they experience feelings of isolation. For the child, it can become a time of deciphering half understood messages. For the parents, it potentially becomes a period of adjustment marked by an irrational feeling that their child can and will adjust to the hearing world normally in time (Goodman, 1971).

The average hearing person has difficulty communicating with those who are deaf. Operating from a preconceived set of expectations about how communication typically takes place, there is a shock in not being able to communicate naturally. Subsequently, hearing individuals frequently become disturbed, irritated, frustrated, or embarrassed when communication does not flow smoothly. As a result, they search for ways to eliminate the cause of their uneasiness and will frequently end the conversation (Garrett & Levine, 1969).

These situations can be unsettling for both parties. For those who can hear, it becomes a blatant reminder that they are unable to express themselves clearly to their deaf child. Furthermore, it becomes apparent that this communication barrier renders them equally handicapped as their child who has the disability. For some, this realization prompts them to explore alternative means to converse with their child to insure that ideas can be shared and that both the communication and the socialization process can be fostered and enhanced. However, for those who are unable or unwilling to accept partial responsibility for the breakdown in communication, they may direct their frustrations outward and place the blame for this failure exclusively on their deaf child. Thus, from these early exchanges that result in misunderstandings, the socialization process is impeded and the child may begin to develop feelings of inferiority.

Furthermore, as deaf children become cognizant of communication problems, their sense of isolation and loneliness is exacerbated as they realize that others may not be comfortable interacting with them. Attuned to the way others view them, they begin to perceive themselves through society's eyes and develop a sense of being outsiders in a hearing world.

As deaf children navigate within Bronfenbrenner's environmental systems, their ability to form relationships and integrate social information becomes a complex process. Bathed in social information, hearing children benefit from direct input from their parents, siblings, peers, and community members. Furthermore, they have the distinct advantage of accessing incidental learning as they become attuned to the events and conversations that surround them. In contrast, hearing parents may struggle from the onset with mastering the skills required to convey key ideas and information. As a result, deaf children may be denied access to direct instruction and may therefore fail to receive pertinent social information. This deficit is further compounded by their inability to hear spoken exchanges that routinely occur in the environment. Denied access to informal social exchanges their opportunities to benefit from incidental learning experiences are thus sharply reduced.

Although deaf children experience the same multiplicity of relationships that hearing children do, their perceptions of the world and the messages contained in the spoken exchanges that occur around them are primarily shaped in their entirety by what they receive through their visual field. Frequently lacking information contained in the multitude of messages and secondary meanings that others receive through audition, they begin to form their perceptions of themselves and the world based on what they see. These perceptions are further influenced by their degree of hearing loss and age of onset when their loss occurred. Figure 6.1 illustrates the impact deafness has on social development within the structure of Bronfenbrenner's environmental system. Although deaf individuals are exposed to the same interactions, an auditory screen surrounds them, filtering out critical information and preventing them from fully interacting with their environment.

A Look at Deafness: The Socialization Process

Deafness encompasses far more than just a hearing loss; it is a complex sociopolitical reality that permeates one's life (Rosen, 1986). If it is present at birth or occurs during the first few years of life, it has far-reaching implications for communication, affecting not only the daily exchange of information but also the vast amount of incidental learning that is embedded in it. Extending into all aspects of one's life, deafness becomes another variable to be considered as the socialization process is explored. Beginning with childhood and continuing through adulthood, this defining characteristic adds another dimension that must be integrated into the total composite as the child forms his or her social identity.

Growing up Deaf: Early Childhood Experiences

Socioemotional development in deaf infants mirrors the developmental pattern exhibited by hearing children. However, when profound deafness is present at birth it drasti-

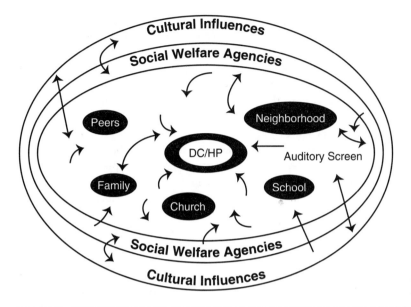

FIGURE 6.1 *Impact of deafness on social development within the structure of Bronfenbrenner's environmental system.*

cally alters the infant's perception of the world. Denied access to auditory information and spoken communication, the child is forced to obtain information primarily through one sense, vision, to glean information from and about his or her surroundings.

Upon entering the world, infants are faced with the task of developing a secure sense of attachment to their primary caregivers. This process begins at birth, intensifies midway through the first year, and when established provides the child with a secure base from which to explore the environment (Ainsworth, 1979). Numerous psychologists have observed the degrees of attachment in young children by applying an observational technique referred to as the Strange Situation. Designed by Ainsworth (1979) it enables professionals to observe a mother and child at play, and the reactions of the child when the mother leaves the room, when a stranger enters the play area, and when the mother reenters the room.

The Strange Situation has also been used with deaf babies to assess attachment formation. Recognizing that verbal exchanges can be challenging between young deaf children and their hearing parents, Greenberg and Marvin (1979) hypothesized that when deaf children were placed in the Strange Situation they would be delayed in their ability to establish secure feelings of attachment. However, the findings of their study revealed the opposite. When reciprocal communication was in place there was no evidence of delay in this being established. This research has been further substantiated by studies conducted by Koester and MacTurk (1991) and Lederberg and Mobley (1990) that reveal the similarities in attachment patterns between hearing and deaf children.

Developing feelings of attachment are dependent in part on the infant's ability to identify and differentiate between emotional expressions that are revealed on the face. According to Kestenbaum and Nelson (1990), hearing infants begin to distinguish differences in facial expressions, (e.g., surprise, anger, sadness) by 3 months of age. However, they do not fully understand the significance of the differences between these expressions until they reach approximately 7 months of age. Additionally, by 9 months of age their perception is heightened and they are capable of recognizing the emotional expressions of others as social signals (Feinman, 1992).

Throughout the first year of life hearing infants continue to discriminate between various facial expressions. However, this ability is not fully mastered until the child becomes much older. It involves an ongoing process throughout childhood that entails developing an understanding of emotions, attaching labels to these emotions, and then matching them to emotive situations (Borke, 1971; Brody & Harrison, 1987; Gross & Baliff, 1991). Furthermore, throughout this time children become attentive to emotional language and begin equating it with the emotions they are observing.

In a comparative study of hearing children and deaf children of hearing parents between the ages of 6 and 11, Russell and Bullock (1985) determined that deaf children could correctly identify and label emotions depicted in photographs of various facial expressions. These results further illustrated that their hearing loss did not impede their ability to match emotions with pictorial expressions and that their perceptions were comparable to those displayed by the hearing children involved in the study.

This study also reported error data indicating that children in both groups confused anger with disgust, and fear with surprise. Furthermore, results indicated that the younger children reflected a tendency to confuse the negative expressions of anger, disgust, and fear with sadness (Gray, Hosie, Russell, & Ormel, 2002).

Gray, Hosie, Russell, and Ormel (2002) have provided additional insights into the ability of deaf children to match facial expressions with emotions. They compared the responses of two groups of hearing and deaf children, ages 7 and 11, as they attempted to match facial expressions of happiness, sadness, anger, fear, disgust, and surprise to the feelings of a protagonist in a series of emotion-arousing vignettes.

Their findings revealed that hearing children were able to assign appropriate facial expressions to pictures more frequently than deaf children involved in the study. The results also suggested that the performance of both groups of students improved with age. However, despite probable differences in their early socialization of emotion, there were no significant differences in their understanding of the facial expressions of happiness, sadness, anger, fear, disgust, and surprise. Both groups possessed a common understanding of the features that differentiated each of these emotions. Furthermore, they were able to apply appropriate labels and associate them with events that would cause the various emotions to occur.

During the elementary years, hearing children begin to move beyond the identification stage and acquire an understanding of when and how to express appropriate emotions. Referred to as display rules, there is evidence to suggest that the extent to which children assimilate these rules is a direct reflection of their general level of social maturity (Ekman, Friesen, & Ellsworth, 1972).

The use of display rules presupposes an awareness of the difference between felt and expressed emotion (Saarni, 1993). Research conducted by Hosie and her colleagues (2000) examined the use of display rules in deaf and hearing children between the ages of 8 and 14. The results of their study revealed that there were no significant differences between the two groups, and that both elementary and secondary school-aged children were able to regulate their expressive behavior appropriately. One interesting contrast cited in the study focused on concealment. When comparing the two groups, significant differences were noted in what the hearing and deaf students chose to conceal. Deaf children were significantly less likely to conceal happiness and anger when compared with their hearing counterparts (Hosie et al., 2000).

Children rely on their ability to develop a sense of emotional intelligence, and employ display rules to socialize effectively with those around them. It becomes their internal barometer as they interact with their parents, and later as they interface with their peers. Furthermore, it assists them as they grow and develop, providing them with insights into their feelings and the feelings of others.

Once children establish a sense of security they feel free to explore the world of play. Play is one of the earliest forms of socialization, and it serves several functions for the young child. It serves a connective function joining children with their peers and thus promoting group interaction. In addition, it is frequently engaged in for pure enjoyment while simultaneously providing the ingredients that are required for the enhancement of cognitive development. Furthermore, it serves as the foundation in the socialization process, providing children with the building blocks they need that are essential as they learn how to relate to each other and develop peer sociability.

Numerous studies have been designed to examine the play behaviors of deaf children. Those conducted by Vygotsky (1978), Casby and McCormack (1985), and Schirmer (1989) indicate that there is a significant relationship between language skills and levels of symbolic play. Their findings consistently indicated that the child's language ability was directly related to his or her ability to substitute one object for another during play.

Research conducted by Gregory and Mogford (1983) has also examined the symbolic play behaviors found in deaf children. Results of their study highlight the differences between deaf and hearing toddlers from 15 to 30 months of age. Data reported indicated that hearing children were involved in significantly greater percentages of play at the "higher, imaginary (or symbolic) levels" than the deaf children. Furthermore, deaf children engaged in more "context-bound" play, and frequently used toys in an inappropriate manner. Gregory and Mogford also observed a difference in the deaf toddlers' ability to plan and structure their play sequences, both skills that have been equated with language abilities. They further surmised that these skills are fundamental to the learning process as children discover how to interact with peers and adults.

The general conclusion from these studies is that deaf children lag behind their hearing peers in cognitive, social, or both aspects of play (Spencer & Deyo, 1993). In addition, deaf children may structure their world of play in a way that is fundamentally different from hearing children. Although current research indicates that deaf children are involved in lower levels of symbolic play, it does not imply that they are not capable of playing at higher symbolic levels (Gregory & Mogford, 1983).

The Function of Play

Mildred Parten (1932) is well known for her study and classification of children's play. She observed children in free play in nursery school settings, and based on these observations developed six categories to describe their activities. She referred to the first category as unoccupied play, which occurs when children stand in one spot, look around the room, and perhaps involve themselves in random movements that do not involve a specific goal. Solitary play is used to describe children who play alone and are independent of others. Her third stage is referred to as onlooker play, the stage wherein children may ask others questions about what they are doing but do not become actively involved in the activity themselves. Parten identified the fourth stage as parallel play; in these instances children play separately from others, frequently using similar toys as their counterparts or mimicking the other child's play behaviors. Associative play occurs when children play together with little if any organization. The focus of these activities is on social exchanges rather than the performance of specific tasks. The sixth category is identified as cooperative play, characterized by a more advanced form of interaction that entails organization and planning whereby children work toward a common goal.

It was once thought that these categories of play were purely developmental and that after children experienced play at one level they would advance to subsequent levels. However, recent longitudinal research conducted by Howes and Matheson (1992) indicates that although these play forms are developmental in nature and children do experience them in the order suggested by Parten, the old forms are not eliminated once new forms are acquired. Rather, children continue to engage in solitary play and parallel play as they enter elementary school.

Research conducted by Higginbotham and Baker (1981) has provided insights into how play develops in deaf children. Using a modification of Parten's social play categories a comparative study of deaf and hearing children between the ages of 47 and 66 months of age was conducted. Results of this study indicated that the deaf children spent significantly less time in cooperative play activities and significantly more time in solitary play than the hearing children. Furthermore, it was also noted that the amount of time the deaf children spent in solitary play was greater than that engaged in by younger hearing children. The authors suggested that these results could be attributed to communication difficulties and a history of failed social attempts.

Additional studies conducted by Vandell and George (1981) further support these findings. In a study comparing deaf dyads with hearing dyads, it was determined that when compared with their hearing playmates, the deaf children initiated more interactions with their deaf playmates than was observed between the hearing youngsters. However, when initiations were made the hearing children in the study responded to one another 75 percent of the time whereas the deaf children responded less than 50 percent of the time. Vandell and George attributed this to the deaf children being oblivious to the other children attempting to initiate dialogue.

Forced to rely on the visual field for communication, deaf children may fail to respond to gestures or signs because their eyes are focused on their objects of play. Furthermore they may experience difficulty dividing their attention between their play activity and their peers, and therefore when they become engrossed in their activity the conversation so prevalent in parallel and cooperative play may fall by the wayside. Unlike their hearing peers, who can listen and respond while simultaneously playing and thus develop their social skills, deaf children must choose one activity over the other. Therefore, there may be reduced peer interaction from the onset, as children become engrossed in their play.

Parten (1932), has provided one avenue for researching play behaviors in children. In addition, contemporary researchers have begun to focus on the cognitive as well as the social aspects of play. Within these domains symbolic, practice, social, and constructive play is examined as further insights are gained into the socialization process.

Social Play, Constructive Play, and Games

Social play involves peer interaction. It increases in frequency throughout the preschool years and continues through middle childhood. Characterized by dramatic play and rough and tumble play, children devote time to running, chasing and wrestling, and play fighting each other. During this time children also become engaged in constructive play.

Constructive play occurs when young people engage in a self-regulated creation or in the construction of a product or a problem solution. It develops during the preschool years and remains a frequent form of play throughout elementary school. Constructive play is incorporated in the classroom to foster academic learning as students solve problems, write creative stories, and express themselves through their artistic endeavors. It is also used outside of the classroom as they draw pictures, put puzzles together, and build with blocks. Used as a vehicle for classroom instruction, constructive play becomes a midway point between play and work.

Preschool children do not limit their activities to constructive play, for at this age games are also initiated. From the onset, young children design games with simple rules that provide for reciprocity and turn taking. However as they enter elementary school their games increase in sophistication and popularity. Games reach their peak between 10 and 12 years of age; at that point they begin to decline as children become involved in conversations and in organized sports (Bergin, 1988). At this point peer interactions become the focal point of socioemotional development.

Peer Interaction and Popularity

Throughout middle childhood and continuing into middle adolescence, children spend an increased amount of time interacting with their peers. During this stage of development, peer acceptance becomes increasingly important. Although some children are readily liked by their peers, frequently nominated as a best friend, and are considered popular, others are rarely nominated as a best friend, are actively disliked by their peers, and are rejected. Still other children are identified as neglected due to the fact that they are infrequently nominated as a best friend but are not disliked by their peers. Social acceptance, or lack of acceptance, is further evident in a group referred to as the controversial children. These young people are frequently nominated as someone's best friend and at the same time are also placed in the category of being disliked (Ladd, 1999; Wentzel & Asher, 1995).

According to Coie, Dodge, and Coppotelli (1982), about two-thirds of the pupils in a typical elementary classroom fit one of these categories. The other one-third are considered average in peer acceptance and therefore do not fit the descriptors of the other categories. Children who are identified as rejected frequently have more serious adjustment problems later in life than those who are neglected (Dishon & Li, 1996). Generally described as being unhappy, alienated, and low achievers, these children frequently display a wide range of emotional and social problems (Coie & Dodge, 1998).

Deaf children enter classrooms with the same expectations and needs as their hearing peers. While some attend residential and day schools where deaf peers surround them, others enter the mainstream where they encounter hearing classmates. Regardless of the school setting, they all arrive with anticipation and an innate desire to be accepted.

Integrating deaf students into the public school environment is not always a positive experience. The class as a group may exhibit negative behaviors toward deaf students, leaving them on the sidelines. When this occurs feelings of rejection, isolation, and indifference may ensue, thus restricting the deaf student's social development (Ladd, Munson, & Miller, 1984).

Developing Friendships

Children's social behavior is a major contributing factor to peer acceptance or peer rejection. In addition, it also plays an integral role in the formation of friendships. Friendships form early in childhood as concrete relationships based on pleasurable activities. These relationships can provide cognitive and emotional resources for children as they grow from childhood into adulthood (Hartup & Stevens, 1997). Although each friendship is unique, friends can promote feelings of self-worth and self-esteem in those closest to them.

According to Gottman and Parker (1987), friendships serve six functions: companionship, stimulation, physical support, ego support, social comparison, and intimacy/affection. Through these relationships children learn to share, to confide in one another, and later, in adolescence, to establish intimate friendships (Berndt & Perry, 1990).

Several researchers have investigated how friendships are formed. This information has been compiled by William Damon (1977, 1988) and is represented according to age in a three-stage sequence. The first level encompasses children between the ages of 4 and 7. At this level friendship is viewed concretely. Children form bonds with each other based on a mutual desire to share in activities. These early friendships are easily dissolved as children tire of sharing or are unavailable to play.

The second level emerges at approximately 8 years of age and continues until the child is about 10. At this point in time, children's perceptions of friendship become more complex. Developmentally they are at a stage where they begin to appreciate others' personal qualities and can respond to their friend's basic needs. Throughout this stage each party conveys a desire to participate in the relationship and a willingness to provide help when needed. Trust becomes one of the defining features, and if broken can destroy a friendship (Damon, 1977).

Between 11 and 15 years of age the third level of friendship becomes apparent. As children enter adolescence, friendships enter a new plane. According to Buhrmester (1996), when adolescents are asked to define friendship they characterize it in two ways. First and foremost they search for individuals with whom they can form an intimate relationship. In this respect they are seeking friends who will provide them with psychological closeness and mutual understanding. Second, they want their friends to be loyal and stay with them. At this level, friends serve an instrumental role in providing mutual understanding and in relieving psychological distress (Sullivan, 1953).

Throughout the adolescent years friendships and peer groups become vitally important. As children transition into teenagers, they spend increasing amounts of time with their friends where their conversations reach a new level of intimacy. At this age, friends depend on their peers for close companionship, and to reassure them of their own self-worth. According to Sullivan (1953), friends play an instrumental role in the shaping of the teenager's emotional well-being. He further contends that when teenagers fail to establish close friendships, they experience painful feelings of loneliness coupled with feelings of low self-worth.

Social development in adolescence is largely dependent on establishing friendships, participating in cliques or peer groups, and establishing a sense of independence. Although communication drives the socialization process, language is taken for granted, with communication being discussed only as it relates to breakdowns in understanding. However, when discussing the social development of young deaf adolescents the issue of language is moved to the forefront, where it is viewed as a critical feature in the socialization process.

There is a plethora of literature within the field of deafness that addresses the development of communication in young deaf children. By comparison, there is a paucity of studies that focus on the social communication and the impact of friendship formation between deaf adolescents and their peers. Available research suggests that while some deaf people enjoy a rich and varied social life, others are extremely lonely at times, experience feelings of isolation, and struggle in their attempt to make and sustain friendships (Gregory, 1998).

Several of these studies have examined the impact of the educational setting on social life. While positive social experiences have been cited in residential school programs (Mertens, 1989), negative feelings of social rejection, isolation, and loneliness have been reported in mainstreamed settings (Davis, 1986; Holcomb, 1996). However, in a recent study conducted by Gregory, Bishop, and Sheldon (1995), a more positive pattern of social development has emerged.

Based on interviews with 82 hearing parents and their young deaf adults, topics concerning language acquisition, communication and family life, and friendship patterns were examined. Responses to the interviews revealed that deaf individuals were successful in engaging in one-on-one communication. However, they further reported that when attending family gatherings they frequently felt left out of the information loop and experienced embarrassment when family members attempted to include them. Furthermore, 80 percent of the young deaf people felt that communication breakdowns created major problems, denying them access to pertinent family information including deaths in the family, pregnancies, and marital breakdowns. Additional results of this study revealed that 77 percent of the deaf individuals surveyed indicated they had formed a close friendship with a special friend or that they belonged to a stable group of friends. Although the topic of loneliness was discussed, it was described as something they experienced occasionally but was not totally encompassing (Gregory, 1998, p. 162).

Deaf individuals develop friendships with those who can hear, those who are hard of hearing, and those who refer to themselves as Deaf. Deaf students who have adopted an oral philosophy and rely on their speech to communicate tend to gravitate toward others, both hearing and deaf, who can speak. Their familiarity with social scripts mastered through incidental learning and their ability to access spoken communication will contribute to the degree of their acceptance by those who can hear. Research conducted by Leigh and Stinson (1991) has revealed that deaf students who embrace an oral philosophy assign a higher rating to the need to establish closer relationships with peers who can speak, rather than those who use American Sign Language (ASL) or simultaneous communication. For those individuals participating in extracurricular activities, establishing a sense of belonging within the mainstream can become an achievable goal.

However, for those with weak oral skills, the socialization process can become daunting. Deaf students who are proficient in sign language and are comfortable using the language generally form bonds with other deaf and hard-of-hearing students, thus establishing a social group based on a shared method of communication. When this occurs they experience fewer feelings of loneliness (Murphy & Newlon,

1987). However, in those settings where the teenager is the only deaf student in the school, the opportunity for forming these bonds may not exist.

Stinson and his colleagues (1990, 1988) and Kluwin (1989) have examined social relationships in respect to the internalization of feelings of social competence. Data compiled from questionnaires completed by deaf and hard-of-hearing adolescents reflect that social competence is significantly related to their social experiences. Those students who enjoyed greater participation in class, in school, and in extracurricular activities and displayed emotional security with hearing peers achieved high ratings of perceived social competence. These results further indicated that students who are comfortable engaging in a variety of activities and feel secure in their relationships tend to feel more confident about their social skills.

Positive social environments during adolescence provide the arena for social growth and development to occur. They afford students opportunities to develop their social skills, express their feelings, establish relationships, and engage in social interactions. Included in these environments is an atmosphere of open dialogue where various modes of communication are recognized and accepted, and where peers speak the same language. With this key element in place, deaf and hard-of-hearing individuals are free to interact with their environment, shaping it as they develop socially.

Summary

The socialization process begins with birth and continues throughout one's lifetime. From the earliest stage attachments are formed and the infant develops a sense of security. Once established, toddlers enter the early childhood stage and play becomes the chief socializing agent. As children progress through middle childhood and into adolescence, play gives way to deepening friendships and peer groups. Thus, at this juncture the individuals enter adulthood and reflect the composite of what they have become.

The majority of deaf and hard-of-hearing infants are born into hearing families. Through their visual exploration of their surroundings, they begin to form perceptions of their identity, of significant others in their environment, and of the role they are expected to play in the family unit. As they progress through the developmental stages they interface with society. For some, their family accepts them, and accepts their preferred mode of communication (either speech or sign), and they master the social script and reflect the behaviors expected by the hearing social majority. For them, life becomes a positive experience as they develop into self-confident and self-assured young adults.

For others, their family and close family friends view deafness as an insurmountable obstacle that cannot be overcome and therefore they form barriers to the socialization process. Establishing lowered expectations for their children, they frequently deny them access to daily conversations and incidental learning experiences. Furthermore, they do not provide them with the scaffolding required for them to

develop into self-confident adults. In addition, by failing to share critical social information with them they hamper their development, instilling in them social behaviors
that are typical of much younger children. Caught in a web of misunderstandings,
these individuals frequently arrive at adulthood searching for a community where they
can establish a sense of belonging.

7

Identifying the Healthy Personality

Over the course of our lifetimes we develop physically, cognitively, and socioemotionally. Although psychologists posit various theories for how this development occurs, all concur that the process encompasses the totality of the individual. Human growth and development lasts a lifetime and is responsible for our physical appearance, our cognitive skills, and our overall mental health. Originating from genetic blueprints, we enter this world with basic needs that must be met in order to survive. In the process of meeting these needs we interface with individuals and events that contribute to the shaping of our identity and the formation of our self-concepts.

How do we form our self-concept? Why do some individuals develop healthy personalities while others struggle to discover who they are and what they want to become? Furthermore, what factors contribute to the shaping of a healthy personality? By exploring the field of phenomenology, one can examine both classic and contemporary theories of growth psychology. In turn, these theories can be applied to deaf individuals so that further insights can be gained into how they develop healthy personalities.

Theories of Healthy Personality

Since its inception, the field of psychology has scrutinized mental processes and external factors that influence behavior. The early contributors to the field studied the mind from both a psychoanalytic and a behavioral approach. Those steeped in psychoanalytic theory placed their focus on examining aspects of the mind concerning instincts, abnormalities, and unconscious thoughts. In contrast, those schooled in behaviorist theory supported the view that behavior is controlled by environmental determinants. Although very different in nature, both schools of thought have directed, and continue to direct, their energies toward examining the problematic aspects of personality development.

From these early beginnings, psychologists began probing the realm of human behavior and mental processes. While some adhered to the original schools of thought, other professionals began to explore another facet of development: humanistic psychology or phenomenology. These individuals began to investigate personal growth, positive personality characteristics, and the capability individuals have to determine their own destinies. Central to this school of thought is the premise that individuals possess the capability to overcome past experiences, and to focus their energies on their talents and creative abilities and develop at a level that exceeds normality.

Growth psychologists delve into the study of the healthy personality. Their view of human nature is optimistic and hopeful. Their theories are based on the premise that we have the capacity to expand, enrich, and fulfill ourselves to become all that we are capable of becoming. Furthermore, they emphasize that a healthy personality is not merely an individual who is free of emotional illness. The absence of neurotic or psychotic behavior does not qualify one as a healthy personality; rather, the absence of emotional illness is merely the required first step toward the beginning of personal growth and fulfillment (Schultz, 1977).

Humanistic psychologists concentrate on what an individual can become. They are not concerned with healing childhood-related conflicts. They recognize that childhood experiences influence personality development, but they further believe that individuals can rise above their past, their biological nature, and the features in their environment. Therefore, they emphasize what a person can become, not what he or she has been, or where the individual is at the moment. Leaders in the field of humanistic psychology include Gordon Allport, Carl Rogers, Erich Fromm, Carl Jung, Viktor Frankl, and Abraham Maslow. By briefly examining these theories, we can gain a broader perspective of what it means to have a "healthy personality."

It should be noted that Erik Erikson has developed an eight-stage model of psychosocial development. Although it is frequently applied to deaf individuals, his work is not cited here. For information regarding his theory and how it applies to deafness refer to *Sound and Sign* (Schlesinger & Meadow, 1972) and *Orientation to Deafness* (Scheetz, 2001).

Gordon Allport

Gordon Allport was one of the first American psychologists to scrutinize the healthy rather than the neurotic personality. By studying normal individuals, he formulated the premise that there are no functional similarities between disturbed and healthy personalities. In essence, he viewed them as separate entities. He further postulated that when one has a healthy personality, one's mental health is forward looking, not backward looking, and that the outlook one has is what the person hopes to become, not what he or she has already become, for this cannot be changed.

Allport characterized healthy personalities as people who are directed toward other individuals. They are depicted as mature persons who are cognizant of whom they are, and are therefore secure in their relationships with themselves and with the world around them. He based his definition of a mature, healthy personality on six criteria:

1. Extension of the sense of self. This is achieved when the welfare of another is identical with one's own. In this instance, strong interests are developed outside of the self and are extended into the critical areas of one's life.
2. Warm relating of self to others. This is characterized by two different kinds of warmth as evidenced in the capacity for compassion and the capacity for intimacy.
3. Emotional security. Included in this is self-acceptance of all aspects of one's personality, including weaknesses and failings, without being passively resigned to them.
4. Realistic perception, skills, and assignments. Included in this criterion is the individual's ability to view the world objectively and a commitment to work. This involvement is reflected in the person's total absorption whereby he or she loses himself or herself in the task at hand.
5. Self-objectification: insight and humor. This involves introspection whereby the person knows who he or she is; it begins early in life and continues throughout one's lifetime.
6. A unifying philosophy of life. This is described as a life that is forward looking, motivated by long-range goals and plans, and a sense of directedness (Allport, 1965).

In essence, Allport theorized that individuals who obtain psychological health are forward looking rather than backward looking, and that they have futuristic goals of what they want to become. Furthermore, he ascertained that when individuals achieve their present goals, they establish new ones as they continuously grow and develop (Allport, 1955).

Carl Rogers

Carl Rogers based his theory on the belief that people are guided by their own conscious perception of their selves and the world that surrounds them, rather than by unconscious forces that they cannot control. Furthermore, he gave credence to the fact that a person must ultimately rely on his or her own experience of the world to construct a sense of reality.

Rogers surmises that past experiences can influence the way that we perceive the present, and this in turn influences our level of psychological health. He acknowledges the fact that childhood experiences are important, but his focus remains on what is currently happening, rather than what has previously transpired. He further states that the primary motivator that drives the healthy person is actualization.

Actualization involves more than the mere act of maintaining a homeostatic balance within the organism. Instead, the goal of self-actualization is to foster growth and enhancement. According to Rogers, this is a continuous process that evolves as individuals move through life with openness to experiences and emotions. Thus, those intent on psychological growth and enhancement direct their energies to those activities that require an increased level of functioning, prompting them to become all that they are capable of becoming. Therefore, once the self begins to emerge, the tendency toward self-actualization appears.

Self-actualization does not occur in isolation, and is dependent on social rather than biological forces. Termed a process, it is aided or hindered by experience and by learning that has transpired, particularly during childhood. This process is ongoing and never finished. At times it can involve difficult and painful experiences as the individual explores his or her full potential. According to Rogers there are five specific characteristics of the fully functioning person:

1. An increasing openness to experience. These individuals have a heightened awareness of their feelings; they are not defensive, but rather are open to the emotions that they experience. Because they are cognizant of how they feel, they are free to experience life subjectively, welcoming the intensity provided by a wide spectrum of emotions.

2. An increasingly existential living. These individuals acknowledge the importance of living fully on a daily basis. They recognize that what one is becoming is contingent upon what one experiences in the present. This implies that individuals become participants in the process of becoming rather than being controlled by it. Furthermore, it denotes an absence of rigidity, and the imposition of structure on experience.

3. An increasing trust in his or her organism. People who have a trust in their own thought processes are capable of weighing the information and constructing their own decision based on their background knowledge and previous experiences. They behave in a way that when something feels right it guides their course of action.

4. The process of functioning more fully. These individuals are able to live fully in and with each and all of their feelings and restrictions. They make optimum use of all of the information their senses can supply and synthesize this knowledge before deciding on a course of action.

5. Creativity as an element of the good life. They espouse creativity and spontaneity, and may not necessarily be adjusted to their culture. Furthermore, because the evolution of the self is vital, these individuals represent the epitome of nonconformity (Rogers, 1961).

Rogers feels strongly that those who possess healthy personalities are self-directed and that they are fully open to all experiences. Furthermore, he believes that they are capable of self-directed change and growth, and that their motivation for self-actualization prompts them to move forward.

Erich Fromm

Erich Fromm's view of the healthy personality differs somewhat from the previous two theorists. He examines the healthy personality in terms of culture and society. He attests to the fact that mental health must be defined in terms of how well society adjusts to the basic needs of all individuals, not in terms of how well individuals adjust to society. Furthermore, he states that psychological health is not so much an individual affair as a social one, and that our mental health is dependent on how sufficiently a society satisfies our human needs.

Fromm believes that all of us possess an inherent striving for emotional health and well-being, and that we have an innate tendency for productive living for harmony and love. He states that when society gives us opportunities this intrinsic tendency will blossom, allowing us to develop to our fullest potential. He further believes that each society establishes their own definition of mental health, and that this definition varies with different times and places.

In essence he states that we possess psychological needs that the lower animals do not have, and that healthy people are motivated by these needs in creative and productive ways. These five basic needs, when satisfied in a productive manner, promote healthy personalities:

1. The need for relatedness is essential to one's psychological well-being. Fromm states that the healthy way to relate to the world is through love. Expressions of love satisfy a requirement for security and allow for a sense of integrity and individuality.
2. The need for transcendence refers to the need to rise above or transcend our passive roles as creatures. Creating is the ideal or healthy means of transcending the passive animal state.
3. The need for rootedness prompts us to establish a feeling of being connected with other members of society. This desire replaces the earlier dependency needs established from infancy within the familial unit. Furthermore, it prompts a sense of involvement within the larger confines of society.
4. The need for a sense of identity stems from our desire to feel like a separate individual. Individuals who experience a well-developed sense of identity feel they have more control over their lives and are less controlled by others.
5. The need for a frame of orientation addresses the fact that each individual must formulate a consistent image of the world. When this occurs the person is better equipped to understand all of life's events and experiences. Fromm indicates that the more objective a person's perception is of reality, the more likely he or she will be able to cope with the world (Fromm, 1947).

According to Fromm, the healthy personality loves fully, is creative, has highly developed powers of reason, is capable of perceiving the world and the self objectively, and possesses a firm sense of identity that is related and rooted in the world. He further believes that we have the capability of achieving a strong sense of self-identity and that it is done within the confines of social reality.

Carl Jung

Carl Jung's theory of personality development places a strong emphasis on the unconscious. However, unlike Freud, he suggests that personality continues to develop throughout one's lifetime and undergoes a "crucial transformation" between the ages of 35 and 50 (Jung, 1954). Jung ascertained that personality development takes place within four stages: childhood, youth and young adulthood, middle age, and old age.

Throughout childhood the child begins to develop an ego, but has no true sense of identity. According to Jung, at this age the child's personality is merely a reflection of the parents. The second stage of development begins at puberty. At this time the individual's personality begins to take shape and form. Termed "psychic birth," Jung characterizes this stage of development of one filled with a multitude of problems, conflicts, and adaptations, as the child is forced to surrender his or her childhood and face the realities of the adult world.

Young adulthood is characterized by an outward focus on education, career, and the establishment of a new family unit. The conscious focus at this time is to achieve and to find one's place in the world. When young adults are successful in their endeavors they become enthusiastic and excited about life. However, the positive nature of the stages changes as one enters middle age. During the third stage, individuals realize that the sense of accomplishment and the sense of adventure has disappeared from their lives. Faced with the realization that the peak of one's career is over, the individual is filled with feelings of despair and a sense of worthlessness. This is followed by the fourth stage, old age, of which Jung wrote very little.

Key to Jung's theory is the belief that the first half of an individual's life is focused on the external world and the second half must be devoted to the inner, subjective world that was previously neglected. During middle age individuals realize that they cannot continue to be guided by the values of youth, and therefore seek a new meaning to life. Through this process they attempt to integrate their unconscious with their conscious in order to achieve positive psychological health, the condition Jung refers to as "individuation" (Jung, 1954).

This individuation process lies at the crux of the healthy personality. It occurs in middle age and is reflected in those who have confronted goals and dreams that they previously suppressed in their unconscious. Furthermore, it is characterized by the person's acceptance and integration of all aspects of the personality into the self. Thus, healthy people are described as those who have contemplated their inner selves, by recognizing both the positive and the negative attributes of their personality. This exploration is followed by an acceptance of the self whereby individuated persons accept their strengths and their weaknesses.

Although Jung does not provide a list of the characteristics to describe the healthy personality, he emphasizes that those approaching this state can be characterized as having fully integrated personalities that are reflected in their general acceptance and tolerance of human nature. Furthermore, these individuals are comfortable accepting the unknown and possess what Jung refers to as a "universal personality" (Schultz, 1977, 98–100).

Viktor Frankl

Viktor Frankl's approach to healthy personality is comprised of three tenants: spirituality, freedom, and responsibility. By attaining and using these components the individual procures the basic tools to discover meaning and purpose in life, for without meaning, there is no reason to continue living. Each individual is responsible for determining his or her own unique meaning for life, and through this search a certain degree of tension is formed. Frankl perceives tension as a prerequisite for psychological health. According to Frankl, the healthy personality contains a certain level of tension between what has been accomplished and what should be accomplished. In essence, this gap provides the individual with the goals that supply meaning to life. Furthermore, he postulates that there are three ways that we give meaning to life: first, in the creations that we share with the world; second, in what we take from the world experience; and third, in the attitude we take toward suffering.

Frankl stresses that our major motivation in life is to search for meaning, which is equated with forgetting oneself. In his terms, the healthy personality has transcended beyond the focus of the self whereby the individual relates to someone or something beyond the person. He states, "To be psychologically healthy is to move beyond the focus on self, to transcend it, to absorb it in one's meaning and purpose. Then the self will be spontaneously and naturally fulfilled and actualized" (Frankl, 1962). Furthermore, he views those who possess healthy personalities as being future goal oriented, aware of the fact that they are free to make choices, and in conscious control of their lives.

Abraham Maslow

The term most frequently associated with Abraham Maslow is "self-actualization." Central to his philosophy of healthy personality is the belief that all individuals possess an innate striving or tendency to become self-actualized. This is accomplished by meeting our basic needs that range in ascending order from basic physiological needs, safety needs, belonging and love needs, to the level of esteem needs. He states that individuals are not simultaneously motivated by all of the needs. Rather as one group of needs is met, the individual is free to move to the next level of the hierarchy. Thus one's physiological needs for food, water, and air must be met before the person can concentrate on safety needs. When safety and security needs are satisfied, people are driven to satisfy the belonging and love needs. This in turn permits the individual to concentrate on a sense of esteem.

Maslow defined two types of esteem needs. He characterized the first type of needs as those that are derived from others. When we perceive that others regard us with high levels of esteem, we are confident and secure in ourselves, and we feel worthy and adequate. This in turn is instrumental in affecting the second type of esteem needs that he termed self-esteem. When individuals lack feelings of self-esteem, they feel inferior and helpless as they attempt to deal with life.

According to Maslow, once all of the basic needs are met, we are then driven by the highest need, and this he termed "self-actualization." Defined as the fulfillment of all of our qualities and capabilities, he ascertained that those who reach this level are not concerned with making up for deficits. At this point these individuals are not in the process of becoming; all of their lower needs have been met. Rather, such people are in a state of being, and are interested in creating a sense of tension whereby they can experience growth and maturation.

Maslow describes those who have reached self-actualization as possessing the following characteristics: an efficient perception of reality; a general acceptance of nature, others, and oneself; a sense of spontaneity, simplicity, and naturalness; and a focus on problems outside of themselves. Furthermore, they have a need for privacy and independence, a preference to function autonomously, a heightened awareness of other's feelings, and a strong desire to establish interpersonal relationships. They accept all people, regardless of ethnic background or social class, and can distinguish between what is morally right and wrong. Those who are self-actualized find humor in humanity in general but never in specific individuals. In addition, they are creative people and are resistant to enculturation (Maslow, 1954).

Maslow believed that self-actualization is dependent on childhood experiences. He stressed that children need to feel loved, especially during the first two years of life when trust and security is being established. Once this is established his supposition was that children acquire the foundation that will allow them to grow toward self-actualization.

Maslow and the other humanistic psychologists tend to agree that psychologically healthy people are in control of their lives, that they know who and what they are, and that they all have a firm anchor in the present. However, they differ in their views of how we arrive at the pinnacle of self-actualization. While one places emphasis on the unconscious, others feel that optimal growth is contingent upon childhood experiences.

Although each of the theories is unique, all have contributed insights into how the personality is shaped at various life stages. When engaging in a discussion pertaining to the healthy personality, it is critical to bear in mind that there is no single definition that describes psychological health; rather, there are multiple ways that one can arrive at this state of mind. However, by examining each of these theories, valuable insights can be gained into this growth process. Table 7.1 provides a summary of the key tenets espoused by each of these theorists.

Identity and self-concept are key elements in the development of the healthy personality. Providing the foundation for psychological growth to occur, these attributes furnish the springboard from which individuals explore uncharted territory and cultivate new ideas. Through this dynamic, ongoing process, unfamiliar plateaus are reached and new goals are established. This accretion in turn stimulates inquiries and promotes cognitive expansion, thus enhancing the self-actualization process.

Healthy Personality and Deafness

Deaf and hard-of-hearing individuals represent a diverse segment of the population. Encompassing a wide array of ethnic and socioeconomic backgrounds this aggregate is further characterized by the contrasting views they hold regarding what constitutes deafness. While some consider their loss as a disability to be overcome, others

TABLE 7.1   *A Comparison of Varying Perspectives of the Healthy Personality*

Gordon Allport	• Psychological health is forward looking, not backward looking.
	• Intentions provide the motivation for the development of the healthy personality.
	• Emphasis is placed on increasing tension for growth to occur.
	• The role of work and the establishment of goals is vital.
	• Responsibility is accepted for others.
	• Healthy personalities see good beyond themselves.
Carl Rogers	• Childhood experiences are important; however, current events play a more critical role in the development of the healthy personality.
	• Self-actualization occurs in relation to those around us and provides the motivating force for healthy personalities to develop.
	• Although no emphasis is placed on work or goals, a state of tension is required for growth to occur.
Erich Fromm	• Culture and society have a direct bearing on healthy personality.
	• Society provides the definition for healthy personalities.
	• Productivity is the driving force behind personality development.
Carl Jung	• Strong emphasis is placed on the unconscious.
	• Self-realization becomes the motivating force that prompts personality development.
	• Individuals develop internally during middle age, when an attempt is made to integrate the unconscious with the conscious—thus achieving positive psychological health.
Viktor Frankl	• Major motivators in life are to seek spirituality and freedom, and to develop responsibility.
	• Tension in one's life must transpire for growth to occur.
	• One must transcend the self to be psychologically healthy.
	• The role of work and the establishment of goals are critical to psychological growth.
Abraham Maslow	• Key to the healthy personality is self-actualization.
	• Emphasis is placed on tension being a necessity for psychological growth to occur.
	• Role of work and goals are of vital importance to the development of the healthy personality.

embrace the philosophy that deafness is a unique, distinguishing feature that unites them with others who cannot hear. Viewed as a defining characteristic, deafness is perceived as comprising an integral part of the individual's persona. In this respect it is valued and not considered a travesty that needs to be "fixed."

Embedded in each of these philosophies is a strong conviction of how deafness should be infused into the personality. For those who foster the belief that it is a handicap that needs to be eradicated, energies are channeled into enhancing spoken communication, investing in amplification (including hearing aids and cochlear implants), and developing techniques and strategies that will foster integration into the larger hearing society. Conversely, those who welcome their hearing loss and view it as an identifying feature of their individuality gravitate toward the Deaf community, where they embrace the values embodied by those who elect membership.

Over the course of their lifetimes deaf and hard-of-hearing individuals become aware of whom they are and determine where they feel they belong. For some, their identity is anchored in the hearing community; for others, it is established within the confines of the Deaf community. Although each of these settings affirms their own values, both provide fertile soil that fosters healthy personality growth and development.

Developing a Healthy Deaf Personality

Within the Hearing Community.   Deaf children born to hearing parents begin their lives in an atmosphere surrounded by sound where speech and spoken communication are valued. From these early beginnings they begin to sculpt their identity based on how their parents react to deafness, how family members elect to communicate with them, and what they perceive they are able to contribute to the family unit. The underpinnings of these early experiences set the tone for subsequent development.

Once a diagnosis of deafness is confirmed parents are faced with the monumental task of determining the mode of communication they will employ with their deaf child. While some embrace a form of manual communication, others rely on speech to engage in interactions with their infants and toddlers. In homes where speech becomes the primary mode of communication, verbal language acquisition is cherished and time is devoted to promoting the development of effective spoken language skills. Originating with these early encounters, children invest hours as they attempt to make their vocalizations clear. Furthermore, this training continues as children reach school age and begin their formal educational training.

Parents who embrace an oral philosophy select educational programs that foster aural and oral habilitation. Within these classrooms children receive support services designed to provide them with equal access to the curriculum. Furthermore, in these settings, deaf and hard-of-hearing students have the opportunity to mingle with those who can hear. While some form close friendships with their hearing peers, others remain withdrawn and aloof from those around them. Their involvement in and out of school activities is largely dependent on their ability to communicate clearly, their acceptance by their peer group, and their desire to become active participants in classroom and extracurricular activities.

Studies conducted by Allen and Osburn (1984) and Pflaster (1980) indicate that deaf and hard-of-hearing students can successfully participate in mainstreamed programs. This can occur if they have good oral communication skills, strong parental support, average or above average intelligence, self-confidence, and adequate support services.

Good communication skills entail learning how to speak clearly as well as becoming adept at speechreading. Degree of loss, age of onset, and early experiences are instrumental in influencing the development of these competencies. After years of intense training those with profound losses are cognizant of their degree of speech clarity. As one young deaf oral adult has stated:

> Mom and I always sat down to practice my speech almost every day. It wasn't easy for either of us to get me to make all my problem sounds like "s," "ch," "sh," "st," "j," "sts." I know we both got frustrated during these practice sessions. I guess all that practice paid off. Today I speak exceptionally well and really don't feel self-conscious about my speech or my language.
>
> To this day I don't fool myself. There is something different about my speech, and I have always known this. But it is not that different, so people usually have an easy time talking with me. Often when people first meet me, they ask what country I come from. I really enjoy this, because some people just think I have a foreign accent! (Altman, 1988).

Strong parental support can extend far beyond the realm of promoting spoken communication skills. In addition, these parents create environments that recognize individual differences, foster independence, and convey a sense of acceptance. Instead of focusing on their child's hearing loss, these parents channel their energies into assisting their children as they develop strategies to interface with the larger hearing world.

> Rather than force me to do things that I could not do, she [mom] simply created a large space in which I could try my luck and if my efforts did not work, go on to something else. She allowed me to be independent. She gave me room to learn how to balance success against failure and accept the results with equanimity (Kisor, 1990).

Supportive parents accept the reality that their children cannot hear, but they refuse to let others set limits for them. Furthermore, they believe that deaf and hard-of-hearing children have the same capacity that hearing children have to acquire language and social and intellectual skills, thus providing the foundation for self-actualization. In addition, they maintain a strong belief that each child's potential needs to be discovered and developed, so that an identity of being "special" is based on who they are or what they can do, rather than what they can't hear.

When supportive parents raise children the stage is set for the healthy personality to flourish. Within these environments deaf children are nurtured and provided with an avenue to develop to their fullest potential. In these instances hearing parents are very instrumental in promoting positive growth and development.

Within the Deaf Community.   According to Byrne (1998), approximately 10 percent of persons with hearing loss in the United States consider themselves members of Deaf culture. However, unlike other cultural groups that identify themselves by ethnicity, race, or geographic location, members of the Deaf community distinguish themselves by three major characteristics: attitude, behavioral norms, and attendance at residential schools (Paul & Jackson, 1993).

These individuals view deafness within the confines of a social construct rather than as a disability that is in need of a cure (Dolnick, 1993). They encourage the use of American Sign Language (ASL) and campaign for its acceptance and implementation in schools, in the workplace, and at public events (Lane, 1995). Furthermore, group members perceive their deafness as a positive identifying feature that distinguishes them and characterizes them as a unique linguistic minority group.

Those ascribing to the cultural belief of deafness contribute to the feeling of cultural solidarity. In this respect, membership into the group becomes an avenue for expression and self-recognition. In this environment community members support the attitudes, language, beliefs, and values of those who belong with no regard to hearing status (Johnson & Erting, 1989). Although individuals who claim membership in this group exhibit varying degrees of hearing, the severity of the loss becomes insignificant and is not considered by those in the in-group as a distinguishing feature of Deafness.

According to group members, the essence of Deafness revolves around the desire to share in the community and the culture based on ASL. For these individuals, deafness represents an affirmation of a cultural characteristic, and becomes a unifying feature that denotes a positive connotation (Dolnick, 1993, p. 43). From infancy, deaf children of culturally Deaf parents begin to form their identity with members of the Deaf community. Born to parents who have experienced life from a Deaf perspective, these children begin their journey to adulthood within an environment that is designed to accommodate shared experiences and communication exchanges.

Unlike deaf children who are born to hearing parents, these youngsters are received into the familial unit by parents who may be thrilled to have a child who is deaf. Frequently these infants are perceived as being the lifeline that will insure the continuation of the Deaf community. As young children they become privy to folklore, stories, and the values and traditions that are cherished by this unique group of individuals.

Membership in the Deaf community is not limited to those who have Deaf parents, or to those who have only attended residential schools. Those who identify with others who are Deaf and who are also committed to working toward the preservation of the ideals upheld by group members may seek entry. Those seeking and maintaining membership support the philosophy that their deafness does not need to be "fixed," that ASL is the preferred language of their cultural affiliation, and that although they must interact with the larger hearing society, their social obligations remain with those who are Deaf.

Although ease of communication is one of the primary reasons deaf adults gravitate toward each other, it is not the sole reason why the community exists. Within these boundaries individuals representing diverse ethnic backgrounds, educational backgrounds (those who have attended mainstreamed programs who later acquire a Deaf identity) and levels, and socioeconomic status come together. Here they share their mutual interests, solve problems, and develop a sense of camaraderie (Jacobs, 1980). Furthermore, it is within the milieu of this community and this social structure that Deaf individuals acquire a self-respecting image of themselves and a productive relationship with others (Schowe, 1979).

Countless vignettes have appeared in the literature throughout the past decade describing feelings of alienation from the larger hearing society and the sense of community deaf individuals experience when they encounter others "like them" for the first time. These reflections highlight the need for shared communication, belonging, and self-acceptance.

> Because I went to a normal school, I was the only Deaf person there. Often I thought I was the only one around. It wasn't until after I finished school that I had the opportunity to meet others with a similar disability. Now most of my closest friends are Deaf people. Why? Because we share common ground. I can relax with them. When I talk with hearing people, I have to concentrate to hear.
>
> My friends and I help each other with difficulties and we teach each other about relationships and life. We've developed into self-accepting more confident human beings. And it is with this confidence that I am beginning to make in-roads into communicating with hearing people. (Harper, 1983)

Deaf individuals who choose membership in the Deaf community form an affiliation with others who recognize them for their individual or unique characteristics rather than for their deafness. In this setting they experience the ease of communication as they discuss issues and express opinions. For some, membership is a reaffirmation of their identity; for others it becomes an entry point from which a Deaf identity is shaped. For both, it provides the arena for self-awareness to flourish, thus providing an avenue for self-actualization and the development of the healthy personality.

Applying the Theories: A Look at Deafness and Healthy Personality Development

The emergence of a healthy personality can be conceptualized as evolving along a continuum that originates with self-identity and expands to include all of life's experiences. Horizontal in nature, it becomes layered with vertical complexities as individuals encounter a myriad of life experiences. Those engaged in this dynamic process have first and foremost determined who and what they are, they are in control of their lives, and they are open to becoming all that they can be. Having developed a sense of security and trust in their ability to make decisions and form opinions, their focus turns to experiences that will enrich their lives.

Before one can begin to develop a healthy Deaf personality, one must first accept the premise that deafness is not a deficit but rather a difference. When this originates in childhood, parents "make the imaginative leap of understanding that will make it possible for them to let their child be deaf and at the same time make him or her a member of the family and the larger culture" (Thomas, 1994). This recognition affords children the opportunity to be raised under the knowledge that their deafness is just another way of being human. Furthermore, when they are allowed to be deaf, their deafness is viewed as just another characteristic of their identity rather than as an affliction. This early acceptance of deafness as a difference allows for the expansion of a healthy self-concept and an identity linked to characteristics that portray this difference as unique rather than dysfunctional.

Deaf infants born to Deaf parents enter this world within the microcosm of the Deaf community. In these families, early acceptance is a natural phenomenon as parents view their children as extensions of themselves. From the onset, raised and nurtured in homes where sign communication flows freely, these children begin to develop a sense of autonomy. Only later, when they encounter and attempt to communicate with hearing individuals who cannot sign, do they realize they are different.

Hearing parents raising deaf children are also capable of providing an atmosphere whereby optimal growth and development can occur. By acknowledging that their deaf infants are complete individuals with unique communication needs, they begin to look for strategies that when implemented will facilitate communication. Once in place, these children are afforded opportunities to engage in experiences and interactions that will ultimately foster and promote the development of a deaf identity and a healthy self-concept.

While some of these children will grow into adulthood and maintain their sense of connectedness with a hearing cultural orientation, others will develop a strong affiliation with the Deaf community, thereby fashioning a Deaf identity. These cultural groups, both hearing and deaf, provide their members with a distinct set of values and beliefs. Although divergent in nature, each one provides fertile ground for the cultivation of the healthy personality. Cultural identity, although deemed important by group members, plays a secondary role in the self-realization or self-actualization process. First and foremost the person must have a positive self-concept that includes a firm grasp of who he or she is, an appreciation for his or her abilities, and a realistic perception of existing or potential shortcomings.

Gordon Allport

Allport characterized healthy personalities as people who are directed toward others and who consider their welfare to be identical to their own. Within his six criteria he emphasized that these individuals develop strong interests outside the self and are motivated by long-range plans and objectives. These forward-looking individuals lose themselves in their work while continuously achieving their goals and establishing new ones.

Deaf leaders, responsible for the establishment of Deaf communities, embody several of the characteristics outlined in Allport's theory. Committed to establishing a haven that promotes the welfare of Deaf individuals, these men and women have extended themselves into meeting several of the critical needs that are evident in Deaf people's lives. Motivated by long-range goals, they have worked diligently to preserve their language and to promote an atmosphere where Deaf people are considered functional, rather than dysfunctional, members of society.

Through the years these individuals have been responsible for establishing numerous proactive Deaf organizations, including the National Association of the Deaf, the National Fraternal Society of the Deaf, and the American Athletic Association of the Deaf. The leaders of these organizations continually evaluate the goals for their organizations and modify them to meet the existing needs of their members.

Carl Rogers

Rogers's theory of psychological health was based on the premise that our experiences of the world are used to construct our sense of reality. Part of this reality is shaped by childhood experiences; however, the majority of it is attributed to what is currently happening. Rogers feels that the self-actualization process is continuous and is dependent on social rather than biological forces. Individuals on the road to self-actualization are cognizant of their feelings; they rely on these feelings to make decisions; and they are comfortable basing their decisions on their background knowledge and previous experiences. He further states that those reflecting a healthy personality are epitomized as being nonconformists, and capable of making self-directed changes.

In March 1988 at Gallaudet University in Washington, DC, the only liberal arts university for the deaf in the world, deaf leaders came to the forefront in what would later be known as the Deaf President Now movement. Prompted by deaf professionals who had been subjected to years of oppression, and supported by deaf students, faculty, and administrators, they joined together to protest the appointment of the eighth hearing president of the University. What followed was a protest that culminated in the installation of the first deaf president at Gallaudet, I. King Jordan. This incident forced professionals in the field to examine their views of deafness and the capabilities of deaf professionals.

In the aftermath of this event, the community became involved in a new social movement. Transformed from being somewhat passive and apolitical, they became mobilized for both traditional political action and nontraditional collective action (Barnhartt & Christiansen, 1996).

Based on Rogers's theory these Deaf individuals would be considered fully functioning individuals. By directing their energies to activities that require an increased level of involvement, they are prompted to evolve into all that they are capable of becoming. Furthermore, Rogers views this process as ongoing in nature, one that is never finished. Thus these Deaf leaders are at the pinnacle of their development, motivated by their desire to become self-actualized.

Erich Fromm

Fromm's view of healthy personality differs considerably from the other theorists. It is based on the premise that mental health must be defined in terms of how well society adjusts to the basic needs of all individuals and not in terms of how well individuals adjust to society; hence one's psychological health becomes a social rather than an individual affair. Fromm emphasized the need for rootedness and being connected. He further stressed that healthy personalities have more control over their lives and are less controlled by others. Recognizing the strong need for identity, he felt that when this was intact the person was capable of perceiving the world and the self objectively.

One can draw direct parallels between Fromm's theory and the establishment of the Deaf Community. Fromm believed strongly that the role of society was to meet the needs of the individual. When this occurred the person was provided with the opportunity to flourish. However, if this did not transpire, the individual's psychological health could be stymied.

Deaf and hearing individuals alike share the same basic needs. However, due to the ramifications of deafness and the accompanying communication barriers that can exist, many of the social needs of the various members of the deaf population were not met. This resulted in the establishment of Deaf communities. In these settings the need for belonging could be satisfied, a firm sense of identity could be formulated, and an objective view of the world could be generated, thus fostering the embodiment of a healthy personality.

Within these communities Deaf individuals are provided with the opportunities to live and love fully while simultaneously exploring their creativity. Expressions of this creativity are reflected in Deaf poetry, artwork, sculpture, and organizations such as the National Theater for the Deaf. Through these venues deaf individuals find avenues for channeling their creative potential. In these instances society (Deaf community) can be characterized as providing Deaf individuals with a sense of social reality while supplying them with the means to acquire a healthy personality.

Carl Jung

Jung based his theory of personality development on the belief that the first half of an individual's life is focused on the external world and the second half must be devoted to the inner, subjective world that was previously neglected. Within this theory he stressed that individuals experience an individuation process that lies at the crux of the healthy personality. Although Jung does not ascribe specific characteristics describing what is entailed in this development, he does describe these individuals as having contemplated their inner selves, both their strengths and weaknesses, and integrating these discoveries into a general acceptance and tolerance of human nature.

Ninety percent of deaf individuals are born to hearing parents. These children frequently find themselves in situations where they are the only deaf family member. Furthermore, they may receive their education in public schools where they are the only deaf student in their grade, or possibly the entire school. In addition, they may have had limited if any contact with other deaf people. Later, when and if these individuals encounter the Deaf community, they are faced with the realization that they are not alone and that there are others like them in the larger hearing world. At this point they are confronted with a Deaf identity and oftentimes engage in the process of defining for themselves who they are.

Glickman's (1993) Deaf Identity Model examines deafness from four different perspectives: culturally hearing, culturally marginal, immersion in the deaf world, and bicultural. Based on individual experiences, Deaf identities are formed with members becoming bicultural only when they affirm Deafness as a cultural difference and feel a profound connection with other Deaf people. Jung's model, although developed with hearing individuals in mind, can be applied to the struggle deaf individuals face as they attempt to determine who they are, where they belong, and how they should identify themselves.

Viktor Frankl

Frankl based his theory of healthy personality development on three tenets: spirituality, freedom, and responsibility. In essence, he postulated that each individual is responsible for determining his or her own unique meaning in life and through this search a certain amount of tension is formed. According to Frankl, tension is a prerequisite to psychological growth. Furthermore, he believed that we give meaning to life in three ways: in the creations we share with the world, in what we take from the world experience, and the attitude we take toward suffering.

Frankl's theory, that tension gives meaning to life, can be broadly applied to those who are deaf. Each day, deaf individuals are placed in situations where they are required to interact with the larger hearing community. Forced to devise and implement communication strategies that will grant them access into the activities surrounding them they fluctuate between a state of tension and one of temporary ease as they successfully navigate each encounter. Through the development of these communication techniques they discover who they are, what they believe, and where they feel they belong.

Once adept at communicating, they are rid of obstructions and can focus on issues that extend beyond themselves, and can use their creativity to determine what they are capable of doing to alleviate these problems. According to Frankl, each individual (deaf or hearing) is responsible for determining his or her own meaning in life. For those who have constructed a positive d/Deaf identity they will be able to apply their energies to enhancing the betterment of the community with which they have formed their strongest affiliation. Once absorbed in these projects they are at liberty to apply their creative talents to problem situations and can thus contribute back to society. These individuals are goal directed, are in conscious control of their lives, and maintain a forward focus in life.

Abraham Maslow

Maslow, noted for his theory of self-actualization, postulated that all individuals have basic needs. These needs can be viewed in ascending order originating with those that are very basic and culminating with the highest level of needs, which he identified as the esteem needs. He ascertained that all people are motivated by basic physiological needs, and that these had to be met before they could advance to the next level of the hierarchy. According to Maslow, once individuals meet all of their basic needs, they are then driven by their highest need, self-actualization. Within these various stages one gains an acceptance of self and others, an ability to focus on external rather than internal problems, and a desire to establish interpersonal relationships.

Deaf individuals have the innate ability to become self-actualized. When raised in environments where financial stability, safety, and security needs are met, they are driven to satisfy their need for love and belonging. In homes where their deafness is accepted and love is conveyed, this need is met and they are then free to concentrate on self-esteem.

Maslow defines two types of esteem needs. The first type is characterized as being derived from others. When we perceive that others hold us in high regard we develop a sense of inner confidence; however, when individuals feel that others do not view them in this manner, they lack feelings of self-esteem and feel inferior. Several factors are instrumental in influencing the development of the deaf person's self-esteem.

Acceptance of the deaf person's preferred mode of communication directly impacts self-esteem. Language becomes synonymous with self, and if one's mode of communication is rejected, it can be perceived internally as a rejection of deafness that is further exacerbated and interpreted as a rejection of the total person. It is at this level of self-actualization that deaf individuals can become stymied. Placed in situations where their language, both signed and spoken, is misunderstood, feelings of inferiority and helpless may ensue as they attempt to deal with life.

Deaf individuals who have overcome the communication barrier engage in conversations freely while developing a sense of self-worth. For some this entails maintaining an identity in the hearing community, for others it results in becoming bilingual and bicultural. However, regardless of the community orientation, when this hierarchical need is met the deaf person is motivated to continue to grow and mature.

Summary

Humanistic psychologists ascertain that we are all born with the innate ability to expand and develop to our fullest potential. Although these theorists each maintain their own separate view of development, they are in agreement that individuals have the capacity to grow and enrich their lives. Based on a school of thought that focuses on the present rather than the past, the process that leads to developing beyond normality is studied.

Deaf individuals engage in the self-actualization process from contrasting perspectives. While some rely on the larger hearing community to become their springboard for growth and development, others form an allegiance with the Deaf community, where they form a Deaf identity and work toward their enhancement and the enhancement of those who are culturally Deaf. Each setting can provide an atmosphere conducive to the development of the healthy personality, for once the individual has formulated an identity and developed a positive self-concept, he or she is free to engage in the self-actualization process.

8

Psychological Assessment of Deaf Individuals

Individual differences are couched within one's cognitive abilities and personality traits. While some people possess the capabilities and motivation to become nuclear scientists and computer gurus, others display strengths in the social service areas and are content to work with the general public on a daily basis. What contributes to these individual differences and how can they be assessed?

Assessment occurs in many contexts and for a variety of reasons. In the broadest sense of the term, it can be defined as a form of examination designed to evaluate the performance and capabilities of an individual. It is conducted on an informal and a formal basis and is implemented in a multitude of settings. Those engaged in the assessment process utilize a wide array of procedures. Through quantitative measures (actual numeric scores on test instruments) and qualitative descriptions (based on observations throughout the assessment procedure), information is obtained regarding the characteristics of the individual.

Psychologists, educators, and vocational evaluators are involved in the assessment process. Psychologists use assessment to measure traits, capacities, or achievements of an individual. Educators incorporate various evaluation techniques to monitor individual learning progress, and to categorize or classify groups of students. Vocational evaluators employ observational techniques, standardized tests, and simulated work samples.

This chapter begins with a brief overview of the origins of psychological testing, followed by a discussion of the assessment process that is conducted outside of the classroom. Test instruments that are appropriate for use with deaf and hard-of-hearing individuals are reviewed, validity and reliability are explored, and techniques for test administration are described. The chapter concludes by presenting the reader with two additional key sections covering the purpose of vocational evaluations, and information on how to effectively utilize the services of a sign language interpreter when tests are administered. This is followed by a discussion of how the skills of these professionals can impact overall test results. Before discussing these topics, a brief historical overview of the tests and an annotated list of the test instruments are included.

Origins of Psychological Testing

Early psychological testing can be traced to the late 1800s and the work of Sir Francis Galton. Considered the "father of mental tests," Galton was an avid researcher and a prolific writer (Santrock, 2000, p. 287). Several of his studies focused on measuring the physical and mental traits of vast numbers of people. To accomplish this task he devised several ingenious tests and measuring instruments while initiating a variety of schemes to obtain the data. Galton was a staunch believer in the theory that one's intellectual level could be gauged by testing the individual's ability to receive information through his or her senses. As a result he designed instruments that could evaluate sensory discrimination. These tests measured both visual and auditory discrimination and were structured to assess kinesthetic abilities. Galton included tests for measuring strength of movement, speed of simple reactions, and other sensorimotor functions.

One of his contributions was the establishment of an anthropomorphic laboratory where, for a small fee, individuals could have their sensory discrimination, motor capacities, and other simple traits evaluated. Those entering the laboratory could manipulate a number of interesting contrivances. While they performed the various functions, one of Galton's assistants would enter data on their abilities. Approximately 9,000 men and women participated in Galton's lab, thus providing the first large sample for an intelligence test (Santrock, 2000).

Galton also initiated the use of free association tests, providing future psychologists with a technique that they would eventually expand and utilize (Anastasi & Urbina, 1997). Furthermore, he was aware of the need to establish mathematical formulas whereby the data on individual differences could be processed. One of these processes included working with the normal distribution curve and correlation, work that would set the stage for the measurement principle of the "coefficient of correlation."

Catell and the Early Mental Tests

Galton was a pioneer in the psychological movement with his simple sensorimotor tests, and another professional recognized for his outstanding contributions was James McKeen Catell. Catell studied at Leipzig under Wilhelm Wundt, a German psychologist. Later he resided in England, where he had contact with Galton. Upon returning to the United States he was active both in the establishment of psychological laboratories and in the development of the testing movement.

Catell is responsible for introducing the term *mental test* to the English psychological literature. In an article published in 1890 Catell described a series of tests that were being administered annually to college students. These tests were developed in an attempt to measure the intellectual level of the students. The battery included a series of tests that measured fitness, sensory discrimination, reaction time, and memory. Catell preferred tests measuring simple functions because of the precision with which they could be measured. He shied away from attempting to measure complex "higher mental processes," fearing that they could not be measured as easily or as accurately.

His series of tests were typical of those being developed during the last decade of the nineteenth century. Although the majority of them focused on sensory functions, some did attempt to evaluate more complex processes by including tests of reading, word association, memory, and simple arithmetic (Anastasi & Urbina, 1997).

Binet's Influence on Psychological Testing

While Catell was developing tests in America, several European psychologists were assembling similar evaluation instruments. However, these tests were not completely embraced by the professional community. Two French psychologists, Binet and Henri, were particularly critical of the nature of the available test designs. Published in an article in France in 1895, their critique disapproved of the popular test series for its emphasis on sensory functions and its undue concentration on simple and narrowly specialized abilities. Binet and Henri argued that simplistic tasks did not require the high degree of precision that was employed to measure these operations. They contended that individual differences could be plotted through more complex tasks and that test instruments should be designed to examine these abilities. The two men further described their own test series that covered such components as memory, imagination, attention, comprehension, suggestibility, and aesthetic judgment. These early tests would later be viewed as the forerunners of the Binet intelligence tests (Anastasi & Urbina, 1997).

In 1904 the French Minister of Public Instruction appointed a commission to study the problem of retardation among public school children. Binet and his student Theophile Simon, under the direction of the commission, prepared the first intelligence scale designed to yield a global index of intellectual level.

The first scale, known as the 1905 scale, consisted of 30 problems or tests arranged in ascending order of difficulty. Difficulty levels were determined empirically by administering the tests to 50 normal children between the ages of 3 and 11, and by testing some children who were mentally retarded. These early tests were designed to evaluate a wide array of functions. Although sensory and perceptual tests were included, a much greater emphasis was placed on verbal content, judgment, comprehension, and reasoning.

The second scale which appeared in 1908, consisted of tests grouped according to age levels and was also designed to evaluate children between the ages of 3 and 11. Compared to the 1905 scale, the revised version had an increased number of tests, and the unsatisfactory items contained in the initial scale were eliminated. Furthermore, within the revised scale only those tests were included that all normal 5-year-olds could pass; the six-year-level tests were those that could be passed by a normal 6-year-old, and so forth.

Due to the grouping of tests by age levels, children's scores could now be expressed as a "mental age," the age of normal children whose performance they equaled. These tests attracted wide attention among psychologists throughout the world. They were translated into several languages and a number of different revisions were prepared. One of the most famous revisions, developed under the direction of L.M. Terman at Stanford University, became known as the Stanford-Binet. It was in this test that the intelligence quotient (IQ) or ratio between mental age and chronological age was first introduced. (Anastasi & Urbina, 1997).

The original Binet tests, as well as the revisions that occurred in 1937 and 1960, were designed as individual scales. Because several of the tests required oral responses from the subject, only one individual at a time could be evaluated. This rendered them unsuitable for use with groups. Furthermore, only highly trained examiners could administer and score these test instruments.

Group Tests

An incident that occurred in 1917 stimulated the development of group intelligence tests. When the United States entered World War I, a committee appointed by the American Psychological Association was given a mandate to address ways in which psychology might be instrumental in assisting with the war effort. Under the direction of Robert M. Yerks, the committee recognized the need to classify the one and a half million recruits in terms of their general intellectual level. In this setting, the first group intelligence test was developed (Anastasi & Urbina 1997).

The original tests, developed by the Army, became known as the Army Alpha and the Army Beta. The Alpha was designed for routine testing and the Beta Scale was employed with individuals who were not literate in the English language. Through the years these tests have undergone several revisions. They have also served as models for most group intelligence tests. Once it became apparent that testing could be conducted in group settings, the entire testing movement experienced a surge of growth. Soon intelligence tests became available for all ages, beginning with preschool children and extending to graduate students.

Aptitude Tests

From the onset, intelligence tests were designed to measure general intellectual level. However, it soon became apparent that these tests were verbally oriented and limited in what they could measure. Psychologists realized that many functions were not being assessed and that the existing instruments did not provide an accurate representation of one's "total intellect." Evaluators began searching for and developing tests that could assess special aptitudes. These special aptitude tests were originally developed for use in vocational counseling and in the classification of industrial and military personnel. However, in the 1920s, the use of both intelligence and aptitude tests became widespread. During that time it became apparent that scores obtained on both types of tests frequently indicted that the ability to complete one task was independent of other traits being evaluated.

Investigations initiated during the early part of the twentieth century merit particular discussion. Due largely to the research of Charles Sperman, T.L. Kelley, and L.L. Thurstone, the concept of "factor analysis" entered the field of psychological testing. The data gathered by these researchers indicated that one's intellectual makeup consisted of a number of relatively independent factors or traits. Based on this information the development of multiple test batteries emerged. These batteries were designed to provide a measure of a person's standing in each of a number of traits. These could then be used to obtain separate scores for one's verbal comprehension, numerical aptitude, spatial visualization, arithmetic reasoning, and perceptual speed (Anastasi & Urbina, 1997).

Standardized Tests

The evolution and maturing of test instruments within the school system have remained abreast of those in the field of psychology. Prior to the mid-1800s, the educational system relied on oral examinations to test the abilities of their students. Then in Boston in 1845, written examinations were introduced into the Boston public school system. After the turn of the century, the first standardized tests for measuring the outcomes of school instruction began to appear. These tests were spearheaded by the work of E.L. Thorndike and utilized measurement principles developed in the psychological laboratory. Tests for evaluating spelling, arithmetic computation, handwriting, and other areas began to appear. These early tests were followed by the publication of the Stanford Achievement Test in 1923.

Throughout the 1930s, statewide, regional, and national testing programs were introduced, and with them test-scoring machines were developed. Achievement tests were rewritten, providing examiners with the tools to measure the broad educational concepts of their students. These revisions have rendered aptitude tests similar to intelligence tests. At this time the difference between the two types of tests is primarily one of specificity of content and the extent to which they are employed.

Personality Tests

In addition to intelligence, aptitude, and achievement tests, psychologists devised personality tests to measure such characteristics as emotional adjustment, interpersonal relations, motivation, interests, and attitudes. Early work in the area of personality testing evolved in the late 1800s. It is attributed to the work of Kraeplin and his free association test that was developed for use with abnormal patients. Later, in the mid-

1950s, Sommer continued work in this area. He also felt that free association tests could be employed to differentiate between the various forms of mental disorders.

Further developments in this field can be traced to Woodworth, who during World War I developed the Personal Data Sheet, a rough screening device for identifying seriously neurotic men who would be unfit for military service. The instrument was designed with a number of questions dealing with common neurotic symptoms, and the score was computed by totaling the number of responses the man indicated. After the war, forms of this questionnaire were included for children and adults outside the military. Woodworth's questionnaire later served as a model for subsequent emotional adjustment inventories.

Other approaches to measuring personality include the application of performance or situational tests. In these tests, the purpose of the task is generally disguised. Tests of this nature were developed in the late 1920s and the early 1930s by Hartshorne, May, and their associates (Anastasi & Urbina 1997). These tests were concerned with relatively complex and subtle social and emotional behavior and had to be administered by trained personnel.

A third approach to assessing personality utilizes what are known as projective techniques. Since its inception, this approach has experienced phenomenal growth. Clinicians are partial to these techniques, which rely on presenting subjects with relatively unstructured tasks.

The assumption that underlies this method is that the individual will project his or her characteristic modes of response onto the task. Although the free association test represents one form of projective techniques, there are several others. Additional tests in this area include sentence-completion tests, as well as those focusing on drawing, arranging toys to create a scene, or interpreting pictures or ink blots.

An Overview of the Assessment Process

Psychological evaluations, academic examinations, and vocational appraisals are conducted on a routine basis, but the information gleaned from these test results comprises only one part of the data required when attempting to measure an individual's aptitudes, intellect, or behavior. Other vital components in the assessment process merit special consideration. However, before examining them, it is beneficial to consider the purpose and the components of the assessment process.

The Purpose of Assessment

Assessment can be defined as a systematic act of acquiring and analyzing information about individuals for some stated purpose; it is usually instrumental in diagnosing specific problems and in planning individual solutions. Initially, information may be compiled in order to determine consumer eligibility for programs. Data that is obtained can also provide insights into the individual's personal attributes, cognitive abilities, environmental status, academic achievement, and health and social competence. This information can then be utilized when selecting program services.

The assessment process can serve as a monitoring device for tracking individual progress. Furthermore, the information can be beneficial when evaluating the quality of stated services and programs. Professionals involved in the assessment process rely on background information, observations, interviews, and test results to assist them in making recommendations (Hammill, 1987).

The Components of Psychometric Assessment

Psychometric testing can be valuable whenever objective indicators are required regarding a client's or a student's level of intelligence, academic performance, vocational aptitudes and interests, personality, and/or other abilities relevant to specific performance areas (Critchfield, 1986). When individuals are referred for assessment, most evaluators adhere to a standard format. Background information is obtained; behavioral observations are noted; tests are administered, scored, and summarized; and recommendations are made.

Background Information.   The assessment process generally begins with an interview. Throughout this initial phase, evaluators endeavor to establish rapport with the individual while generating feelings of mutual trust. Interviewers must remain empathetic yet objective, flexible yet organized, and alert yet nonjudgmental in order to obtain the information that is needed.

Through a series of questions the professional strives to form a composite of how the individual perceives himself or herself in conjunction with the environment in which he or she resides. These questions elicit responses that depict the person's hopes, problems, and coping mechanisms. In addition, they reflect the interplay of those events, experiences, and attributes that contribute to the shaping of the individual. Gathering this information provides insights into how one's personality has developed, what behavioral or familial problems exist, and what interventions might be appropriate.

Interviews may be highly structured and follow an orally administered questionnaire covering specific predetermined areas. Other interviews are nondirective whereby the interviewer provides the backdrop for the interviewee to express freely his or her feelings. Although both types of interviews are implemented, those utilizing a structured interview protocol are currently employed in the majority of clinical and research settings (Anastasi & Urbina, 1997).

Throughout the interview process clinicians observe the individual's expressive speech and language patterns, poise, and response to interacting with a stranger. Furthermore, the clinician elicits the life history of the individual. Background information can offer insights into what the person might do in the future, as well as how the individual perceives various life events and how they currently evaluate their present life experiences.

The interview process can provide the clinician with critical information. However, in the event that important information is overlooked or is not solicited, the interview may conclude with the clinician forming an inaccurate composite of the individual's concerns or behaviors.

In some instances, as in the case of adults with limited language skills, the examiner is required to gather pertinent information through interviews with parents or significant others. In these situations clinicians should be cognizant of the fact that although the background information they receive can be beneficial, it is relayed though the eyes of someone other than the client. Thus, these responses may reflect parental perceptions, concerns, and interests rather than those of the individual being tested.

In other instances parents or significant others related to young children become the primary individuals engaged in the interview process. In these situations it is critical that the clinician make every effort to ensure that the parent or significant other feels comfortable with the interview process. Once rapport has been established the interviewer usually focuses on gathering information from four major areas. The four major areas of interest include obtaining both a family and a developmental history, as well as gathering information pertaining to the child's academic and social histories (Pierangelo & Guiliani, 2002).

Behavioral Observations.   During the interview phase and continuing throughout the assessment process, the examiner pays particular attention to behaviors that are exhibited. Because test instruments alone cannot be used as predictors of human behavior, it is critical to observe the interaction of individuals as they respond to the examiner's questions (Levine, 1981). Test scores provide pertinent data; however, impressions formed through observation and information obtained from interview protocols are equally important. By integrating test data with behavioral observations and interview findings, skilled evaluators are able to gain a more comprehensive understanding of the internal phenomena that generate external responses.

Psychometric Testing.   Psychometric testing is administered to compare particular individuals with a specific population. These instruments evaluate a diverse number of attributes. In general, they examine those areas pertaining to individual intelligence, visual/motor coordination, academic achievement, communication skill, vocational aptitude, adaptive functioning, and personal/vocational interests (Critchfield, 1986). Candidates for assessment include infants, children, and adults. Some are referred for neuropsychological evaluations while others enter the testing situation to determine their vocational interests and aptitudes.

When the psychometrist or evaluator has completed administering the test battery, the process of summarizing and reporting the results begins. Background information, observations, and test results are all included in the final report. Special consideration is given to factors that ultimately influence the overall composite. Particular attention is focused on the individual's cultural and language origins and the environment in which the person resides. Any known physical or mental disabilities are considered, and any difficulties in communicating test directions are noted.

Although language and communication are only two of the factors considered in the assessment process, they are two of the most critical ones when planning to evaluate deaf and hard-of-hearing individuals. Other pertinent issues must also be considered in order to insure accuracy when testing this population. Evaluators must understand the ramifications of deafness, and must become familiar with test instruments that are appropriate for use with this population.

Assessment and the Deaf Population

When considering the implications of deafness, certain factors are imperative to consider. It is important to know the cause of the hearing loss, the age of onset, the severity of the loss, the incidence of familial deafness, the person's visual acuity, and whether there are any additional handicapping conditions. (See Chapter 1 for types and causes of deafness.) Furthermore, attention must be given to the mode of communication used in the home, the method of facilitating communication that was (or is) used in the educational environment, and the clarity (or lack thereof) of speech produced by the deaf person. It is also important to note the individual's involvement in or contacts with the Deaf community. All these factors have a significant impact on the assessment process and must be taken into account before appropriate tests can be selected (Ziezula, 1982; Elliott, Glass, & Evans, 1987).

The communication methods employed by members of the Deaf community are as diverse as the population itself. Some are very articulate and possess exceptional speechreading skills, and others rely on gestures and home signs for conveying information. There are those who prefer to converse through the use of written communiqué; while others embrace the language of the Deaf community, American Sign Language (ASL). ASL has been, and continues to be, developed by and for members of the Deaf community. It is a distinct language, and its grammar and syntax differ from the grammatical and syntactical features of English (Quigley & Paul, 1984). While this mode of communication is used by a segment of the deaf population, others rely on an English-based signed system (SEE I, SEE II, SE, CASE, and so on) or cued speech. (See Chapter 9 for a detailed description of ASL and the English-based sign systems.)

In order to obtain valid test results from any deaf or hard-of-hearing individual, the issue of communication must be addressed. It is crucial that the examiner ascertain whether the person fully understands what is expected during the test situation. Upon determining the mode of communication the deaf person prefers, every attempt must be made to facilitate communication by incorporating the language or that communication system. Once the mode of communication is established and the evaluator has obtained background information, the initial selection of appropriate test instruments can be initiated. Based on the specific needs of this population, several factors are considered when this selection is made.

Factors to Consider When Selecting Appropriate Test Instruments for the Deaf Population

According to Ziezula (1982), four major questions must be asked when selecting a test for deaf or hard-of-hearing individuals. First, does the test consist of verbal test items or performance items? Second, do the instructions for the test require verbal communication? Third, do any of the test items discriminate against an individual with a hearing loss? And fourth, are people with hearing disabilities included in the normative sample provided by the test examiner?

It is imperative that the instructions be carefully scrutinized prior to selecting a test. This consideration applies to both verbal and performance instruments. Although many performance tests require nonverbal tasks, the examiner must know if the use of verbal instructions is mandated and if the test developer presents or permits alternate instructional procedures. In the event that the individuals being tested cannot fully comprehend the tasks that are required of them, the validity of the test results must be questioned.

Several of the tests administered to this population do not contain standardized instructions for administration procedures. This is particularly true of tests designed with verbal instructions. When this problem arises, the validity of the results becomes a major issue. The problem becomes even more obvious when one compares the test results of two deaf or hard-of-hearing individuals who have been given directions differently. If one is instructed "by the book" and the other is given the same test with a different type of instructions, the results may reflect marked differences.

Administration of test directions is only one factor that must be considered when selecting a test instrument. The evaluator must also thoroughly evaluate the test items. It is essential that those test items that relate directly or indirectly to an individual's ability to hear and function in a hearing world be examined carefully. It is not uncommon to discover test items that discriminate against individuals with hearing losses, especially in the areas of intelligence, personality, and vocational interest items.

Once the instructions and the test items are examined, the population upon which the test was normed must be considered. Does the test being considered have normative data on deaf and hard-of-hearing people similar to the person being tested? Are deaf and hard-of-hearing people included in the general normative sample? These factors are of paramount importance when determining the selection of test instruments.

Compiling an appropriate battery of tests is only one component in the total assessment process. Although these instruments can provide the examiner with valuable information, in order to have any merit the results must be interpreted by a competent professional, otherwise they remain meaningless data on a printed page.

Assessing Deaf Individuals: Evaluator Characteristics

There is a common misconception among the public that test instruments, used in and by themselves, render psychological assessments. Although these diagnostic techniques provide avenues for gathering information, the examiner must know which instruments to select and how to interpret the results. This background information, coupled with a thorough knowledge of the ramifications of deafness, is critical. Without this understanding, misdiagnosis frequently occurs.

At the heart of the assessment process lies the need for clear communication, which provides psychologists with a vital link whereby they can gain insights into the functioning abilities of their clients. When communication ceases to function effectively, psychological practice suffers a "crippling handicap" (Levine, 1981). Most prelingually deaf people, and many who are hard-of-hearing, lack a mastery of the syntax and vocabulary of English. Research indicates that by age 6, hearing children have learned most rules of syntax and have a vocabulary of 8,000 to 14,000 words (Carey, 1977). However, most deaf children of the same age have difficulties constructing complete sentences, and their sign vocabulary may include only around 500 words (Griswold & Commings, 1974). Additional studies conducted by Quigley and his colleagues suggest that even when deaf students understand the vocabulary and the concepts in reading material, they still have difficulty understanding simple declarative sentences (Quigley & Kretschmer, 1982). Therefore, it is imperative that clinicians master the language forms used by deaf persons or employ the skills of an interpreter who is trained in this area. They must be able to "think deaf" conceptually, and pose their questions accordingly, thus ensuring that they will be understood.

In addition, evaluators planning to work with deaf persons need to become thoroughly familiar with those social experiences that are altered due to the impact of deafness. Bridging the communication gap is only one component that merits consideration. Other factors include a thorough understanding of the social/cultural differences, the significance of the Deaf community, the effects of environmental deprivation, and the perceptual differences that occur as a result of the individual's inability to comprehend spoken concepts. Clinicians must be attuned to these factors in order to provide quality psychological services. Practitioners must understand how mental, scholastic, social, and emotional development is affected by the ability to hear. If environmental influences are not understood and if behaviors are not examined within the confines of deafness, grave misunderstandings can occur.

These characteristics must be considered in tandem with valid test results when psychological examinations are conducted. Based on these findings the psychologist can then obtain an assessment reflective of the individual's unique characteristics. When accurate information is provided the Deaf population can be viewed as the widely diverse, heterogeneous people they are, instead of the stereotypic group they are often thought to be.

Assessment can begin in infancy and continue through the senior citizen years. It can be used to identify secondary handicapping conditions or personality disorders. It is employed in the schools to assess aptitudes and abilities and in the rehabilitation setting to determine vocational interests. Which instruments provide the examiner with the most valid profiles of their client's abilities? What types of information can be generated from these instruments, and how valid is this data when compared with results procured from similar groups of hearing individuals?

Infant and Child Assessment

Assessment of infants is a relatively new phenomenon. Traditionally, evaluations were conducted when the child entered school and placement was considered. In 1986 Congress passed P.L. 99-457, an amendment to P.L. 94-142. This legislation focused on children from birth to five years.

P.L. 99-457 is designed to provide funds for states to identify and serve developmentally delayed and at-risk children. However, even with this legislation the majority of preschoolers are not being served. The reasons for this are twofold: first, the age at which the hearing loss is detected, and second, the restricted number of services available for infants under six years of age, which limits the number served (Bradley-Johnson & Evans, 1991).

When a child is suspected of having a hearing loss, a team of multidisciplinary professionals intervenes. The specialists responsible for evaluating the child may include pediatricians, otologists, audiologists, educators, psychologists, and rehabilitation counselors (Gerber, 1984). They employ intervention strategies designed to accommodate the developing child and to assist the family in ensuring that language and educational growth can be facilitated.

When infants are referred for psychological testing, practitioners focus on the developmental behaviors of the child, rather than on the traditional measures referred to as the IQ. During this period of rapid development the fundamental purpose of assessment is to determine if the child is capable of successfully engaging in the tasks of environmental exploration, interplay, and incorporation that underlie enculturation. Despite the fact that one of the tenets of assessment is to predict how the child will perform during the school years, the use of IQ testing with infants is not recommended before the child reaches age 2. By the time children become 2 or older their cognitive development has become fairly stable, thus permitting IQ tests to be administered. Research indicates that at this time the results will have a certain degree of predictive validity. Furthermore, it should be noted that although testing by age 2 is more reliable, the most reliable results do not occur until after the age of 5 or 6.

Prior to age 2, intelligence can be conceived as a broad category reflective of the child's functioning ability rather than as a specific number. Developmental schedules or developmental scales are administered in an attempt to determine the child's cognitive functioning ability. Although there are a variety of instruments designed to accomplish this purpose, only part of them are appropriate for use with deaf and hard-of-hearing infants. Certain scales lend themselves better to the assessment of deaf infants than do others. Several of them have been normed on deaf preschoolers, thereby providing additional data for the evaluator.

Table 8.1 summarizes the infant development scales. Following this table is a general description of each of these instruments. Although this descriptive listing is not all inclusive, it does provide a fairly comprehensive representation of those instruments available for and utilized with this population. As with all assessment devices, it is imperative that the child understands what is expected of him or her. If

TABLE 8.1 *Infant Development Scales*

Test	Age Group	Type of Assessment
Bayley Scales of Infant Development, 2nd ed. (1993)	1 month–42 months	Mental, motor, behavior
Cattell Infant Intelligence Scale	2–36 months	Perception, motor, manipulation
Columbia Mental Maturity	3 years, 6 months–9 years, 11 months	Mental age
Smith-Johnson Nonverbal Performance Scale (1977)	24 months–48 months	Nonverbal performance scale
Leiter International Performance Test, Revised (1997)	2–20 years, 11 months	Individual performance scale
Merrill Palmer Scale of Mental Tests	19 months–6 years	Screening evaluation for developmental functioning ability
Adaptation of the Wechsler Preschool and Primary Scale of Intelligence (WPPSI-R, 1989)	3 years–7 years, 3 months	Performance test
Denver Developmental Screening Test	2 weeks–6 years	Individual
Slosson Intelligence Test	5 months–adult	Individual screening instrument
Peabody Individual Achievement Test	5 months–18 years	Wide range screening measure of achievement
Vineland Social Maturity Scale	Birth–35 years	Developmental schedule; assessment of ability to take responsibility for practical needs
Peabody Picture Vocabulary Test	29 months–18 years	"Use" vocabulary

this is not communicated, the validity of the results must be questioned. Although many of these instruments overlap and include the school-aged population, all of them extend downward to include infants and preschoolers. They all measure the cognitive ability of the age group and are presented in alphabetical order.

Infant and Child Development Scales

Bayley Scales of Infant Development
Author: N. Bayley
Publisher: Psychological Corporation
Copyright: 1969; 2nd Ed., 1993
Age Level: 1 month to 42 months

The original Bayley Scales tested infants from 1 month to 25 months. The Bayley II, a revision of the first edition, can be used with infants between 1 and 42 months. These scales are designed to provide a three-part evaluation of the child. Test results yield a mental scale, a motor scale, and an infant behavior record. All items on the scales are arranged in developmental order.

Use with Deaf and Hard-of-Hearing Children.   These scales can be used with deaf and hard-of-hearing infants. Approximately 12 percent of the items on the Bayley require auditory language skills. Many deaf and hard-of-hearing children will fail most of the auditory language items. However, because the items are arranged in developmental order, if the child passes a developmental task at a higher level than one that is language based, the language item should be credited that precedes the successfully completed performance item (Vernon & Andrews, 1990).

Cattell Infant Intelligence Scale
Author: P. Cattell
Publisher: Psychological Corporation
Copyright: 1960
Age Level: 2 to 36 months

This instrument is a downward extension of the 1937 Stanford-Binet, Form L. In addition to Stanford-Binet items, the Cattell scale utilized material from the Gesell Developmental Schedules and from other available infant tests, together with some original items. All items in the Cattell scale are administered without a time limit. Scales require no more than 20–30 minutes to give. At the youngest ages, the tests are largely perceptual, comprising such activities as attending to a voice or a bell, or following a dangling ring or a moving person with the eyes. A few motor items are also included. With increasing age, more complex manipulatory tasks are introduced and increasing use is made of verbal functions.

Use with Deaf and Hard-of-Hearing Children.   This instrument employs a sophisticated English language component. However, several of the subtests are deemed appropriate for use with deaf and hard-of-hearing children: the tests for visual sequential memory, visual reception, manual expression, visual closure, and the visual association subtest.

Columbia Mental Maturity Scale
Author: B.B. Burgemeister, L.H. Blum, and I. Lorge
Publisher: Psychological Corporation
Copyright: 1972
Age Level: 3 years, 6 months to 9 years, 11 months

Originally developed for use with cerebral palsied children, this scale is comprised of 100 items, each consisting of a set of three, four, or five drawings printed on a large card. The subject is required to identify the drawing that does not belong with the others, indicating the choice by pointing or nodding. Scores are expressed as mental ages and ratio IQs.

Use with Deaf and Hard-of-Hearing Children.   This test can be employed with deaf and hard-of-hearing children if they understand what is expected of them. However, it is generally only used as a second measure when motor problems are suspected. The child is instructed to look at all the pictures presented on the card and to point to the one that is different. Items that are incorporated do not discriminate against hearing loss. However, it is critical that the examinee understand what is required so that random pointing does not occur.

Smith-Johnson Nonverbal Performance Scale
Author: Smith and Johnson
Publisher: Western Psychological Services
Copyright: 1977
Age Level: 24–48 months

This is a systematic nonverbal developmental measuring instrument designed to be used with deaf and hard-of-hearing preschool children between the ages of 24 and 48 months. The scale consists of 14 categories of tasks, with several subtasks within each category. No global score is provided. A performance summary allows the clinician to compare the child's overall performance in all 14 categories to the performance of children in his or her age group in the normative sample in terms of chronological age equivalent (Spragins, 1999).

Use with Deaf and Hard-of-Hearing Children.   Norms are available for both hearing and deaf children between the ages of 2 and 4. The format for the test includes simple gestures or pantomime instructions and there is no time restriction. The scale is brief and provides a fairly broad clinical picture without the use of language. As a measure of general cognitive function, the Smith-Johnson has utility.

Leiter International Performance Scale–(R)
Author: R.G. Leiter
Publisher: Western Psychological Services
Copyright: 1969 (Revised, 1997)
Age Level: 2–20 years

This is an individual performance scale whose distinctive feature is the complete elimination of instructions, either spoken or pantomime. Each test begins with a very easy task representing the type of task that will be encountered throughout that test. The Leiter-R consists of two nationally standardized batteries: a revision of the visualization and reasoning domains, and new attention and memory domains. Task comprehension is treated as part of the test. The materials include a response frame with an adjustable cardholder. All tests are administered by attaching the appropriate card, containing printed pictures, to the frame. The examinee chooses the blocks with the proper response pictures and inserts them into the frame. The Leiter scale was originally designed to cover a wide range of functions similar to those found in verbal scales. Performance items contained in this test include matching identical colors, shades of gray, forms, or pictures; copying a block design; picture completion; number estimation; analogies; series completion; recognition of age differences; spatial relations; footprint recognition; similarities; memory for a series; and classification of animals according to habitat. Administered individually with no time limit, these tests are arranged into year levels from 2 to 20. This evaluation instrument has an extensive nonverbal cognitive scale and a separate nonverbal attention and memory scale.

Use with Deaf Individuals. The Leiter-R has potential for use within the field of deaf education. Although no norms for deaf and hard-of-hearing individuals are available on the revised edition, the test may prove beneficial for identifying deaf students with attention/memory deficits, independent of their nonverbal "intelligence" or reasoning.

Merrill-Palmer Scale of Mental Tests
Author: Rachel Stutsman
Publisher: Stoelting
Copyright: 1931
Age Level: 19 months to 6 years

This is primarily a performance test and has been employed widely as a supplement to the more highly verbal Stanford-Binet. Tests are grouped into 6-month age levels from 19 months to 6 years. The order of administration within each level is flexible. Tasks included in this general intelligence test are block building, color sorting, matching puzzles, and so forth.

Use with Deaf and Hard-of-Hearing Children.   In order for this test to be used with those who are deaf or hard-of-hearing, the examiner must possess a thorough under-standing of deafness and what effects it has on psychological assessment. Subtest in-structions can be given in pantomime or through Total Communication. Adjustment in the scoring can be made for items that are refused, omitted, or failed because of lan-guage difficulties. Many of the items are timed, thus creating a problem for some deaf and hard-of-hearing children. These test results can best be used as a screening eval-uation for developmental functioning ability.

Wechsler Preschool and Primary Scale of Intelligence (WPPSI-R)
Author: S. Ray and M. Ulissi
Publisher: Steven Ray
Copyright: 1982
Age Level: 3 years to 7 years, 3 months

This test is designed as a standardization of the WPPSI Performance Scale for use with deaf and hard-of-hearing children. The adaptation uses the same performance scale items and materials as the WPPSI. There are no standardized instructions for deaf and hard-of-hearing children. The adaptation contains two sets of modified instructions. The alternative instructions are WPPSI instructions with less complex syntax and vocabulary. These linguistically modified instructions are signed or spoken. The sup-plemental instructions provide additional demonstration and practice items for four of the five performance subtests to ensure comprehension of task requirements. The supplemental instructions are spoken or signed and are intended for deaf and hard-of-hearing children with limited communication skills. Used as part of a cognitive assessment, this evaluation yields composite scores for verbal IQ, performance IQ, and full-scale IQ.

Use With Deaf and Hard-of-Hearing Children.   This is one of the best known and widely researched scales for children, and is one of the three most popular tests for deaf and hard-of-hearing students. The Performance Scales of the WPPSI-R can be used with younger and older deaf populations. However, it is suspected of underrating the abilities of young deaf children.

Denver Developmental Screening Test
Author: W.K. Frankenburg & J.D. Dodds
Publisher: Lacoda Project and Publishing Foundation
Copyright: 1975
Age Level: 2 weeks to 6 years

The DDST is designed to be administered as an individual test. It consists of 105 items and is arranged in four sections: personal-social tasks, which indicate how well chil-dren are able to care for themselves and how well they can get along with others; fine motor-adaptive tasks, indicating how well children can use their hands to draw and pick up objects; language, assessing the ability to hear, carry out commands, and speak; and gross motor tasks, which reflect the child's ability to sit, walk, and jump (Ziezula, 1982). Children continue with the test until they experience three failures in each of the sections.

Use with Deaf and Hard-of-Hearing Children.   Although this instrument has not been normed on deaf and hard-of-hearing children, all segments with the exception of the language section can be administered to this population. Directions can be signed, pantomimed, or demonstrated.

Slosson Intelligence Test
Author: R.L. Slosson
Publisher: Slosson Educational Publications
Copyright: 1981 (revised)
Age Level: 5 months to adult

The Slosson is designed to be a brief individual screening instrument for use when assessing intelligence. Test items are designed for three age-levels: infants (5 to 24 months), preschoolers, (2–4 years), and children above 4 years old. Test items administered at the preschool level and above require verbal responses. The Slosson is designed to be given individually and can be administered in 10–30 minutes. There are different performance requirements for each of the various age groups.

Use with Deaf and Hard-of-Hearing Children.   No specific procedures have been established for administering the Slosson to deaf children. Although it has been used with this population under the age of 2, its heavy verbal emphasis at the older levels prohibits it from being used with older age groups.

Peabody Individual Achievement Test–R
Author: L.M. Dunn
Publisher: American Guidance Service
Copyright: 1989 (revised)
Age Level: 5 months to 18 years

The purpose of the PIAT is to provide a wide-range screening measure of achievement in the areas of mathematics, reading, spelling, general information, and written expression. The five subscores and the total score can be converted into a variety of norms: grade scores, percentile ranks within ages, and normalized standard scores. The PIAT-R test materials include two volumes of test plates on rings. This is a power test that can be administered by well-trained para-professionals.

Use with Deaf and Hard-of-Hearing Children.   This test lends itself to ease in administration and should be administered through American Sign Language or by employing whatever sign system the child feels most comfortable utilizing. The PIAT-R is a useful screening device to compare the achievement of the deaf and hard-of-hearing with the scores of their hearing peers. However, it is not designed to be used as a diagnostic instrument in any of the content areas it covers.

Vineland Social Maturity Scale
Author: E.A. Doll
Publisher: American Guidance Service
Copyright: 1965
Age Level: Birth to 35 years

This developmental schedule is concerned with the individual's ability to look after his or her practical needs and to take responsibility. Although covering a range from birth to over 25 years, this scale has been found most useful at the younger age levels, and particularly with the mentally retarded. The entire scale consists of 117 items grouped into year levels. The information required for each item is obtained not through test situations but through an interview with an informant or with the subject himself or herself. The scale is based on what the subject has actually done in daily living. The items fall into eight categories: general self-help, self-help in eating, self-help in dressing, self-direction, occupation, communication, locomotion, and socialization.

Use with Deaf and Hard-of-Hearing Children.   This scale is useful in assessing the social maturity of the deaf and hard-of-hearing population. However, some of the test items are dated and normative information is only provided for deaf and hard-of-hearing residential students between the ages of 6 and 13. Parts of the tests contain language-related questions, making them difficult to adapt for use with deaf adolescents. Even when a well-trained examiner administers this instrument, scoring consistency may vary due to differences in examiner's interviewing styles.

Peabody Picture Vocabulary Test (PPVT-III)
Author: L.N. Dunn
Publisher: American Guidance Service
Copyright: 1997 (3rd Ed.)
Age Level: 29 months to 18 years

This test permits the utilization of a simple pointing response and provides a rapid measure of "use" vocabulary, especially applicable to persons unable to vocalize well. The original test was created in 1965. It consists of 150 plates, each containing four pictures. As each plate is presented, the examiner provides a stimulus word orally; the subject responds by pointing to or in some other way designating the picture on the plate that best illustrates the meaning of the stimulus words. Although the entire test covers a range from 2½ to 90 years, each individual is given only the plates appropriate to his or her own performance level, as determined by a specified run of successes at one end and failures at the other. Raw scores can be converted to mental ages, deviation IQs, or percentiles. The PPVT-III is untimed and is available in two parallel forms that utilize the same set of cards, but different stimulus words.

Six new features were added to the third edition, including an increased number of test items, extended national norms, new illustrations and packaging, and the grouping of items into 17 sets.

Use with Deaf and Hard-of-Hearing Children.   This test is only effective for use with deaf children if the child is adept at speechreading. The test manual states that the examiner must not spell, define, or show the words to the person being tested. Therefore, it is not appropriate for use with those who rely on sign language or sign-supported speech as their primary mode of communicating.

Assessment of School-Aged Deaf and Hard-of-Hearing Children and Adolescents

Although many deaf preschoolers are screened in infancy, more formalized assessment begins as the child enters elementary school. At this time, professionals employ test instruments to determine intellectual functioning abilities, aptitudes, personality characteristics, and the existence, if any, of neuropsychological problems. Assessment continues throughout the school years, with results depicting the unique psychological characteristics of the individuals.

When selecting tests, the psychometrist must pay particular attention to the amount of verbal communication required on the part of the examiner. In addition, the psychologist must be sensitive to the amount of verbal content included in the tests. Several of these instruments require language experiences that are uncommon to the majority of deaf individuals who have experienced prelingual hearing losses. Whenever possible, tests should be employed that have been standardized using samples that include deaf subjects, or those in which norms for the deaf have been established. When this is not possible and hearing standardized tests must be used, it is imperative that experiential responses are matched to the subject's experiential background. As a rule, the greater the experiential gap between a subject's background and that of the test's standardization group, the greater the likelihood of meaningless responses.

Several tests are deemed appropriate for use with deaf school-aged children. Some are used individually for initial assessment purposes; others are administered as part of an overall test battery. Tests are selected based on the type of information the psychologist is attempting to secure. In certain situations only intelligence is assessed. On other occasions information must be gathered that reflects the student's maturity level, aptitudes, and personality characteristics while determining if any additional disabling conditions exist.

As children advance to the secondary level, the assessment process expands to include a vocational component. In addition to intelligence, achievement, and personality, vocational aptitudes and interests are also explored. At this stage, post-secondary training opportunities are explored and career goals are established.

Table 8.2 presents a list of tests that are frequently administered to the deaf school aged population. Following this are descriptions of these instruments. Although not comprehensive, this list is representative of several of the instruments commonly administered when testing this population.

General Assessment Tests

Detroit Tests of Learning Aptitude-2
Author: H. Baker and B. Leland
Publisher: Bobbs-Merrill Company
Copyright: 1935; revised 1967
Age Level: 6–18 years

This multidimensional test battery is designed to measure intellectual abilities. Scores can be reported for subtests, composites, and the general intelligence quotient. The 11 subtests in the battery are grouped into eight separate composites, four domains, and one overall composite: word opposites, sentence imitation, oral directions, word sequences, story construction, design reproduction, object sequences, symbolic relations, conceptual matching, word fragments, and letter sequence.

Use with Deaf and Hard-of-Hearing Children.   The five subtests that comprise the nonverbal composite are beneficial and can be used with deaf and hard-of-hearing individuals. These subtests are design reproduction, object sequences, symbolic relations, conceptual matching, and letter sequences.

Gates MacGintie Reading Tests
Author: Gates and MacGintie
Publisher: Riverside Publishing Company
Copyright: 1972
Age Level: All ages and categories of deaf and hard-of-hearing children, 6 years to adult

This test is designed to assess the child's average reading level. It is comprised of tests focusing on vocabulary and comprehension. Although the manual states that the vocabulary subtests require 20–30 minutes and the comprehension subtest requires 30 minutes, there are also speed tests for grades three and above. The test may be administered individually or in a group.

Use with Deaf and Hard-of-Hearing Children.   There are no special directions for administering the GMRT to deaf students and no norms on this population have been established. When administering this test it is imperative that the examiner present the instructions through the primary mode of communication utilized by the examinee. In addition, ample time must be provided for the completion of sample test items.

TABLE 8.2 *Assessment of School-Aged Children*

Test	Age Group	Type of Assessment
Detroit Tests of Learning Aptitude-2	6–18 years	Multidimensional test battery, intellectual abilities
Gates MacGintie Reading Tests	6 years–adult	Average reading level assessment; vocabulary and comprehension
Metropolitan Achievement	6–16 years	Group-administered achievement test
Stanford Achievement Test for Deaf and Hard-of-Hearing Students	5–18 years	Group-administered achievements
Test of Syntactic Abilities	10–18 years	Group-administered achievements
Wechsler Intelligence Scale for Children-Revised	6–16½ years	Verbal, performance subtests
Wide Range Achievement Tests	5 years–adult	Intelligence and behavior adjustments
Bender Visual Motor Gestalt	Child–adult	Screening device for visual-motor perceptual problems related to brain damage
Benton Revised Visual Retention Test	8 years–adult	Visual motor coordination and visual memory
Graham-Kendall Memory for Designs Test	8½ years–adult	Screening for brain damage
Test of Nonverbal Intelligence (TONI-3)	5–85 years	Test of nonverbal intelligence
Bruininks-Oseretsky Test of Motor Proficiency	6–14 years	Scale of motor development
Goodenough Harris Drawing Test	5 years and above	Accuracy of observation; development of conceptual thinking
Make A Picture Story	6–12 years	Thematic projective technique
House-Tree-Person Projective Technique	3 years and above	Personality
Draw-A-Person Projective Technique	5 years–adult	Personality
Strong-Campbell Interest Inventory	13 years–adult	Vocational interest battery
Kuder Interest Inventory	12–18 years	Vocational interest battery
General Aptitude Test Battery	No specific ages given	Aptitude
Differential Aptitude Test	13–18 years	Aptitude

Metropolitan Achievement Test
Author: Durost, Bixler, Wrightstone, Prescott, and Belaw
Publisher: Harcourt Brace Jovanovitch
Copyright: 1971
Age Level: Grades K–9 (6–16 years)

This group-administered achievement test is normed on deaf and hard-of-hearing children. Subtests include reading, language, spelling, math, science, and social studies.

Use with Deaf Individuals.   Even though the Metropolitan has been normed on both hearing and deaf and hard-of-hearing children, it has been criticized for having an inadequate normative sample. With achievement tests this becomes a critical issue, since the purpose of these instruments is to compare individuals with their peers. If this cannot be done, the test measure loses some of its effectiveness.

Stanford Achievement Test
Author: Madden, Gardner, Rudman, Karlsen, and Merwin
Publisher: Harcourt Brace
Copyright: 1995; 9th Ed., Form S, 1996
Age Level: Grades 1–9

This group-administered test measures the abilities and skills of individuals in reading, language, spelling, mathematics, social studies, and science. It reflects the curriculum content commonly taught in grades one through nine throughout the United States. The Stanford 9 is available in eight levels of difficulty. The test administered to deaf students is exactly the same as the one administered to hearing students. However, when testing deaf students a school typically orders screening tests from the Gallaudet Research Institute (GRI). On the basis of the screening tests the school assigns the appropriate Stanford 9 level to each student and then orders materials from the Research Institute.

Use with Deaf and Hard-of-Hearing Students.   The Stanford 9 is administered in group settings. It contains a new mathematics component designed to test math within a context of realistic problems. Both mathematics subtests rely on verbal information and have been modeled on recommendations made by the National Council of Teachers of Mathematics. Some advanced students may "top out," leaving a question as to their true achievement level. For this reason the test may prove more beneficial for "middle-of-the-road" achieving students, but it does not give enough information for high-achieving students in the areas of math or science.

Test of Syntactic Abilities
Author: Quigley, Steinkamp, Power, and Jones
Publisher: PRO-ED
Copyright: 1982
Age Level: Deaf students, 10–18 years; hearing students, 8–10 years

This test was developed to assess the abilities of deaf and hearing students to recognize correct English syntax when presented with written reading material. There are two forms of the test and it can be administered to groups or individually. One form is used as a screening test and the other is employed as a more in-depth diagnostic battery. The screening test provides an overall assessment of syntactic skills. The diagnostic battery consists of 20 assessment instruments designed to provide scores on each of the nine syntactic structures: negation, conjunction, determiners, question formation, verb processes, pronominalization, relativization, complementation, and normalization.

Use with Deaf and Hard-of-Hearing Students.   The TSA was primarily designed for use with deaf students. The manual states that this test is not appropriate for use with students whose reading levels are above the sixth grade, because the skills examined with this instrument would already have been mastered.

Wechsler Intelligence Scale for Children (WISC–III)
Author: D. Wechsler
Publisher: Psychological Corporation
Copyright: 1974
Age Level: 6–16½ years

The WISC-III is an instrument designed to be administered as an individual assessment for use as part of a cognitive assessment. The scale yields composite scores for verbal IQ, performance IQ, and full-scale IQ. However, the performance scale is generally the only recommended instrument for use with deaf individuals. The WISC-III performance scale provides three performance-based measures of intelligence: an overall Performance Intelligence Quotient (PIQ), a Perceptual Organization Index (POI), and a Processing Speed Index (PSI).

Use with Deaf and Hard-of-Hearing Individuals.   The verbal scale cannot be considered a valid measure of any deaf or hard-of-hearing individual's intelligence. However, when administered by a skilled professional it can be used to ascertain information pertaining to a student's level of verbal achievement relative to that of hearing peers. One of the best-known and well-researched scales for children, the WISC-III is one of the three most popular tests for deaf or hard-of-hearing students. This instrument is best used as one part of a multifactored evaluation to obtain an overall measure of the student's performance.

Wide Range Achievement Tests
Author: J.P. Jastak, S. Bijou, and S.R. Jastak
Publisher: Jastak Associates
Copyright: 1978
Age Level, Level I: 5 years, 0 months to 11 years, 11 months; Level II, 12 years,
   0 months to adult

According to the authors, this test is designed to be administered in conjunction with other tests of intelligence and behavior adjustment. It is a brief test, individually administered, that provides a rough indication of three limited components of educational achievement. The components are spelling, decoding isolated printed words and pronouncing them correctly, and carrying out computational exercises in arithmetic and algebra. The items in each part are timed, if not speeded, and in the word-pronouncing test the task is stopped after a specific number of failures.

Use with Deaf and Hard-of-Hearing Children.   This instrument can be used as a quick screening device to determine grade level, sight word recognition, spelling abilities, and arithmetic computation skills. The reading and spelling subtests should only be used if the examiner is fluent in simultaneous communication. In addition, this instrument should be administered in conjunction with other instruments to garner an assessment of achievement.

Wide Range Achievement Test-3 (WRAT-3)
Author: Gary S. Wilkinson
Publisher: Jastak Associates/Wide Range
Copyright: 1993
Age Level: 5–75 years

This is the new edition of the Wide Range Achievement Test. This instrument provides two forms; however, the two previous levels have been combined into a single-level format. The two forms can be used as a pretest/posttest, or they can be administered together in a combined test format. There are three subtests in this edition: reading, spelling, and arithmetic.

Use with Deaf and Hard-of-Hearing Individuals.   This instrument provides a very quick screening device. The reading subtest measures word recognition only, and the mathematics subtest measures computational math only. The revised edition can be used with deaf and hard-of-hearing individuals if the test administrator is fluent in the communication mode used by the individual being tested.

Test of Nonverbal Intelligence (TONI-3)
Authors: L. Brown, R.J. Serbienou, and S.K. Johnson
Publisher: PRO-ED
Copyright: 1997
Age Level: 5–85 years

The Test of Nonverbal Intelligence (TONI-3) is designed to assess the nonverbal intelligence of individuals who are deaf, bilingual, or speak a language other than English. Furthermore, it can be administered to those who are socially or economically disadvantaged as well as those who are language disordered, motor impaired, or neurologically impaired.

Use with Deaf and Hard-of-Hearing Individuals.   This test is easy to administer and is very appropriate for use with individuals with multiple disabilities. When responding to the test items, gestures are sufficient when indicating a response.

Special Clinical Tests

Bender Visual Motor Gestalt
Author: Bender
Publisher: Western Services
Copyright: 1938
Age Level: Child–Adult

The Bender (also known as Bender-Gestalt) is primarily a screening device for visual-motor perceptual problems related to brain damage. This instrument is used most effectively with children 9 years or older with evidence of IQs above 80. When administered to younger children or to those known to have degrees of retardation, it may be difficult to differentiate intellectual deficits from visual motor pathology created by other etiologies.

Use with Deaf and Hard-of-Hearing Individuals.   Although this instrument has been used extensively with deaf subjects, it is most effectively used with children 9 years and older. Currently, no norms provided are for the deaf and hard-of-hearing population, and little research is available to indicate whether deaf or hard-of-hearing children respond similarly to hearing children when taking this test.

Benton Revised Visual Retention Test
Author: Benton
Publisher: Psychological Corporation
Copyright 1974
Age Level: 8 years to adult

The Benton has been designed to evaluate visual motor coordination and visual memory. The test utilizes 10 cards, each containing one or more simple geometric figures. Each card is exposed for 10 seconds and then removed. Immediately following its removal, the subject is instructed to draw the geometric figure represented on the card. The test requires spatial perception, immediate recall, and visuomotor reproduction of drawings.

Use with Deaf Individuals.   This test, in conjunction with other screening devices, can be useful in identifying individuals exhibiting symptoms of brain injury. Although useful with children, it produces even more striking results when administered to adults.

Graham-Kendall Memory for Designs Test
Author: F.K. Graham and B.S. Kendall
Publisher: Psychological Tests Specialists
Copyright: 1946
Age Level: 8½ years and above

The Graham-Kendall was primarily developed to screen for brain damage; however, some clinicians utilize it as a projective technique. Structured to be administered in approximately 15 minutes, the test consists of 15 five-inch cardboard squares printed with geometric designs. The subject is given a plain sheet of white paper and is instructed to reproduce each design. Each card is viewed for five seconds and removed, then the examinee draws what he or she remembers. This test can be useful in detecting a perceptual dysfunction.

Use with Deaf and Hard-of-Hearing Individuals.   The nonlanguage design of this instrument permits easy administration with deaf people through sign language or gesture without affecting the standard administration procedures. No reading or verbal skills are required to complete this test; therefore, it appears to be very appropriate for use with deaf and hard-of-hearing people. When visual acuity or manual dexterity problems are apparent, the instrument should not be utilized.

Bruininks-Oseretsky Test of Motor Proficiency
Author: Sloan
Publisher: Stoelting
Copyright: 1978
Age Level: 6–14 years

The Bruininks-Oseretsky is a revision of the original Oseretsky test, first designed as a scale of motor development for use with mentally retarded youngsters. This scale was intended to cover all major types of motor behavior. The current test battery is designed to be administered in 45 to 60 minutes. The complete battery is comprised of 46 items grouped into eight subtests. This instrument yields three scores: a gross motor composite, a fine motor composite, and a total battery composite.

Use with Deaf and Hard-of-Hearing Individuals.   Instructions for this test are given orally and through demonstration. When evaluating deaf and hard-of-hearing children, directions that cannot be demonstrated may need to be expressed in the language most familiar to the child.

Projective Techniques

Goodenough Harris Drawing Test
Author: Harris
Publisher: Psychological Corporation

Copyright: 1926; revised 1963
Age Level: 5 years and above

Individuals completing this test are instructed to make the very best picture of a man that they can. Emphasis is placed on accuracy of observation and on the development of conceptual thinking rather than on artistic skill. Credit is given for the inclusion of individual body parts, clothing details, proportion, perspective, and similar features. There are a total of 73 scoreable items based on age differentiation. Subjects are also asked to draw a picture of a woman and of themselves. The woman scale is scored in terms of 71 items similar to those in the man scale.

Use with Deaf and Hard-of-Hearing Children. The directions for this test are not designed to be given to young children in a standardized fashion. Furthermore, scoring is less objective than would be desired. However, it does have merit when employed to gain insights into the deaf child's personality (Vernon & Ottinger, 1981).

Make A Picture Story (MAPS)
Author: Schneidman
Publisher: Teacher's College Press
Copyright: 1951
Age Level: 6–12 years

This is a thematic projective technique that involves 67 figures and 22 backgrounds upon which to place them. Subjects must choose figures and backgrounds and design stories around them. This test is usually incorporated as part of a group of psychological tests.

Use with Deaf and Hard-of-Hearing Children. When using this test with deaf individuals, the examiner must be fluent in sign language, or both the client and the examiner must be skilled in oral communication. This test has been used with deaf children and has proven to be a valuable assessment tool when used with them (Vernon & Andrews, 1990).

Draw-A-Person: Screening Procedure for Emotional Disturbance (DAP:SPED)
Author: W. H. Urban
Publisher: The Psychological Corporation
Copyright: 1963 (1991)
Age Level: 6 years and above

In this test, the examinee is provided with paper and pencil and told simply to draw a person. The individual is also asked to draw a person of the opposite sex. Then the person is instructed to draw a picture of himself or herself. This can be followed by a series of questions pertaining to the drawings. Scoring of the DAP:SPED is essentially qualitative, involving the preparation of a composite personality description from an analysis of many features of the drawings.

Use with Deaf and Hard-of-Hearing Individuals. This instrument is analogous to the Draw-A-Person test. It can be used effectively with deaf individuals. It can also be used as a gross screening device for identifying children and adolescents who may have emotional or behavior disorders. However, it must be used in conjunction with other instruments to make a definitive diagnosis. There are no norms provided for drawings by deaf or hard-of-hearing children.

House-Tree-Person Projective Technique (H-T-P)
Author: J.N. Buck
Publisher: Western Psychological Service
Copyright: 1948
Age Level: 3 years and above

In this evaluation examinees are told to draw the best picture of a house that they can. The same instructions are repeated with the drawing of a tree and a person. The pictures are followed by an oral inquiry. The drawings are analyzed both quantitatively and qualitatively, chiefly on the basis of their formal or stylistic characteristics.

Use with Deaf and Hard-of-Hearing Individuals. The first phase of this test is nonverbal and can be administered with a minimum of communication; thus it is appropriate for use with deaf and hard-of-hearing individuals. However, if the evaluator is not skilled in the communication mode used by the client, then the second phase of the test should not be administered. If communication has been established, this portion of the test can be incorporated and used as a measure of personality. This instrument is widely used with deaf and hard-of-hearing children, although there has been little research data documenting its use.

Vocational Interest Batteries

Strong-Campbell Interest Inventory
Author: E.K. Strong and D.P. Campbell
Publisher: Stanford University Press
Copyright: 1981; revised scoring, Form T325
Age Level: 13 years and above

This test can be used with persons from 13 years of age through adulthood. Because interests begin to solidify for most people at age 17 or 18, the results are more appropriate for career planning at this age level. The SCII booklet reads at approximately the sixth-grade level.

This test consists of 399 items grouped into eight parts. In the first five parts the examinee records his or her preference by circling one of the letters L, D, or I, signifying "like," "dislike," or "indifferent." Each of the five parts is concerned with one of the following categories: occupations, school subjects, amusements, activities, and types of people. The remaining three parts of the Strong require subjects to rank given activities in order of preference, compare their interests in various pairs of items, and rate their present abilities and other characteristics.

Use with Deaf and Hard-of-Hearing Individuals.   This instrument relies totally on the individual's ability to comprehend written English at a sixth-grade level. The median reading level of deaf individuals graduating from high school is at or below the fourth-grade level. According to Quigley and Paul (1984), the average deaf student performs at the same level as the average 9- or 10-year-old hearing student. As a result, this instrument is generally not appropriate for use with the deaf and hard-of-hearing population. In the event it is administered, extreme caution should be taken in interpreting the results.

Kuder Occupational Interest Inventories
Author: G. Frederic Kuder
Publisher: Science Research Associates
Copyright: 1956; revised 1985
Age Level: 12–18 years

The various forms, versions, and editions of the Kuder Interest Inventories can be regarded as a family of related instruments that approach the measurement of interests from different perspectives. Each of these forms is designed for somewhat different purposes. Best known of these inventories is the Kuder Preference Record—Vocational. This instrument allows individuals to indicate their relative interest in a small number of broad areas, rather than in specific occupations. The items in the Kuder-Vocational are of the forced-choice triad type. The interest scales include outdoor (agricultural, naturalistic), mechanical, computational, scientific, persuasive, artistic, literary, musical, social service, and clerical. Separate gender norms are available for high school, college, and adult groups.

Use with Deaf and Hard-of-Hearing Individuals.   This test provides information pertaining to an individual's vocational preference. However, the client must have a reading level above the sixth grade (Levine, 1981). Deaf individuals reading at or above this level are able to comprehend the test questions. However, without an understanding of the questions, the test becomes invalid.

General Aptitude Test Battery (GATB)
Author: U.S. Employment Service
Publisher: Specialty Case Manufacturing Company
Copyright: 1979
Age Level: No specifics are given; cut-off scores given for ninth- and tenth-grade students and for adults

Factor analysis underlies the development of this battery, which consists of 12 tests and nine factors. The factors covered by the GATB are G, General learning ability; V, verbal aptitude; N, numerical aptitude; S, spatial aptitude; P, form perception; Q, clerical perception; K, motor coordination; F, finger dexterity; and M, manual dexterity. The four tests used to measure factors F and M require a simple apparatus; the other eight are paper-and-pencil tests. Alternate forms are available for the first seven tests that are designed to measure factors G through Q. Administration of the entire battery requires approximately 2½ hours.

Use with Deaf and Hard-of-Hearing Individuals.   There are no special instructions in the manual for administering the GATB to deaf and hard-of-hearing individuals. This instrument may be considered inappropriate for many deaf individuals because the majority of the subtests require verbal and reading skills. However, it is possible to administer this test through a qualified interpreter.

Differential Aptitude Test (DAT)
Author; G.K. Bennett, H.G. Seashore, and A.G. Wesman
Publisher: Psychological Corporation
Copyright: 1975
Age Level: Grades 8–12

This battery was designed principally for use in the educational and vocational counseling of students in grades eight through twelve. The DAT yields the following eight scores: verbal reasoning, numerical ability, abstract reasoning, clerical speed and accuracy, mechanical reasoning, space relations, language usage I-spelling, and language usage II-grammar. The complete battery is available in two equivalent forms L and M. With the exception of clerical speed and accuracy, all tests are essentially power tests.

Use with Deaf and Hard-of-Hearing Individuals.   It is critical that the examiner be aware of the language level of the examinee prior to administering this test. Because many of the subtests as well as the administration procedures are verbal in nature, this test may be inappropriate for the majority of deaf and hard-of-hearing clients. In the event it is administered, extreme caution should be taken in interpreting the results.

Assessment of Adults

Psychometric screening of adults is usually scheduled for one of two reasons: either the individual is seeking further training and/or employment, or a dramatic change has occurred in the person's personality, thus signaling the need for an evaluation. As with younger members of the deaf population, it is imperative that pertinent personal data be compiled prior to engaging in the assessment process. A review of the client's biographical data is helpful, with particular attention being paid to those characteristics associated with deafness. In addition to determining the etiology of one's deafness, background information pertaining to the educational, vocational, and family history of the individual is compiled. The reason for the assessment is noted and some measure of the person's language skills is obtained.

Although there are no specific tests that all deaf and hard-of-hearing individuals should take, a number of them can be administered to this population to obtain valuable information regarding the client's overall functioning abilities. Included in the adult test battery are those instruments that might focus on perceptual and intellectual functioning, personality, achievement, vocational interests, and aptitudes. There are several major factors that are considered when selecting tests: the vocational goals of the client; the presence, if any, of behavior problems; the communication mode preferred; the client's language level; the purpose for which the test was designed; and whether it is compatible with the other instruments selected for the battery.

Table 8.3 provides a list of appropriate tests that can be administered to adults. A discussion of these instruments follows the listing. Tests that are appropriate for adults but were previously discussed at the secondary level are not included here. They are listed in alphabetical order according to the purpose for which the test was designed.

Evaluation of Memory and Perceptual Functions

Wechsler Adult Intelligence Scale–III
Author: David Wechsler
Publisher: Psychological Corporation
Copyright: 1989
Ages: 16–89 years

One of the best indicators of the intellectual functioning level of deaf adults can be found in the performance scale of the WAIS-III (Spragins, 1998). Instructions can be demonstrated and pantomimed so that clients with no communication skills can be evaluated. The test yields a verbal IQ, a performance IQ and a full-scale IQ. When assessing the abilities of low-achieving deaf clients, only the performance scale is administered. However, when testing higher-achieving deaf persons contemplating postsecondary training, the verbal scale can be administered.

TABLE 8.3 *Assessment of Adults*

Test	Age	Type of Assessment
Weschsler Adult Intelligence Scale	16–89 years	Intelligence
Rorscach Ink Blot Test	School age–adult	Personality
Thematic Apperception Test	4 years–adult	Personality

Use with Deaf and Hard-of-Hearing Individuals.   The verbal scale of this instrument is an inappropriate intelligence measure for many deaf and hard-of-hearing adults. The vocabulary has not been standardized to incorporate sign language, so it cannot be utilized for this purpose. The performance scale can be used as an excellent predictor with most deaf and hard-of-hearing clients. Instructions can be presented through pantomime or sign to ensure the reception of valid responses occurs.

Personality-Projective Assessment

Rorschach Ink Blot Test
Author: Rorschach
Publisher: Grune and Stratton
Copyright: 1942
Age Level: school age to adult

Of all the projective techniques, the Rorschach is probably the most popular. The test consists of 10 cards, or plates, each representing a bilaterally symmetrical inkblot. Five of the blots are printed in shades of gray and black; two contain additional touches of bright red, and the remaining three combine several pastel shades (Anastasi & Urbina, 1997). As the person is shown the inkblot, he or she is asked to describe what the blot could represent.

Use with Deaf and Hard-of-Hearing Individuals.   Although this instrument can be administered to deaf individuals who are able to communicate fluently, they must also be of above average intelligence for the test to have much value. It can be used in conjunction with other clinical methods. However, no norms for the deaf have been developed.

Problems with administering the Rorschach to deaf individuals include giving the instructions to the client while attempting to pay attention to their signing and simultaneously recording their responses. Changing the instructions from "Tell me what it might mean" to the ASL expression "What does it look like?" and employing the skills of a qualified interpreter are recommended in order to obtain optimum results (Elliott, Glass, & Evans, 1987, p. 102).

Thematic Apperception Test (TAT)
Author: Murray and others
Publisher: Harvard University Press
Copyright: 1938
Age Level: 4 years to adult

The TAT consists of 20 cards, 19 of which contain vague pictures in black and white and one that is completely blank. The individual being tested is asked to make up a story pertaining to each picture by responding to three directives: describe what precipitated the event in the picture, describe the event itself with an explanation of what the characters are thinking and feeling, and describe what the outcome of the situation will be. When the blank card is shown, the individual is instructed to imagine a picture on the card, describe it, and then tell a story about it. The test was originally designed to be given in two one-hour segments, with 10 cards being shown in each hour.

The examiner interprets the TAT stories, first by determining who the hero is in the story and then by analyzing the content in reference to Murray's list of needs. This test has been used extensively in personality research, and although normative data is available, most clinicians rely on subjective norms built from their own experience with the test (Anastasi & Urbina, 1997).

Use with Deaf and Hard-of-Hearing Individuals.   This highly verbal test can be employed with deaf adults when the clinician can effectively communicate with the client. However, when the client does not possess an effective communication base, answers are often concrete, superficial, and few in number (Watson, 1976).

What Test Results Show

The purpose of assessment is to determine the functioning abilities of the individual at a particular point in time. Characteristics are identified, behaviors are studied, and individual differences are analyzed. When evaluations are conducted with deaf individuals, the examiner tries to determine the effect deafness has on the person's intellectual, emotional, and social development. Furthermore, the psychological examination strives to distinguish between the innate abilities of the person and the impact the environment has on fashioning these qualities and behaviors. Through the use of appropriate test measurements, the evaluator is able to provide a profile of the individual's strengths and weaknesses.

Test Results and the School-Aged Population

Hearing infants do not have to be taught how to comprehend and use their spoken linguistic system. They reside in an environment where they are exposed daily to spoken language. They acquire a verbal system that is governed by sets of rules that are phonological, syntactic, and semantic (Myers, 1987). They incorporate this system as they grow and are never formally taught the rules until they enter school. Because prelingual deafness usually delays the development of verbal language, it slows the pace of all learning based on language mastery. Research indicates that the loss of hearing sensitivity in children produces a significant impact on their linguistic intake, thus affecting their ability to comprehend English syntax. In addition, verbal association studies imply that deaf and normal-hearing individuals differ with respect to the manner in which they organize and acquire lexical information. Furthermore, word-sorting data indicates that the difference in the semantic organization between deaf and hearing adolescents appears to lie primarily in the semantic domains for which the deaf have little experience, such as those words associated with auditory imagery (Tweney, Hoeman, & Andrews, 1975).

Test data also suggests that reading achievement of deaf students is far below that of their hearing peers, placing them at a tremendous disadvantage. However, the poor performance on reading tests is attributed to linguistic deficiencies rather than pervasive cognitive or intellectual defects (Quigley & Paul, 1984).

Research conducted by Trybus and Karchmer (1977) indicates that reading achievement levels of approximately half of the deaf high school population is below that of an average 9½-year-old hearing child (below fourth-grade level). However, this cannot be interpreted to mean that an average 18-year-old deaf student scoring at the fourth-grade level on a standardized reading or vocabulary test is performing at the same level as fourth-grade hearing students. The reason this assumption cannot be made lies in the fact that these standardized tests measure educational achievement rather than linguistic ability per se, and therefore they presuppose a level of linguistic proficiency lacking in most deaf children (Moores, 1970).

Reading is only one area affected by this linguistic deficit. There are further indications of deficiencies in the area of writing. Although the performances of deaf teenagers resemble that of younger children when producing writing samples, the two groups are not on par with each other. Attempting to equate scores obtained from deaf adolescents with those from hearing elementary school children should therefore be avoided (Bochner, 1982). Even though deaf individuals frequently select words from appropriate syntactic categories (nouns, verbs, prepositions, and so forth) to complete their sentences, the words they select are often inappropriate. Furthermore, their vocabularies are limited, thus affecting their compositions. They may have a difficult time incorporating articles, prepositions, verb endings, and words associated with time referencing (Ivimey & Lachterman, 1980).

The reading difficulties experienced by most of the prelingually deaf school population necessitate the administration of nonverbal instruments when intelligence is being assessed. When performance IQ tests are given, the results for deaf students appear to be relatively stable and to demonstrate respectable concurrent validity with other nonverbal intelligence measures (Vernon & Andrews, 1990).

Over the past two decades researchers have increased their efforts to standardize intelligence tests with deaf children. Tests such as the CID Preschool Performance Scale, the Smith-Johnson Nonverbal Performance Scale, the WISC-R Performance Scale, and the WPPSI Performance Scale have been normed on deaf students. Standardized administration procedures specifically for use with deaf students have been developed and data has been collected.

Although several of these tests have been renormed, the fairly recent standardization of the WISC-R merits special consideration. This effort was conducted by Anderson and Sisco (1997) in conjunction with the Center for Assessment and Demographic Studies in Washington, DC. To accomplish this task Anderson and Sisco collected protocols of 1,228 students from residential schools and day schools throughout the country. The students ranged in age from 6 to 16 years and all had hearing losses of 70 decibels (dB) or greater in the better ear. Of the sample collected, 77 percent were tested through the mode of total communication, 2.2 percent using speech only, 4 percent using fingerspelling and speech and the remainder using gestures, pantomime, or other unspecified methods. This sample resembled the original WISC-R hearing sample adhering to the same percentage representation of sex, race, urban/rural residence, geographic region, and parental occupation variables (Blennerhassett, 1990).

Although the deaf students scored significantly higher on the object assembly subtest, performance IQ was significantly lower (deaf mean was 95.70). Lower performance was also noted on the following subtests: picture arrangement, coding, block design, and picture completion. However, Anderson and Sisco (1997) concluded that this difference was attributed to the younger, lower-scoring children in the sample and in most cases deaf children performed comparably to hearing children in all subtests except coding and picture arrangement (Blennerhassett, 1990).

Data collected on this sample was also analyzed with special attention given to the differences between deaf students of deaf parents and deaf students of hearing parents. Sisco and Anderson (1980) reported significantly higher performance IQs for deaf students of deaf parents (mean of 106.7) compared to deaf students of hearing parents (mean of 96.0). Additional studies conducted by Kusche, Greenberg, and Garfield (1983) concur with these findings, reporting that the IQ among residential school students with deaf parents exhibited a mean of 111.89 compared with 100.74 reported for deaf students of hearing parents (Blennerhassett, 1990).

Wechsler subtest comparisons are also instrumental in identifying learning-disabled deaf and hard-of-hearing students. This population accounts for the largest percentage of deaf students with additional handicapping conditions. Indications of learning disabilities occur when the individual's test score on the Wechsler reflects average intelligence accompanied by an atypical subtest scatter. In a study conducted by Rush, Blennerhassett, Epstein, and Alexander (1989), atypically low scores were discovered on the picture completion, picture arrangement, and arithmetic subtests. Although the arithmetic subtest from the verbal scale is not generally administered to measure intelligence with deaf students, when low scores occur they may indicate the possibility of an underlying learning disorder.

Even though the performance scale of the Wechsler may be an indicator of the child's intellectual abilities, it may not be the most valid indicator for predicting academic achievement. Researchers are divided regarding the use of the nonverbal IQ. While some are very supportive of its use, others question its predictive validity. Due to the implications of language, the verbal scale may never be a valid predictor of intelligence.

Intellectual development and academic achievement are only two of the components inherent in the assessment process. Attention is also directed to those factors contributing to the emotional and behavioral characteristics of the individual's personality. Screening devices are routinely administered within the school setting with more in-depth evaluations being provided by mental health professionals.

Mental Health Assessment and the
Deaf Population

Deaf individuals are referred to mental health professionals for assessment for various reasons. At times discrepancies between intelligence and academic achievement merit the need for further testing. On other occasions, inappropriate behaviors or emotional outbursts warrant additional study. Frequently, a secondary handicapping condition is suspected and the person is referred for a neuropsychological evaluation. This type of assessment is conducted to determine if there is evidence of an organic brain disorder. Four of the five major causes of childhood deafness may also contribute to other impairments. Frequently they are of a neurological nature, requiring that the etiology and the concomitants be clearly identified early in the assessment process. Research indicates that approximately one-third of all deaf persons have some type of secondary disability (Gallaudet Regional Institute, 1998) and it is critical that these be delineated.

The deaf and hard-of-hearing population presents a unique challenge for mental health professionals. Due to the ramifications of deafness the signs and symptoms of brain dysfunction may go undetected. When deaf individuals with limited English language skills and/or those who are lacking a well-organized lifestyle are referred for testing, the characteristics they project are often attributed to linguistic deprivation and lack of socialization. However, deafness can mask brain pathology, and if it is unidentified and left untreated, it can become a potential cause for life-threatening consequences. Even in cases in which the undiagnosed and untreated brain disorder poses no threat to life, it can severely impair the individual's ability to function and can limit the quality of and satisfaction with life (Wisniewski, DeMatteo, Lee, & Orr, 1985).

Poor performance by a deaf client on a task that depends on English for directions and instructions may indicate a brain dysfunction; however, it can also signal that the individual is experiencing difficulty understanding the task or the requirements. Similarities exist between the potential impact of deafness on psychosocial development and learning and certain neurological syndromes. When these similarities are confused, a misdiagnosis can occur and administered treatment may be inappropriate.

Deaf individuals may exhibit characteristics that reflect limited language skills, short attention span, and aggressive behavior. These characteristics may be caused by a neurological dysfunction or may be attributed to familial or environmental influences. Deaf individuals raised in families without communication or sufficient socialization may exhibit functional developmental deficits that make it difficult for them to monitor their feelings or develop good relationships. These individuals may present the same symptoms and problems of those who are emotionally disturbed due to a neurological dysfunction. Although these two individuals may present a very similar picture in terms of their patterns of behavior, the origins of their actions are quite distinct, thus requiring that diverse treatments be provided (Wisniewski et al.,

1986). Results obtained from neuropsychological assessments have proven especially useful in discriminating between psychiatric and neurological symptoms and in identifying brain dysfunction not associated with structural abnormality.

The deaf population is as vulnerable as the hearing population to the causes of brain dysfunction. Head trauma, cerebral tumors, toxic disorders, and alcoholism are all common causes. Moreover, when deafness is caused by maternal rubella, Rh incompatibility, prematurity, or meningitis, there is an increased risk of brain dysfunction (Isselbacher et al., 1980). Research conducted by Schlesinger and Meadow (1972) and Wilson, Rapin, Wilson and VanDenburg (1975) indicates that deafness caused by an insult to the central nervous system rather than by hereditary etiology yields a larger proportion of individuals labeled as severely disturbed. The behavioral deficits commonly observed in the clinical deaf population (impulsivity, low frustration tolerance, difficulties with cause-and-effect relationships) may be signs of neurologically based learning disabilities. It is imperative that these developmental psychosocial problems not be attributed to functional linguistic deafness.

Mental health personnel confronted with deaf and hard-of-hearing clients are often faced with the arduous task of making a valid assessment. Early surveys of deaf patients housed in psychiatric hospitals indicated that proportionally there were three times as many deaf as hearing patients. However, the reasons for this soon became apparent. When psychiatrists were confronted with "mute persons gesticulating wildly" they were more likely to make a mistaken diagnosis than with hearing persons whom they understood well. Frequently the most common diagnosis was "psychosis with mental deficiency" (Altshuler & Abdullah, 1981, p. 101).

However, more recent research by Myers and Danek (1989) indicates that mental health disorders in the deaf population are proportionally equal to mental health disorders in the hearing population. Borderline personality disorders occur on average in 3 to 5 percent of both the general and the deaf populations. This type of disorder is one of 13 personality disorders listed in the Diagnostic and Statistical Manual of Mental Health Disorders. It may originate early in childhood, stemming from the child having a frustrated relationship with parental figures. As children grow they may have a difficult time integrating good and bad experiences into a whole, thus becoming overwhelmed with the complexities of external situations. As a result, children adopt a developmental pattern where everyone is viewed as either all good or all bad (Farrugia, 1988).

Frequently, borderline personality disorders manifest themselves in behaviors that appear to be inflexible to the point of seriously impairing the person's capacity for love and work (Meyer, 1998). Approximately 20 percent of the population in psychiatric treatment facilities experience this disorder (Grinspoon, 1987).

Of all the psychotic disturbances, schizophrenia is the largest category. It is characterized by a loosening of the thought processes, a high frequency of hallucinations and delusions, and a blunted or otherwise inappropriate emotion mismatched with ideas being expressed. A study conducted by Altschuler and Abdullah (1981) of deaf psychiatric patients in the state hospitals in New York indicated that half of the inpatients, both hearing and deaf, were schizophrenic. Psychosis with mental deficiency was a more frequent diagnosis of deaf than of hearing patients, due to brain damage caused by varying etiologies of deafness.

Additional findings indicated that there was a relative absence in deaf patients of certain depressive signs found commonly in hearing patients. Although both groups were found to have symptoms of clinical depression, the manner in which each group displayed the symptoms was different. Among the hearing patients, those who were severely depressed tended to show signs of self-recrimination, delusions of guilt, and a slowing of movement. However, among the deaf population with a corresponding diagnosis, patients tended to show signs of anxious agitation, activity levels near or above normal levels, and often bodily preoccupations (Altshuler & Abdulah, 1981). Other deaf patients in the hospital portrayed primitive behaviors, suggestive of individuals who have been hidden at home and become overly dependent on their families. However, once these factors were considered, accurate diagnoses could be made.

Strategies for Interpreting for Psychological Assessments

Interpreting for psychological evaluations can be both a demanding and a rewarding process. As with other interpreting assignments, it is critical that the professional use discretion when accepting assignments of this nature. In the event that you are called upon to interpret in a testing situation, consider the following points prior to your arrival:

- Generally more than one standardized test will be administered.
- These instruments may be used to evaluate intelligence, reasoning, personality factors, aptitude, memory, neurological functioning, motor skills, and cognitive functioning.
- Several of these instruments require verbal responses, so you should be prepared to voice.
- It is acceptable and appropriate to ask questions (test instruments that will be administered, length of time for test battery) prior to accepting the assignment.
- If the deaf consumer misunderstands the interpreter, a faulty diagnosis can occur.
- Become familiar with the tests and the procedures before the designated test time.
- Recognize that when severe mental illness manifests itself in deaf consumers, their thoughts may be distorted and it is not the role of the interpreter to make coherent sentences from the language that is produced.

Summary

A great deal of current research strongly suggests that many of the cognitive, emotional, and behavioral problems of prelingually deaf persons are not the result of deafness per se, but of "superimposed environmental vicissitudes associated with deafness" (Heller, 1987, p. 5). The deaf person's major problem is not the inability to hear, but the difficulty in understanding and being understood.

Problems associated with prelingual deafness influence the psychological examination. As a result, the examiner must be attuned to the characteristics of this population, and be sensitive to the implications that loss of hearing can have on individuals. Special attention must be given to the parent-child relationship, the environment in which individuals were raised, and the community in which the majority of the interaction has occurred. Furthermore, the practitioner must be familiar with the abilities and disabilities associated with deafness. Then and only then can an accurate diagnosis be made and the potential for stigmatization reduced.

9

Counseling Techniques and Therapeutic Models

Counseling can be defined as a helping relationship comprised of one party who is seeking help, a facilitator, and a setting that allows a helping process to occur (Cormier & Hackney, 1987). It involves more than just a set of techniques. Individuals participating in counseling engage in a series of purposeful actions, thus permitting specific preselected goals and objectives to be achieved (Purkey & Schmidt, 1987).

Closely akin to and sometimes overlapping the field of counseling is guidance and psychotherapy. According to Mowrer (1988), these should be viewed as activities on a continuum rather than as well-defined, distinct practices. Guidance, which appears at the origin of the continuum, is less formal than either counseling or psychotherapy and consists of influencing another person's thoughts or behaviors. Those looking for or in need of guidance receive information, advice, and suggestions from professionals whose training is less formalized than that of mental health counselors or psychotherapists. The individuals who seek the services of a guidance counselor generally experience problems and/or concerns that can be resolved in a relatively short amount of time.

Counseling expands beyond the realm of information giving. Individuals requesting these services are generally mentally healthy. However, they may feel the need to make personal adjustments or may be compelled to examine their methods or styles of interacting with others. Counseling can help them take an in-depth look at their positive and counterproductive behaviors. Further, it enables them to evaluate and face their values and beliefs, increase their personal awareness and self-knowledge, and achieve self-development (Shipley, 1992; DeBlassie & Cowan, 1976).

In contrast, those requiring psychotherapy frequently exhibit characteristics of mental illness and require professional intervention to eliminate these psychopathological feelings and behaviors. By engaging in treatment with trained professionals (psychiatrists, clinical psychologists, and other mental health professionals), those receiving services are afforded the opportunity to eliminate negative personality traits and enhance their behavior. Regardless of the setting, it is imperative that all consumers are provided with the opportunity to receive services from skilled practitioners. The therapist's training, philosophy, and skills, combined with the client's cultural, familial, and educational background, will influence the dynamics of how problems are resolved within the counseling setting. By examining the characteristics of mental health professionals as well as the clients they serve, specific strategies and techniques that foster behavior change can be discussed.

Mental Health Professionals

Mental health professionals must be spontaneous, flexible, open, emotionally stable, and have the ability to concentrate. Furthermore, they must exude a sense of trustworthiness, honesty, and belief in the client's ability to change (Shipley, 1992). Counselors must be versatile and proficient in selecting techniques from a variety of sources. They must draw from their own clinical skills as well as from the experiences their clients bring into the counseling setting. Counselors are as unique as the population they serve. However, all must be committed to the dignity and worth of humanity before they can effectively engage in the counseling process.

Clients Seeking Mental Health Services

In the helping profession, clinicians primarily encounter individuals or family units who are concerned about the problems they are experiencing. Although some recognize that problems exist and actively seek therapy, others are resistive and present the counselor with a difficult and challenging encounter. Clients may become uncomfortable when topics become intense. They may fear change or new situations and begin questioning the treatment suggested by the clinician (Okun, 1987).

Frequently clients will enter the counseling setting feeling frustrated, afraid, or threatened. They may feel that daily situations are out of control, thus sensing that they are powerless. Sometimes they respond to these feelings with anger, thus projecting an image of a person with a "short fuse" (Cormier & Hackney, 1987).

Others seeking help exhibit characteristics of those who have been raised in an overprotected environment. Typically they have been shielded from opportunities to experience life, become independent, and make optimal progress. When there is evidence of overprotection, a variety of strains and imbalances occur within the existing family structure (Cunningham & Davis, 1985).

Periodically clinicians will encounter clients who are insatiable. Regardless of what transpires they are never completely satisfied with what is occurring or what has previously taken place. While some are hostile, others attempt to conceal their unresolved feelings by intellectualizing everything. Occasionally clinicians encounter patients exhibiting paranoid behaviors. These individuals portray unhealthy fears, suspicions, and feelings of persecution. They can be chronically angry, suspicious, and distrustful. Upon entering the counseling setting it is easy for them to believe that other people and agencies are "out to get them." It is common for paranoid patients to distrust the motives of the clinician.

While discrepancies in behaviors may be observed in some clients, others convey mixed messages when they speak. They may resort to conversational shifts when the topic becomes too painful or they feel they are revealing too much. When this occurs the counselor must confront these behaviors, thus assisting their clients in gaining insights into their feelings and the role they play in their environment.

The Counseling Process: Facilitating Change

When mental health professionals meet new clients, they generally conduct interviews, gather background information, and determine what difficulties exist. A case history is collected whereby autobiographical information is noted, observations are recorded, and testing (if needed) is conducted. Information and preliminary observations generated during the initial interview set the stage for the interactions that will follow. According to Dillard and Reilly (1998), there are three significant dimensions to an interview. First, the interview must be viewed as a serious conversation. Second, it should be conducted with a specific purpose in mind; and third, it must involve a plan of action that entails communication. They further state that inadequacy in any of these areas will preclude optimal effectiveness of the interview.

During the interview basic facts are obtained and insights are gained into people's feelings, thoughts, and beliefs. The process is interactive in nature, providing both the client and the clinician with the opportunity to ask questions and contribute information. Knowledge gained from this session is instrumental in prioritizing problems and concerns while determining the counseling techniques that will be implemented. It is imperative that the counselor remains attentive to the vital information that is communicated both verbally and behaviorally during the initial interview and throughout subsequent counseling sessions.

What happens when counselors encounter individuals with communication disorders or find themselves in situations where the exchange of information is restricted or in the traditional sense, nonexistent? What issues do clinicians address when they find themselves faced with clients whose identity and values are rooted in a culture foreign to the larger society where they reside? What is the result when the therapist sits face to face with a deaf or hard-of-hearing client for the first time? Do the issues vary? Do traditional counseling techniques work effectively, and how is communication achieved? Figure 9.1 illustrates factors that must be considered in the counseling process.

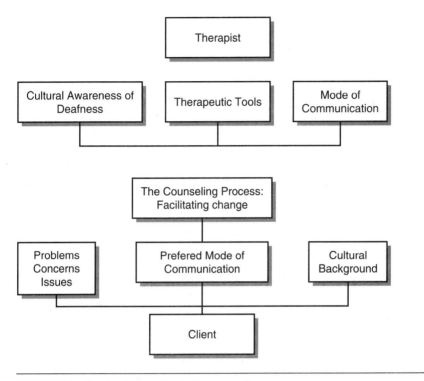

FIGURE 9.1 *Factors to consider in the counseling process.*

Meeting the Needs of Deaf and Hard-of-Hearing Clients

In recent decades increased attention has been focused on the field of mental health and the role professionals play when providing services to deaf and hard-of-hearing consumers. From the early works of Myklebust (1964), Sussman and Stewart (1971), Rainer and Altshuler (1966), and Schlesinger and Meadow (1972), to the more recent works of Vernon and Andrews (1990), Harvey (1989), Glickman (1993), Lane (1992), and Marschark (1993), the field has undergone a metamorphosis. As a result, the pathological view of deafness has been transformed into a healthier perspective that portrays individuals who are deaf as potential members of a distinct cultural group.

This cultural group is as diverse as the larger majority that encompasses it. Membership is based on a desire to join; an appreciation of shared values, experiences, and beliefs; a willingness to support group-sponsored activities; and a conviction that one wants to remain deaf. Through American Sign Language (ASL) these beliefs are shared and a sense of camaraderie is fostered.

Although this cultural group represents a unique segment of society, there are those who are deaf and hard of hearing who refrain from seeking membership. These individuals prefer to remain in the mainstream, where they affiliate with those who can hear. They may or may not sign, they frequently prefer written or spoken communication, and they perceive their hearing loss as something to be overcome.

Those seeking counseling services may reflect the beliefs and values indicative of Deaf culture or display characteristics of the deaf or hard-of-hearing population. In order for psychologists to work effectively with all these individuals they must become familiar with the diverse nature of this group. Furthermore, they must examine their own cultural assumptions about clients who are Deaf and hard of hearing and then consider the cultural differences between the two groups.

Within the field of counseling psychology the importance of recognizing cultural differences became apparent in the early 1980s. At that time, the American Psychological Association (APA) became sensitive to cross-cultural counseling. This resulted in the establishment of a task force to delineate the dimensions of the "culturally competent counselor" (Sue & Sue, 1981). In essence, the APA determined that the counselor should:

1. Be aware of his or her own worldviews in order to prevent ethnocentrism.
2. Actively attempt to understand the worldview of his or her culturally different clients without making negative judgments.
3. Actively develop and practice appropriate relevant and sensitive intervention strategies and skills when working with culturally different clients (p. 13).

These tenets have become important for counselors who deal with clients from a wide array of cultural backgrounds. As a result, individuals both inside and outside the field of deafness have developed paradigms of cross-cultural counseling (Locke, 1991), systemic models of psychotherapy with Deaf, deaf, and hard-of-hearing persons (Harvey, 1989), and techniques for engaging in culturally affirmative psychotherapy with Deaf persons (Glickman & Harvey 1996).

When therapists assume the responsibility for providing quality counseling services across cultural boundaries it becomes a formidable task, entailing the professional developing an awareness of self (values, beliefs, opinions, and attitudes that represent a consistent part of the dominant culture), as well as an awareness of the clients' values, beliefs, opinions, and attitudes. The process itself is complex and the variables that must be considered are multitudinal. Figure 9.2 illustrates a hierarchical tree depicting the multilateral factors that are linked to the cross-cultural counseling process. By examining these components one can gain a deeper understanding of the skills and competencies required when providing services to Deaf, deaf, and hard-of-hearing people.

According to the 1990–1991 National Health Interview Survey (National Center for Health Statistics, 1990–1991 [NCHS]), 20 million people in the United States experience some degree of hearing loss. Data indicates that of the total population, 10 percent of the males, 7 percent of the females, 9 percent of white Americans, and 4 percent of African Americans comprise this population. Additionally, people who are deaf and hard of hearing within the U.S. population comprise 12 percent of those with family income under $10,000, 11 percent in the $10,000–$25,000 income range, 7 percent of the $25,000–$50,000 income range; and 6 percent in the income range greater than $50,000. Additional statistics indicate that 9 percent of the high school graduates in the United States are deaf or hard of hearing, and 17 percent of them have fewer than 12 years of education.

Moreover, the NCHS has revealed that hearing loss is more common in rural than in urban areas. Information collected from this survey indicates that 8 percent of the urban population and 11 percent of the people in rural areas have some degree of hearing loss. Additional findings from the 1990–1991 data also reiterate previous studies indicating that there is a higher incidence of hearing loss among the elderly. Statistics reflect a loss in 29 percent of people over 65 years of age, 13 percent in people between the ages of 45 and 64, 4 percent in individuals between the ages of 18 and 44, and 2 percent of the population between the ages of 3 and 17 (Henwood & Pope-Davis, 1994).

Of those who are deaf and hard of hearing, 4 percent have a congenital loss (present at birth), 12 percent stated they had a lost their hearing due to ear infections, 5 percent experienced ear injuries, and 23 percent lost hearing due to other noise. Although 28 percent indicated "getting older" as the cause of their problem, 18 percent listed "other" for the etiology of their hearing loss (Henwood & Pope-Davis, 1994, p. 491).

Upon entering the counseling setting it is imperative that clinicians be attentive to how the client identifies his or her loss (Deaf, deaf, or hard of hearing), and that they ascertain when the loss occurred. These two characteristics, age of onset and severity of loss, are ancillary factors in the communication process. Furthermore, these two components contribute to the amount of experiential deprivation that may occur, the type of educational placement that is or has been selected, and the person's cultural preferences. Each of these attributes is instrumental in shaping social, psychological, and emotional development, is influence the personality characteristics displayed by those who enter the counseling setting.

Characteristics of Congenitally Deaf Individuals

Of all of the ramifications of congenital deafness, the inability to engage in communication with significant others during one's developmental years is the most detrimental, for it severely impedes all facets of psychosocial development (Lane, 1984; Mindel & Vernon, 1987; Moores, 1982; Schlesinger & Meadow, 1972, all cited in Glickman & Harvey, 1996, p. 157). These individuals, with or without amplification,

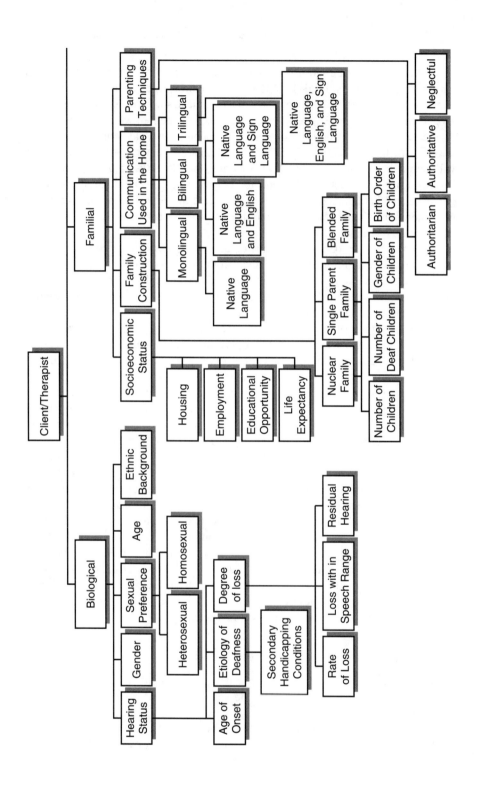

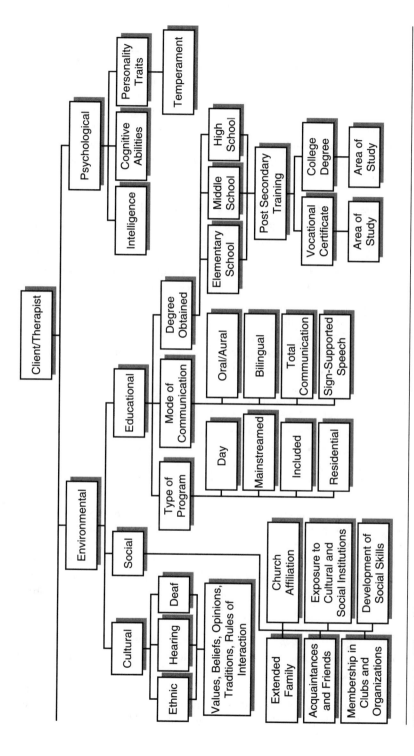

FIGURE 9.2 *Hierarchical tree depicting the complexity of cross-cultural counseling.*

receive fragmented acoustic messages or no acoustic messages at all. This in turn limits the number of conversational exchanges that can and do take place and affects the quality and quantity of information that is delivered and received. Research indicates that 90 percent of deaf babies are born to hearing parents, therefore the immediate challenge facing the family is how they will communicate with their deaf child. Early in life these families must decide whether they will try to channel their children into the world of audition or whether they will permit them to access language and concepts through vision. This decision will influence their child's social, emotional, and academic development.

Developing Language: Oral versus Manual Methods. Parents who support the oral method encourage their children to receive information primarily through the aural/oral channel. Emphasis is placed on speechreading, utilizing residual hearing, and clarifying articulation. Supporters of oral communication focus their attention on amplification and assisting individuals as they attempt to comprehend spoken communication. Some parents initially embrace an oral approach and later become frustrated if spoken communication becomes strained or unclear. At that point they may turn to a form of manual expression. Although the selection of a mode of communication frequently presents a dilemma for hearing parents, deaf parents (approximately 10 percent of deaf children have deaf parents) generally prefer to communicate with their children using American Sign Language (ASL).

American Sign Language. American Sign Language (ASL) is a language in its own right and can be viewed as a separate communication system complete with its own vocabulary and syntax. One of the most striking differences between ASL and English is that English is an aural/oral language developed by a community of hearing and speaking individuals, while ASL is a visual/gestural/conceptual language that has been developed within a community that relies on its sight and body movements for communication (Scheetz, 1993).

Viewed as a foreign language, ASL's vocabulary and syntax separate it from other languages. Signs represent words and concepts, while nonmanual cues such as facial expression, head tilts, body movements, and eye gazes can be incorporated to express specific grammatical functions in the language. Mastery of the language can be difficult, if not altogether impossible for those who are not culturally Deaf. Therefore, many of these signs have been incorporated or modified for use in English-based signing systems.

English-Based Signing Systems. Communication systems that incorporate ASL signs in an English word order are referred to as forms of manually coded English. When English-based signing and speech are delivered simultaneously, Simultaneous Communication or sign-supported speech occurs. There are several forms of manually coded English systems. Those developed to present English in a manual manner include Seeing Essential English (SEE I), Signing Exact English (SEE II), Signed English (SE), and Pidgin Sign English (PSE).

Seeing Essential English (SEE I).   Developed in the 1960s by a deaf man named David Anthony, SEE I is a system whereby English is presented visually to deaf children the way hearing children hear it. Within this system, Anthony proposed that every English word and morpheme would have a sign.

Signing Exact English (SEE II).   In the early stages of developing SEE I, a group of individuals worked together with David Anthony. However, due to various philosophical differences the group divided. Later three of the members worked together to develop a signed system with one basic objective in mind: they wanted to ease the basic acquisition of English by deaf children. Developed by Gerilee Gustason, Donna Pfetzing, and Esther Zawolkow, this system introduced initialized signs into the sign system and also added signs where none were previously available. Signing Exact English, or SEE II, is a result of the culmination of their efforts.

Contact Signing or Pidgin Sign English (PSE).   A pidgin language is typically devised when two speakers who are not fluent in each other's language want to communicate. As a rule, a pidgin contains vocabulary from both languages, but it generally adheres to the syntactical structure of the majority language. Wide variations in language use may occur when a pidgin is employed, which can be attributed to the competency and fluency possessed by the language users in conjunction with the topic being discussed (Cokely, 1983). Contact signing, previously referred to in the literature as Pidgin Sign English (PSE), incorporates American Sign Language (ASL) within the confines of the syntax of spoken English (Wilbur, 1979). A variety of sign systems fall under the category of PSE. Terms used to identify these systems are American Sign English (Ameslish), Sign English (Siglish), Signed English, and manual English (Bragg, 1973). Two additional forms of communication merit discussion, the Rochester method and cued speech. Unlike the manually coded English systems, these modes of communication rely on fingerspelling and signs (Rochester method) or oral English with speechreading supported by hand positions (cued speech) to facilitate communication.

Rochester Method.   The Rochester method originated 1919 and was developed by Zenus Westervelt. At that time he was the superintendent at the Rochester School for the Deaf in Rochester, New York. The Rochester method was originally called the Great Innovation, a system based on fingerspelling spoken or written English words. Fingerspelling, also referred to as dactylology, provides an avenue for expression whereby one hand shape is incorporated for each of the 26 letters in the alphabet. As a manual representation of the language that is spoken, fingerspelling has no separate syntax, morphology, phonology, or semantics; rather it is dependent on the linguistic structure of the language it is representing (Wilbur, 1979). As words are formed and messages are conveyed they are spelled out in much the same way as one would spell words incorporating Braille or a Morse code system.

The original Rochester method relied exclusively on fingerspelling. However, today it has been modified and is used in conjunction with a signed vocabulary system. It serves as a means of communication and is in use at the school today.

Cued Speech.   Cued speech is used in conjunction with speech. Eight handshapes are utilized in four positions on or near the face to supplement the spoken signal (Martin, 1987). By incorporating the handshapes, one is able to distinguish between speech sounds that look similar when produced orally. See Table 9.1 for an illustration of how ASL, the sign systems, the Rochester method, and cued speech relate to one another.

Socialization and Language

In all societies the family functions as a cultural unit, a microcosm that reflects family-specific cultural beliefs and values (Henry, 1965). This process occurs as the parents communicate cultural norms through language. In turn, language provides the vehicle for transmitting culture and is instrumental in the development and maintenance of one's identity (Coleman, 1985). Based on what children hear and observe, they begin to develop norms for social behavior.

When deafness occurs at birth or early in life, it interferes with the linguistic means of transmitting culture, and the rich cultural content of the socialization process is lost (Becker, Heimberg, & Bellack, 1987). Although some aspects of this process may occur as language is acquired, the bonding that transpires between the parent and the child is often absent. Furthermore, if this communication barrier persists, the child may not have the opportunity to begin developing socially or emotionally until he or she enters the educational setting. As Becker states:

> The language barrier thus significantly interferes with relationships between parent and child. This phenomenon has few parallels cross-culturally. Lack of parent-child socialization coupled with poor communication and fragile emotional bonds has created a weak link between the deaf person and his or her family of origin that has culminated in further separating the deaf individual from the hearing world in adulthood (Becker et al., 1987, p. 61).

When deaf children are excluded from information sharing that originates in the home, their socialization process is hampered. This exclusion may extend to breakdowns in communication, thus affecting the way these children perceive themselves. At a young age they may sense that they are different and struggle with many unanswered questions. During this time parents may be dealing with guilt feelings because they have produced an "imperfect" child. As they grapple with these feelings they may convey negative attitudes and feelings toward and about the child. Deaf children in turn may internalize the idea that they are devalued members of the family unit and become sensitive to the stigma attached by both family and society.

As children reach school age, feelings of rejection, inferiority, and isolation may accompany them into the educational setting. If the youngster remains at home and attends a mainstreamed or included program, these feelings may intensify, creating problems that continue into adulthood. Deaf children find themselves competing with those who obtain information both auditorily and visually. Hearing children are knowledgeable in the cultural traditions and values of the larger hearing society, and

TABLE 9.1 A Comparison of Modes of Communication Used by Deaf and Hard-of-Hearing Individuals

	ASL Syntax and Grammar	English Syntax and Word Order	Used in Conjunction with Speech	Designed to Present Visual English	Incorporates Finger-spelling	Incorporates Gestures	Relies on Handshapes rather than Signs	Recognized as a Foreign Language	Classified as a Sign System	Invented in Homes for Communication
Home Signs						●				●
American Sign Language	●		●		●	●		●		
Contact Signing/Pidgin Signed English	●	●	●	●	●	●				
Signed Supported Speech		●	●	●	●					
Signed English		●	●	●	●				●	
Signing Essential English (SEE I)		●	●	●	●				●	
Signing Exact English (SEE II)		●	●	●	●				●	
Manually Coded English (MCE)		●	●	●	●				●	
Rochester Method		●	●	●	●					
Cued Speech		●	●	●				●		

213

oftentimes can compete with ease in the educational setting. Deaf children frequently find themselves on the outside looking in as clubs, sports, and other activities bustle around them. Excluded from daily verbal exchanges, their experiential base is weakened, their socialization process delayed.

Although some deaf students remain at home, others attend residential facilities designed to meet the needs of the deaf. In these settings deaf peer groups are formed and children rely on other children for emotional support and information about the world. This early bond provides the foundation for the Deaf community, a place where deaf individuals can go for ongoing nurturance and positive reinforcement of identity.

Residential schools have a strong influence on their inhabitants. Employees who reside at the school nurture the child, and these people become the child's surrogate family. Deaf children become part of the group and view themselves as members of the group rather than as individuals. In turn, the group becomes an organizing element in the social world of Deafness (Becker, 1987).

Upon emerging from residential schools deaf children may reflect a "group mindset" rather than reflecting a strong sense of individualism. However, within the larger hearing community individualist and independent thought are character traits that are valued. This places the deaf individual's value of "group thought" in direct conflict with the need for individuality, a value that is espoused by the larger, dominant society. As a result, deaf children of hearing parents may find they must adjust their core values once they leave school. Whereas most hearing adolescents graduate from high school and are ready to integrate the various aspects of their lives, deaf teenagers may emerge with limited knowledge of their familial background, including their parents, values, and beliefs. As they reach the brink of adulthood, their behavior may reflect delays in language acquisition, often leaving them ill prepared to function in adult roles in society.

Characteristics of Adventitiously Deaf Individuals

Those who lose their hearing after age 2, when the fundamentals of spoken language are in place, are referred to as the adventitiously or postlingually deaf. Generally the later the individual incurs the loss, the more closely his or her language pattern will reflect the features of English syntax. The degree of loss can also be instrumental in influencing the mode of communication the person will employ. Those experiencing a profound loss in childhood are faced with challenges that are not necessarily experienced by older adults who lose their hearing due to the aging process.

Although both must learn to communicate with the hearing world again, the child is faced with an additional daunting task. Children who experience an acquired loss must find a way to master those prerequisite and essential language skills that will render them competitive within the educational setting. Both children and adults quickly discover that their loss has denied them access to verbal exchanges. As a result, voids in the information received become prevalent and a sense of social isolation can develop. This ensuing barrier to communication can in turn become the catalyst for a multiplicity of social and psychological problems. Frequently, individuals prefer to remain functioning as if they can hear and will attempt to compensate for their hearing loss by relying on speechreading and forms of written communication. This can be very taxing and frustrating for those who experience a loss. Furthermore, it forces those around them to adapt to their specific communication needs, often creating an extremely stressful situation. Deafened individuals may feel they are missing important parts of verbal exchanges and may ultimately feel embarrassed and detached from those around them.

Communication difficulties and feelings of isolation can manifest themselves outwardly into expressions of anger. Furthermore, while they try to cope with the frustrations of comprehending what is said, they may also be struggling with trying to maintain a sense of dignity. Because they cannot hear, they may feel that the hearing community is rejecting them. As a result, they may formulate perceptions that everyone is talking about them.

Although these individuals may enter the counseling session with a better command of the English language than their prelingually deaf counterparts, the concerns they have and the problems they experience may be similar. As they enter the counseling setting they bring with them their individual needs, coupled with their unique personalities. This prompts those who will work with them to rely on a wide array of counseling techniques. By becoming sensitive to these needs and implementing effective strategies this unique population is afforded the opportunity to benefit from the counseling process.

Counseling within the School Setting

Counseling services are provided in the schools, vocational rehabilitation offices, mental health facilities, doctor's offices, and psychiatric hospitals. Although the nature and the severity of the problems may vary and the techniques and methods utilized may be diverse, the ultimate goal is to enhance the individual's mental health.

Within school settings students frequent counselors' offices with a myriad of problems and concerns. Many of these concerns permeate auditory boundaries and are expressed by students of all ages. To determine the most frequently expressed concerns of deaf and hard-of-hearing students Ziezula and Harris conducted a national survey of school counselors who work with deaf students. They wanted to determine what types of concerns the students shared with them on a daily basis. Throughout the course of a semester the counselors identified the following eleven concerns: peer relations, aggressive behaviors, parental relations, communication issues, career decisions, strategies for interacting with hearing individuals, issues surrounding sexual involvement, dating, sexual abuse, suicide, and withdrawal (Ziezula & Harris, 1998).

This study is reflective of the issues counselors are faced with daily. On a routine basis these counselors help students resolve family conflicts, develop interpersonal communication skills, and find solutions to dating problems. However, occasionally, they are faced with behaviors and/or issues that extend beyond the realm of their professional expertise. When this occurs they frequently make referrals to mental health agencies. There, students as well as other individuals with varying mental health needs receive therapy from professionals who work within the confines of outpatient clinics, private offices, and state mental hospitals. For a discussion of mental illness and mental health facilities see Chapters 10 and 12.

Counseling Techniques, Theories, and Strategies

While some enter therapy with clear communication skills and appreciation for the counseling process, many more arrive at the therapist's door filled with trepidation. They may have little or no understanding of why they are there, what role it is assumed they will play, and ultimately what is expected of them. These individuals represent the products of a society that has denied them basic communication, a quality education, and access to the community. Thus, when they are referred for services the therapists are faced with individuals who have been geographically isolated, environmentally and/or language deprived, chronically mentally ill, withdrawn, socially inept, impulse disordered, or mentally retarded (Zitter, 1996).

Furthermore, those who arrive for services may have had limited access to the hearing world and thus believe that the issues they are struggling with are unique, therefore assuming that because they need counseling they must be "crazy."

> Like those who are hearing, clients who are deaf worry about the stigma of having an emotional problem . . . some deaf clients become so isolated, they do not realize the commonality of their life experiences both happy and painful (Isenberg, 1996).

As a result, throughout the counseling process they are surprised to discover that not only do other deaf people share similar problems to those they are experiencing, but they also share similar feelings. All these factors can have a direct bearing on the outcome of the counseling process. Thus it is critical for the therapist to become cognizant of the client's mode of communication and cultural identity, as well as how the individual receives and conceptualizes information (Leigh, Corbett, Gutman, & Morere 1996).

The implementation of the Americans with Disabilities Act (ADA) in the 1990s prompted the field of psychotherapy to provide equal access to individuals with disabilities. As a result, the field has experienced an increase in articles and texts that provide therapists with strategies and techniques that can be utilized with the special needs population.

Although the ADA has been instrumental in promoting equitable services for all disability groups, the changes that have occurred in regard to the deaf population can be traced to a much earlier date. When reviewing the literature it becomes apparent that the 1970s marked a pivotal point in providing mental health services for this population. Prior to 1970, any research that was done in the area of counseling in relation to deaf patients was conducted in mental hospitals. At that time, very few counselors were trained to work specifically with those who were deaf, and very little information was reported in the literature. Throughout the 1960s, research conducted by Rainer and colleagues (1963) and Rainer and Altshuler (1966) involved inpatients in mental hospitals. The nature of this research and the theoretical orientation of these practitioners dealt primarily with the application of essentially psychoanalytic principles. As a result, very few articles were published that pertained to counseling approaches that could be used successfully with deaf clients (Sussman & Stewart, 1971).

Beginning in the mid-1970s the counseling field expanded and numerous articles pertaining to deafness began to surface in the literature. Early research cited by Vernon (1978), Sussman and Stewart (1971), and Brauer (1978) indicated that frequently when deaf clients expressed themselves in the counseling setting their behaviors reflected what appeared to be inherent psychological problems. However, when the clinician was knowledgeable about the ramifications of deafness, it became apparent that these behaviors were not indicative of deep-seated problems, but rather were the outward manifestations of behaviors that transpire when one's environmental experiences are restricted.

Individuals who have experienced an isolated childhood void of communication and varied experiences may have a difficult time adjusting to the problems of daily living when they begin to function independently. Due to their experiential limitations they may find themselves unable to cope with society and thus are faced with multifaceted challenges. When deaf individuals encounter difficulties in solving problems, they may turn to a counselor for help. Oftentimes they will seek a counselor upon whom they feel they can unload their burdens, a counselor who will take responsibility and make decisions for them.

> [M]any clients will be dependent upon the counselor and will often look to him for immediate, sometimes "magical" solutions to their problems. Overcoming dependency and unrealistic expectations requires that the counselor help the client to understand the purpose of counseling, the responsibilities of the counselor and the client, and how the two can work together to achieve their goals . . . The counselor must be prepared to repeatedly explain and clarify what is happening in counseling and why. The dependency of many deaf people is often not of the type characteristic of individuals who are emotionally dependent upon others. Rather, this dependency is engendered by the fact that the deaf individual has a more restricted range of experience to guide him in his behavior, has had fewer opportunities to make decisions on his own, and has generally had others help him most of his life (Sussman & Stewart, 1971, p. 28).

Deaf individuals may have had fewer opportunities for social involvement, thus rendering their decision-making skills weak and underdeveloped. As a result they may strive to establish a dependency relationship. These inadequacies all contribute to the situational barriers that may hamper the counseling process.

Although social contacts are instrumental in shaping behaviors and contributing to personality development, the interrelationships that occur between members of society are equally important. This interrelating will influence what those who are deaf are permitted to experience, and will also determine if they are acknowledged as exhibiting acceptable behaviors. The way in which the environment views deafness will affect the psychosocial development of the deaf individual.

> [E]nvironment is a major factor in the psychological development of all of us. Corollary to this, when environment is systematically altered in a significantly consistent way for any given group of people those individuals will tend to be different in some shared ways from those whose environment has not been altered in this systematic manner . . . Deafness changes one's perceived environment so that people who are deaf share some common factors in their psychological development which people who are hearing do not experience (Vernon, 1978, p. 12).

The way that society relates to deaf individuals will influence their development. Due to the hearing loss, certain lags in psychosocial development may occur as a result of the limitations placed on individuals within the environment in which they live.

> [D]eafness does not necessarily create development or adjustment problems. Rather, it is the people in the deaf person's world, through omission, or commission, who impose limitations on him. Because most people know so little about deafness and how to communicate with deaf people, a host of adjustment problems are created.
>
> [D]eafness often isolates the deaf person within the family circle, cuts him off from free interaction with his peers, restricts the input of information from the world about him, curtails learning of behavior that will permit independence as an adult, and makes his ability to adjust to his world significantly less (Sussman & Stewart, 1971, pp. 73–74).

This feeling of isolation is critical in the development of any individual. If, in fact, deaf individuals are eliminated from family and social conversations, their knowledge base of the world around them will be minimal. They will not benefit from the social learning experience of nonformal conversations, but rather will express themselves in behaviors that are viewed as maladjusted and unacceptable. When society imposes the barrier of noncommunication upon deaf individuals and refuses to accept them as equal members of society, adjustment problems occur. Deaf people may be viewed as "different" and thus regarded as second-class citizens, incapable of functioning in society.

The importance of environmental influences on personal/social development cannot be overemphasized. How society relates to any given individual will have a bearing on that person's development and self-concept. If people grow up believing they are different and therefore inferior to those around them, they will develop negative self-concepts. As Harlan Lane has so succinctly stated: "Deafness is not in itself a significant issue in the lives of culturally Deaf people. Hearing people have created deafness as an issue. White people have created Blackness as an issue" (Lane, 1992, p. 59). Barbara Brauer's writings in the 1970s reflect that even during that time period these same sentiments were shared:

> The most pervasive mental health problem confronting deaf Americans is "handicapism" akin to what other ethnic groups experience as "racism." From childhood they feel different from other members of their own families. Throughout their lives they encounter significant persons who view them with distress, ignorance, conflict, with "attitudinal apartheid," or with distorted expectations. Handicapist attitudes that have assaulted deaf Americans are now being viewed by several mental health professionals as a major factor in the development of negative self-concepts. This is manifested in the pathological denial of deafness found in some deaf persons and also in deaf men and women learning to hate themselves and each other because they are deaf. This self-devaluation is seen as stemming from their identification of themselves with negative and defective body parts, thoughts and feelings, and materializes, as a result, from their finding themselves treated in ways similar to the treatment of their "defectiveness" (Brauer, 1978).

Consequently, when these negative feelings are internalized the effect on the self-concept is damaging. Those involved have little regard for them and feel they are unable to function as useful members of society. The hearing community's acceptance or lack of acceptance of deaf people contributes to their psychosocial development. In order to work effectively with the deaf population, counselors must comprehend the complexities of the communication differences. They must be sensitive to the issues surrounding experiential deprivation and the effect this has on psychosocial development. Frequently, members of the hearing community view deafness as an extremely disabling condition. Therefore, they deny deaf individuals the opportunity to participate in routine social events. When this occurs on a regular basis, deaf individuals begin to perceive themselves as "different" in a negative sense. Consequently, their preoccupation with what hearing people say about them may not be reflective of an emotional problem, but rather an accurate insight into reality.

When examining the problems deaf people experience, one must keep in mind the characteristics that influence the overall development of the individual. In view of these considerations problems can then be viewed objectively and effective techniques can be employed. Furthermore, prior to the onset of the initial session the counselor should adopt the tenets found in cross-cultural counseling models. By broadening their perspectives they can become attentive to those potential factors that can alter the dynamics of the therapeutic process.

Once sensitivity to the client's cultural diversity is established, techniques and strategies can be modified that will insure that optimum effectiveness is obtained. Recognizing that the nature and principles of counseling with deaf people are no different than those that characterize counseling with hearing people, the focus can be directed toward how these principles are applied and implemented, thus accommodating the deaf client. Of all of the modifications, the most significant lie in the areas of cultural identity and communication.

Ramifications of Communication within the Counseling Setting

Communication is the underlying force that drives the counseling process. When it functions smoothly, it provides an avenue for problem resolution. However, when communication becomes ambiguous or breaks down altogether, it stymies progress and prohibits personal growth. Therefore, before any counseling techniques can be successfully implemented, it is imperative the therapist insure that the mode of communication he or she selects to use is mutually acceptable to the consumer. Particular attention should be given to sign/spoken communication as well as the reading/writing level of the client. This will assist in determining whether spoken communication will be utilized, whether the services of a sign language interpreter will need to be solicited, or whether the therapist's sign or other communication skills will be sufficient. Once this information has been gleaned, appropriate counseling techniques can be selected, and any necessary modifications can be made.

Spoken Communication Strategies

When therapists encounter clients who prefer to communicate through spoken exchanges there are several strategies they can implement to insure maximum communication effectiveness. First, it is essential that the client be in a position directly facing the therapist to facilitate speechreading. Bright light sources (windows, lamps, and the like) located behind the clinician should be avoided to minimize eyestrain.

Second, questions and comments should be expressed in a conversational manner, free from excessive mouth movements and exaggerations. Homophonous words should be avoided and statements should be rephrased rather than repeated when obvious misunderstandings have occurred. Third, statements or questions that are brief and specific may be understood better than those that are complex and open ended. When it becomes apparent that clients cannot decipher what is being said, they should be asked to indicate what part of the message they experienced difficulty comprehending. This will assist the therapist in restructuring the question. Clients should be encouraged to inform therapists if they are experiencing extreme difficulty speechreading, because the services of an oral interpreter may need to be employed. Furthermore, therapists have a responsibility to inform their clients when they are having difficulty understanding their speech. When this occurs, the services of an oral interpreter should also be requested.

Interpreters

Interpreters are employed in the counseling setting to facilitate communication. These professionals may be trained as oral interpreters (equalizing communication between those who rely on spoken exchanges), sign language interpreters (interpreters and transliterators), or certified deaf interpreters (those whose expertise can be invaluable when faced with clients who rely on home signs, gestures, and mime for the majority of their expression). Certified by the Registry of Interpreters for the Deaf, these professionals are skilled in a minimum of two languages (English and ASL). They can assess the client's communication needs, adjust their communication to adhere to the preferences of the consumer, and provide translations between the therapist and the client (Leigh et al., 1996).

When employing interpreters in the counseling setting it is critical that the practitioner remain sensitive to the dynamics involved. This is particularly true when employing an interpreter for oral clients, who generally take great pride in their communication skills. Hence a therapist's recommendation that an oral interpreter be added to the counseling team may be met with mixed emotions. On the one hand clients may be cognizant that they are struggling with understanding, yet by accepting the services of an oral interpreter they may feel they are admitting that their skills are inadequate. This in turn can affect their self-esteem, thus impacting the overall outcome of the counseling session. Therefore, broaching the subject of interpreters should be done tactfully and with the understanding that the client will have the ultimate say as to whether these services are desired.

Once cultural and communication factors have been addressed, specific techniques and strategies can be implemented to foster behavior change. These techniques can involve role-playing, storytelling, and the incorporation of Deaf role models, or they can implement strategies that utilize visual aids and videotape replay. Furthermore, interventions can be integrated that stem from the visual/spatial linguistic features of ASL.

Techniques and Strategies

Role-Playing.   Role-play can be used with children as well as adults, in both individual and group sessions. It provides clients with an avenue of expression when they are lacking the language skills necessary for appropriate social interaction and/or the expression of emotions. By providing clients with structured situations whereby they can simulate various roles, they are afforded the opportunity to increase their social skills while heightening their awareness of how to express emotions appropriately (Swink, 1985).

When inappropriate behaviors are exhibited during role-play situations, the "mirror" technique (Moreno, 1959) can be introduced. In these instances the counselor asks the client to step out of the scene. Then the counselor will play the part, or substitute another person to play the part. This person duplicates the inappropriate behavior. When the client develops a sense of why it is wrong a new behavior is substituted and then reinforced by "social feedback or other more tangible reinforcers" (Swink, 1985).

Role-play can be used to help clients gain insights, learn appropriate behaviors, and grasp abstract concepts. Stein (1976) has used the word "pride" to illustrate how abstract conceptualization can be fostered using pictures, signs, and words:

> A boy is instructed to play baseball and to be the batter. Another person pitches an imaginary ball, which the batter hits over the fence. A person taking the role of the father comes up and, with a big smile and nodding head, hugs the batter (son) while signing the word *proud*. Other similar situations are shown until the client is able to create one of his or her own, showing an understanding of the concept (Stein, 1976, as cited in Swink, 1985, p. 276).

Storytelling.   Storytelling can be used as a therapeutic tool in a variety of ways. Through this narrative process clients reveal how they make sense of their lives by "storying" their experiences. Problem areas are divulged and the consumer's solution and/or reactions to the scenario are disclosed. This provides the therapist with insights into the client's perception of the problem. It also sets the stage for the clinician to describe alternative stories, thus furnishing the consumer with other ways to view his or her problem.

Storytelling can also be incorporated as a powerful tool to highlight creative solutions to difficult problems. Because Deaf "success stories" play an integral role in the Deaf community (Padden, 1989) these examples can be utilized to illustrate various problem-solving behaviors that can be adopted by the client. In these instances the Deaf role models that are depicted in the narratives serve a very important function. Because they have encountered difficulties and overcome them, they may alleviate some of the anxieties the client is experiencing to realize that deafness need not be equated with worthlessness. On the other hand, when deaf individuals discover that other deaf people face the same types of problems, such as language deficiencies and experiential encounters, they realize that they are not hopelessly ignorant. They become aware that when others have been faced with similar dilemmas, they have confronted and successfully solved them.

Videotape Replay.   Videotaping can be integrated in counseling sessions in a variety of ways. It can be used to capture role-plays, and to illustrate incongruities between what is said and what is communicated nonverbally. Furthermore, taping individual counseling sessions and replaying them provides the client with the opportunity to reflect upon what transpired during the interaction. Clients are often busy "watching" the content of what the counselor is saying and do not have the opportunity to think about its real meaning. By using videptaping, after the exchange clients can view the conversation, stop the tape, and relate to it. This is also an excellent way to give the opportunity to observe their own behavior.

Visual Aids. Additional strategies that can be beneficial when used within the counseling setting include drawing, writing, and incorporating pictures, graphs, and diagrams to illustrate emotions. Often, providing a sign for a concept and utilizing the written word simultaneously offers clients the needed vocabulary to express their feelings more adequately. Sequencing pictures that depict cause-and-effect relationships are also highly beneficial. Effective use of this technique draws attention to events that have causal relationships; this in turn can be useful when highlighting problems that arise in interpersonal relationships. Pictures illustrating various human emotions are also valuable and can be used with deaf individuals who may not have the wide range of vocabulary needed for self-expression. When deaf clients are permitted to point to pictures that project various emotions, they are able to express their feelings more accurately.

Techniques Involving the Visual/Spatial Linguistic Features of ASL

ASL is a rich and powerful language comprised of spatial features that provide a mechanism for clients to externalize, examine, and resolve problems. Through externalization, clients can learn that problems they previously considered inherent and unchangeable are actually due to an outside influence that can be confronted.

The therapeutic process of externalizing problems can be traced to the pioneering work of two family therapists, Michael White and David Epston (1990). This process encourages clients to view problems as outside influences that can impact negatively on individuals or relationships. Thus, the problem rather than the individual becomes an object that can be dealt with. According to White and Epston, the client should be encouraged to engage in relative influence questioning, which allows the client to map out the influence of the problem and of the person or persons in the "life of the problem," and therefore distance himself or herself from the problem.

By externalizing emotions such as anger, loneliness, or embarrassment, clinicians can direct clients to examine how these feelings have impacted them and their relationships with others, thus mapping the influence of the problem. This is followed by a series of reflexive questions designed to determine when the individual took control of a problem, thus allowing them to generate new strategies for resolving old issues.

This technique lends itself nicely to ASL. By using sign space, problems can be identified, objectified, and manipulated to represent whether the problem was overcome, whether the person was overcome by the problem, or if it is still in the process of being resolved (Freedman, 1994). As clinicians observe sign placement, they can question their clients to determine if they have been able to keep the specific problem at a distance and if so, what strategies they have used to take control of the problem.

Current Psychotherapies and Their Use
with Deaf Individuals

All psychotherapies are methods in learning intended to change people. Their aim is
to enable individuals to think differently (cognition), to make them feel differently
(affection), and to make them act better (behavior) (Corsini, 1984). Although there has
been a wealth of information published within the field of psychotherapy, there has
been very limited research in the area of counseling theories that can be utilized with
deaf clients. However, the conclusions drawn from the research state that approaches
employing a high degree of abstract thinking and extensive verbal interaction are the
least effective.

The present state of knowledge concerning the applicability of various
approaches in counseling with deaf clients does not permit us to draw meaningful
conclusions other than that the approaches requiring intricate mental manipulation
and prolonged verbal exchanges between the counselor and the client will, in most
cases, be of limited applicability. However, this fact may not be as limited as it may at
first appear, since evidence from counseling hearing persons suggests strongly that the
relationship between the counselor and the client is the agent of personality change,
rather than the method or techniques used by the counselor (Sussman & Stewart,
1971).

If a quality counseling relationship exists and if there is a viable means of
communication, several of the techniques may be employed. The pages that follow
present a brief overview of several of the theories. All of these can be implemented
and utilized when counseling Deaf, deaf, and hard-of-hearing individuals.

Reality Therapy.   William Glasser developed reality therapy during the 1950s and
1960s. According to Glasser, this type of therapy is applicable to individuals exhibiting a variety of psychological problems, ranging from mild emotional upset to
complete psychotic withdrawal (Glasser, 1984). In essence, this type of therapy focuses on the present and upon making people cognizant of the fact that they make
choices involving actions in an attempt to fulfill basic needs.

Based on the concept that our brain works as a control system and that all of
our behavior is to fulfill needs built into the genetic structure of that system, this theory purports that all of our behaviors are internally motivated. According to Glasser,
this means that individuals spend their lives attempting to act upon or, more accurately, to control the world around them. By doing this they are more effectively able
to satisfy their basic needs (Glasser, 1984).

According to Glasser, all therapy is teaching, and to the extent that this teaching leads to fulfillment, it is therapeutic. Therapists engaging in reality therapy focus
on the present and strive to assist their clients in examining their behaviors as they
relate to their own value systems. Individuals are asked to determine if the behaviors
they exhibit are instrumental in assisting them in achieving their desired goals.
Throughout the therapeutic process, reality therapists carefully instruct their clients,

providing them with better ways or better behaviors to deal with their world. The intention of the therapist is to help the consumer control the world more effectively. For this control to be more effective individuals must examine their choices, evaluate the choices they make, and eventually choose a better behavior. When this occurs, clients take more effective control of their lives, allowing them to gain better control of the world around them. In this eight-step process, the therapist always focuses on the part of the world that is directly related to the individual's own life. The eight steps can be summarized as follows:

I. The therapist establishes rapport with the individual and determines what the client wants to control.
2. Existing behaviors and actions are identified.
3. Clients are asked to evaluate their current choices to determine if they are generating sought after results.
4. If it is determined that the present course of action is not adequate, a plan is designed to achieve the desired outcome.
5. The client is asked to commit to follow the plan established in step 4.
6. Emphasis is placed on when the behavior/action can be implemented and how it is working.
7. No punishment is given for failed attempts.
8. The client is instructed never to give up (Glasser, 1984, pp. 333–337).

Using Reality Therapy with Deaf Individuals. In reality therapy counselors teach clients better ways to fulfill their needs within the confines of reality. This can be a useful tool in helping deaf clients deal with their deafness. Oftentimes deaf individuals have experienced years of rejection and isolation. Because of this they may have a tendency to blame their problems on other individuals. Reality therapy forces them to take the responsibility for their feelings and actions and deal with them constructively. This theory places an emphasis on learning to maintain a satisfactory standard of behavior and can be viewed as an asset when working with deaf individuals who are experiencing behavioral problems. In these instances, learning what is deemed appropriate behavior and becoming acquainted with ways to maintain it can be very useful skills for the deaf client to develop. The major drawback to this theory lies in the element of involvement. In schools for the deaf where the caseload may be small, the time factor may not be crucial and adequate time may be available to become involved with the clients; however, in most rehabilitation agencies the caseloads are so large that this element may be missing, and therefore the theory remains minimally effective.

To date, only a few articles in the literature pertain to the use of reality therapy with deaf clients. Although articles by McCrone (1983), "Reality Therapy with Deaf Rehabilitation Clients," and Norton (1978), "Reality Therapy: A Practical Approach to Troubled Youth" exist, the evidence of the effectiveness of this theory with deaf clients is purely anecdotal at this time (McCrone, 1983).

Cognitive-Behavioral Psychotherapy.   Cognitive-behavioral psychotherapy has increased in popularity throughout the past decade. Designed to provide a systematic model of intervention, it is deemed useful when assisting clients in establishing a more "active, responsible, and competent role in problem-solving, personal management, and goal attainment" (Loera, 1994, p. 159). Attributed to the work of Meichenbaum (1977), this technique has been found to be effective with diverse populations.

The major goal of cognitive-behavioral psychotherapy is to equip clients with skills that can be applied to both current and future problems. Strategies are provided that enable the client to develop new skills, monitor existing behaviors, modify those thought processes that may be distorted, and reduce the amount of stress they experience when encountering new or difficult situations.

Throughout the therapy process clients engage in a three-phase process of change. In phase I the problem is conceptualized, information is gathered, and the therapist and client work in tandem to gain a mutual perspective of the existing problem. During this phase it is critical that both the client and the therapist have a clear understanding of the problem. Clients are frequently given homework assignments that help them focus on their thoughts and feelings that lead to problematic behavior.

Phase II focuses on the reconceptualization process. During this phase the emphasis is placed on recognizing that the individual's problems can be solved. Therapy sessions may incorporate role-plays, problem-solving therapy, and/or imagery rehearsal to assist clients in developing problem solving strategies. Additional homework assignments are made whereby clients indicate which assignments they are willing to complete and the frequency with which they will complete the tasks. Clients are directed to attend to self-statements and document the difficulties and positive experiences that they encounter. The goal throughout this stage is to reduce resistance and noncompliant behaviors, thus enabling supportive and collaborative relationships to be formed between the therapist and his or her clients.

During Phase III clients are provided with in-depth problem-solving and goal-oriented strategies (Loera, 1994). Emphasis is placed on acquiring new behavior patterns that can be applied to existing and future problems. Furthermore, internal dialogues are examined and individuals are encouraged to replace maladaptive behaviors with alternative coping responses. The overall goal of this phase is to assist clients in determining if their coping behaviors will produce positive outcomes, and if not, to monitor their behaviors to insure that a successful outcome can be achieved.

Cognitive-behavioral psychotherapy can be used in individual and group counseling settings. Although the therapist provides the primary source of support and information in individual sessions, group members serve as role models and are instrumental in providing feedback in group sessions. Both settings afford individuals the opportunity to experience personal growth and development.

Using Cognitive-Behavioral Psychotherapy with Deaf Individuals.   Deaf clients frequently enter mental health settings ill prepared to participate in the counseling process. They may be experiencing difficulties in solving problems and struggle with effective problem-solving solutions. Furthermore, they may respond impulsively when problems arise, rather than thinking through possible solutions. In these instances they fail to recognize the consequences of their behavior.

Although the literature does not reflect extensive research in the effectiveness of applying this form of psychotherapy with deaf individuals, those researchers (see Greenberg, 1985, Greenberg, Kusche, Gustafson, & Calderone, 1984, Harris, 1978, O'Brien, 1987) who have implemented these strategies have found them to be beneficial. By providing deaf individuals with the opportunity to focus on their thought processes when problems arise, they are afforded an avenue to explore the how and why of their behavior. As they gain insights into their behaviors they can establish an internal locus of control and develop proactive life problem solving skills.

Family Therapy.   Today, family therapy may be broadly defined as an attempt to modify relationships in a family in order to achieve harmony. The focus is placed on the family as a whole rather than on a specific individual, and within this type of therapy the task of the family therapist is to change the relationship between members of the troubled family so that symptomatic behavior disappears. Tenets basic to family therapy include placing emphasis on the family constellation, stressing the here and now, putting responsibility for behavior on the person or family unit, and viewing the family's problem as a response to a system (Foley, 1984). A family is seen as an open system created by interlocking triangles, maintained or changed by means of feedback. Therefore, in family therapy there reside three basic concepts: the system, or the family itself; interlocking triangles, the basic building blocks of the family relationship system; and feedback, the process whereby the system adjusts itself (Foley, 1984).

When family therapists work with the family unit they not only examine each member of the unit, but how each interacts with the other. Emphasis is placed on what is happening within the family, rather than why it is happening. The therapist believes that if they can observe what is going on, they can ameliorate the problem. Therefore, emphasis is placed on interactions between family members rather than on internal thought processes. Throughout the course of family therapy, the therapist strives to engage the family in identifying or relabeling their problems and discovering alternative solutions to ameliorating them. The initial interview sets the tone for the therapy, which progresses according to the following phases:

1. *Warm up:* The family has the opportunity to see the therapist's personality.
2. *Relabeling:* Family members are asked to identify the problem.
3. *Spreading the problem:* The therapist points out alternative ways to define the problem.
4. *Need for change:* The therapist asks the family what solutions have been tried. The issue is getting the family to focus on change, which is directed to occur among all the family members.
5. *Changing pathways:* The therapist intervenes into the family by making suggestions (Foley, 1984, pp. 465–467).

Using Family Therapy with Deaf Individuals.   The problems that revolve around the nucleus of the family can create the foundation for many of the problems that will be exhibited by deaf individuals throughout their lifetimes. From the time a child's deafness is diagnosed the counseling process should begin.

> Attitudes of family members toward deafness may represent a very real situational barrier for the deaf person . . . When a family first discovers it has a deaf child the reaction is generally traumatic. Grief, guilt, and overwhelming helplessness are normal responses . . . Effective counseling at this critical time would enable parents to work through their feelings and direct their efforts and anxieties toward constructive endeavors for the deaf child. It is the lack of appropriate parent counseling at this crucial time, when deafness in the child is first discovered, that lays the groundwork for much of the later family pathology and related difficulties faced by parents and their deaf child (Sussman & Stewart, 1971, p. 30).

By engaging the parents and siblings in early counseling sessions many of the misunderstandings may be corrected and attitudes toward the deaf child altered. The counselor must have a thorough understanding of both the social and psychological ramifications entailed in a hearing loss, and be able to provide the parents with realistic expectations. If the parents and other family members are made aware of the problems and needs of deaf or hard-of-hearing individuals, the disability can be dealt with in a constructive rather than in a handicapping manner. The importance of family therapy cannot be overemphasized, since if the family feels it has a reliable source to turn to for information when problems arise, many of the problem areas will be alleviated.

Articles cited in family therapy literature that focus on serving deaf individuals and their families include Harvey (1982), "The Influence and Utilization of an Interpreter for Deaf Persons in Family Therapy"; Robinson and Weathers (1974), "Family Therapy of Deaf Parents and Hearing Children: A New Dimension in Psychotherapeutic intervention"; and Shapiro and Harris (1976), "Family Therapy and Treatment of Deaf: A Case Report" (Scott & Dooley, 1985).

Person-Centered Therapy.   Person-centered therapy, previously known as client-centered therapy, was originally developed in the 1940s by Carl Rogers. In 1974 Rogers and his colleagues changed the name of this approach because they felt "person-centered" more accurately reflected the tenets of this theory when working with the individual (Meador & Rogers, 1984). It was initially developed as an approach to counseling troubled individuals, which today remains the most widespread application of the theory. It can be applied to any relationship in which people want to understand each other and to be understood.

The central hypothesis of this theory is that the growthful potential of any individual will tend to be released when a relationship exists in which a helping person experiences and communicates "realness, caring, and a deeply sensitive, nonjudgmental understanding" (Meador & Rogers, 1982, p. 142). The role of the therapist in therapeutic situations is to provide an "if-then" hypothesis. In this way, the person designated as therapist provides congruence, positive regard, and empathetic understanding, thus enabling the client to experience "growthful change."

The underlying hypothesis of this theory is that humans have a tendency toward self-actualization. Individuals are viewed as having an inherent tendency to develop all their capabilities to the fullest, thus enhancing the organism. When people "bump into" significant others and those significant others relate to them that they are loveable and acceptable, feelings of self-worth develop. According to Rogers, this is one of the primary tenets in the self-actualization process. When this occurs, people have the potential to become self-actualized and can overcome the restrictions they have placed on themselves in relation to their feelings of self-worth.

When establishing a therapeutic relationship, it is critical that three conditions be present: a sense of genuineness and congruence, accurate empathetic understanding, and unconditional positive regard. Although these conditions can be defined individually, they are interdependent and logically related. It is essential that the therapist accept the other person; furthermore, these helping professionals must be in touch with their own inner feelings so they can understand and relate them to the problems being experienced by the client. When this transpires, feelings of genuineness and congruence are conveyed and the client perceives a caring therapist. Clients must sense that their therapist believes they have the ability to become self-actualized. Rogers purports that when clients perceive the attitude of a caring therapist, their personalities will begin to change. They will become more aware of their inner experiences and will move away from their state of "rigid, static repetitive behavior to behavior that is characterized by the change and flow of (their) inner experiences" (Meador & Rogers, 1984, p. 144).

Person-centered therapy has been referred to as nondirective therapy. Rather than examine past experiences, this technique focuses on the moment-to-moment interaction of the therapeutic relationship. The therapist is not put in the role of the expert. Instead, the focus is placed on enabling clients to become aware of, and trust in, their own actualizing process. Thus, the inner experiences of the client dictate the pace and direction of the therapeutic relationship.

Using Person-Centered Therapy with Deaf Individuals.   When deaf individuals are highly verbal, the therapist may find that this approach can be very beneficial. However, if the client possesses less than a fourth-grade language level, it will be nonproductive. The goal of this therapy is to promote "growth, change, and flexibility in the person, rather than focusing on the fixed, limited, and rigid experiences of the neurotic" (Harmatz, 1978). Although the aim of this therapy is to assist clients in establishing a sense of worth and a positive self-regard for themselves, it can also be employed to combat the inherent negativism that is instilled in the self-concept of so many deaf clients. The largest drawback to this technique lies in the fact that the therapist functions primarily as an agent who rephrases and reflects upon the client's statements. If the client does not possess the verbal skills required to express his or her emotions adequately, the reflective process merely becomes confusing to the client.

The other drawback in attempting to incorporate this therapeutic technique lies in the fact that the client is responsible for the direction the counseling process takes. Hearing-impaired individuals who have been raised in a directive environment where they were continuously told what to do may find the responsibility of expressing themselves overwhelming. However, for those who are capable of expressing their feelings adequately, this can be a very advantageous type of therapy.

Gestalt Therapy.   Founded by Frederick (Fritz) S. Perls and Laura P. Perls in the 1940s, Gestalt therapy has subsequently been developed by several others (Simkin & Yontef, 1984). Gestalt therapy is a form of phenomenological-existential therapy. Phenomenology here refers to a systematic exploration of the perceiver's sense of knowledge. Genuine knowledge is defined as that immediate body of information that comprises a person's experiential basis. Thus, in Gestalt therapy one trusts immediate awareness. The objective is to examine significant realities that are apparent and determine how they fall into place with respect to the whole. In existentialism, emphasis is directed to the act or the perceiving person. The primary focus is placed on the individual as he or she experiences joy, suffering, anger, or other feelings. However, the key phrase is "as he or she experiences it."

Gestalt therapy directs its attention to helping the individual resolve internal conflicts. Emphasis is placed on becoming aware of one's behavior. The goal for clients is to become aware of what they are doing, and how they are doing it, while at the same time developing feelings of esteem in themselves (Simkin & Yontef, 1984).

During the therapy hour the clinician observes the development of behavior that occurs. Emphasis is placed on what is rather than on what was or what could, might, or should be. Attention is further given to the process: the patient, the therapist, and the interaction between them. Based on the premise that people exist in relation to their environment, which is comprised of other individuals, the Gestalt therapist emphasizes relationships in its personality theory and in its therapeutic methodology.

The primary tools employed in Gestalt therapy consist of awareness and dialogue. Emphasis is placed on what the individual is experiencing at that point in time. The person is taught the difference between talking about what happened previously and experiencing what is happening now. Throughout the counseling session the therapist conveys a warm, caring relationship through an "I-thou" dialogue. In essence the client and the therapist speak the same language with the dialogue focusing on the direct experience of both participants.

According to Gestalt therapy, people are the primary agents in determining their own behaviors. In addition, they are responsible for making their own moral choices. Those who blame outside forces (genetics, parents, or environment) for what they choose engage in self-deception. Therefore, Gestalt therapists attempt to get their clients to learn to be aware of and responsible for their choices, thus gaining the tools to explore their beliefs and behaviors more fully. Through this multidimensional form of therapy, the emphasis is placed on holism. Because people manifest their distress in their behaviors, thought processes, and feelings, Gestalt therapy views the entire environment as important.

Using Gestalt Therapy with Deaf Individuals.   When this approach is used, the clinician concentrates on instilling a "sense of responsibility" in clients for their behavior. One of the tenets of Gestalt therapy is that if individuals become aware of what they are doing, they will have the option to continue that activity or to change it. Through this awareness people begin to own their actions and take responsibility for what they choose, or do not choose, to do. Emphasis is placed on "how" individuals are acting and what they choose to do about it. Deaf individuals frequently experience problems involving interpersonal relationships. When these types of problems arise, strategies incorporated in this therapy can provide an effective method for discussing the problem areas. Coupled with role-playing, these strategies serve as useful techniques, thus opening a valuable avenue for comprehending one's actions and feelings. By getting in touch with the various components in one's personality, deaf individuals are able to deal with their behavior more effectively.

Transactional Analysis.   Eric Berne originated transactional analysis (TA) in the 1950s. It is viewed as a complete theory of personality and also incorporates a diverse range of treatment techniques specifically designed to meet the needs and goals of clients. The premise for TA is based on the presence of three active, dynamic, and observable ego states referred to as the parent, the adult, and the child. Each is thought to exist and operate in each individual. In addition, each person has a basic, innate need for recognition, or "strokes." In order to receive these strokes, individuals design a plan or a life script, formed during childhood and rooted in one's early beliefs about oneself and others. These beliefs are then reinforced as the person engages in social interactions or repetitive, stereotyped games with others (Dusay & Dusay, 1984). Through a lifetime of these interactions, personality is formed and remains fixed unless one actively decides to change one's behavior. TA perceives the role of the therapist as a potent catalyst, capable of facilitating change and promoting growth in clients.

Basic terms associated with transactional analysis include parent, adult, and child; ego states; transactions; games; strokes; scripts; and egograms. The Child ego state, also known as the archaeopsyche, represents the regressive ego state of the individual. At times it manifests itself in our creative and emotional attributes; at other times it is responsible for our rebellious or conforming attitudes.

The adult ego state or neopsyche represents the realistic or logical part of us and is referred to as the computing and data processing part of our being. The third state, the parent or exteropsyche, is thought to be an introjection from and identification with one's biological parents (Dusay & Dusay, 1984).

These three ego states are dynamic and are symbolized by three connected, distinct circles to represent unique, separate, and independent entities. As individuals interact and communicate with one another, these ego states manifest themselves on the social level while influencing the individual on a covert or psychological level. When one individual (stimulus) triggers a related response in another, a transaction is said to occur. In addition, when a series of transactions occur simultaneously on both the social and the psychological level, a game is usually underway.

The goal of transactional analysis is to manifest changes in the client's behavior. Although the therapist provides the specific tools for growth, the client is ultimately encouraged to make his or her own explanations and interpretations. The client is directed toward replaying early emotions and feelings about a problem rather than talking about said emotions. Clients also are encouraged to engage in a redecision process whereby they trace their early experiences and determine the reactions they experienced in early childhood that made them feel like a "not OK" person. Then they are asked to restructure their behavior by making new decisions about self and life (Dusay & Dusay, 1984, p. 400).

By directing clients to examine their previous experiences and the behaviors they have elicited, the therapist gains insights into the present behavior patterns that have been established. By focusing on these "rackets"—repetitive behavior with corresponding emotions that originated in early script messages—the therapist can help clients to redirect their reactions and behaviors.

Using Transactional Analysis with Deaf Individuals.   Transactional analysis can be used with deaf individuals who have a good command of the English language, or with a therapist who is a skilled signer, working within a group of clients who are all fluent users of ASL. Furthermore, it is essential that both communication groups can be engaged in the art of role-playing. Because transactional analysis is frequently used in group situations and the focus is on transactions between the individuals in the group, the participants must be able to interact freely with the other members of the group. In working with deaf clients, the strength of this theory lies in clients being taught "to distinguish their ego states, to consistently identify the source of distorted ideas, and to change to the state that is appropriate for the present purpose" (Harmatz, 1978, p. 503). Transactional analysis supports the premise that the way children perceive themselves is determined between the ages of 3 and 7. When individuals examine the perceptions they have of themselves, they can deal more effectively with their behavior. In order for counselors to engage in this type of therapy with deaf individuals, they should have not only a thorough understanding of transactional analysis, but a grasp of the impacting factors on deafness as well.

Rational Emotive Therapy.   Albert Ellis developed rational emotive therapy (RET) in the 1950s, based on the premise that when a highly charged emotional consequence (C) follows a significant activating event (A), that event may seem to have caused the consequences but actually does not cause (A). Instead, emotional consequences are largely created by (B), the individual's belief system. In essence, when an undesirable consequence occurs, such as severe anxiety, this can usually be traced to the person's irrational beliefs. Therefore, when these beliefs are effectively disputed (at point D) by challenging them rationally, the disturbed consequences disappear and eventually cease to recur (Ellis, 1984).

Concepts basic to rational emotive therapy include the following:

- People are born with a potential to be rational as well as irrational. They have the capacity to be creative and to be interested in others, and the capability to learn from their mistakes. In addition (within their realm), they have the propensity toward self-destruction, procrastination, and the ability to engage repeatedly in making the same mistakes.
- Their family and the culture in which they reside frequently exacerbate people's tendency toward irrational thinking. These sources provide their greatest influence during the early years of development.
- Individuals tend to perceive, think, emote, and behave simultaneously. When people respond to any situation or stimuli, they rarely act without engaging in these behaviors. Therefore, when problems arise, it is generally beneficial to employ a variety of perceptual-cognitive, emotive-evocative, and behavioristic-reeducative methods.
- RET incorporates highly cognitive, active-directive techniques that tend to yield effective therapeutic results within short periods of time.
- RET therapists do not believe a warm relationship between the counselor and the counselee is necessary in order for an effective change in the counselee's personality to occur.

Using Rational Emotive Therapy with Deaf Individuals. RET is based on the assumption that what individuals say to themselves determines the way they feel and act. The thrust of the therapy is to identify why clients have negative feelings about themselves and to help each of them establish a better self-concept. This can be particularly valuable in working with deaf clients. It is especially beneficial for use with those who assume that when they exhibit obnoxious behavior, others responding to them are not projecting feelings of dislike because of their deafness, but rather because of the behavior they have exhibited. Because of the communication difficulties, deaf individuals often misinterpret what others say about them; thus misconceptions occur and a negative self-concept may develop. It is important that the counselor be able to perceive the difference between the client who has misunderstood the context of the conversation and the one who is being attacked for his or her behavior. This type of therapy can aid the counselor in getting to the crux of many of the problems that are frequently expressed by members of the deaf population.

Summary

Deaf individuals seeking counseling services frequently find themselves in the presence of mental health professionals who can hear. Although some of them possess sign skills, others rely on the services of an interpreter to facilitate communication. Whether clinicians sign for themselves or employ interpreters, it is imperative that they comprehend the subtleties of style and the affective state communicated in the articulations of the signs themselves.

10

Mental Illness and Deafness

There are an infinite number of illnesses prevalent in the world today. Of all of them, perhaps one of the most feared is the diagnosis of mental illness. Misunderstood by many and hidden by others, it remains a topic shrouded in a cloak of mystique and discussed in hushed tones of foreboding. Mental disorders know no social, ethnic, or socioeconomic boundaries. They indiscriminately permeate the lives of individuals, rendering them in need of psychological or psychiatric services. What constitutes mental illness? What factors contribute to abnormal behavior? What are some of the prominent categories of mental disorders? How prevalent is mental illness within the deaf and hard-of-hearing population? Do deaf individuals experience mental illness differently?

Defining Abnormal Behavior

Mental illness manifests itself through some form of abnormal behavior. Although the term "abnormal behavior" is difficult to define and the distinction between what is normal and what is abnormal is not always clear cut, certain criteria can be considered when forming a definition. According to Santrock (2000), abnormal behavior is "behavior that is deviant, maladaptive, or personally distressful" (p. 448). Although he makes the distinction that only one of the criteria needs to be met for the classification of abnormal behavior, he further indicates that two or three may be present.

Deviance refers to atypical behavior that deviates from what is acceptable from a cultural perspective. While maladaptive behaviors are distinguished as those behaviors that interfere with the person's ability to function effectively in the world, personal distress can be equated with the individual's bleak outlook on life. Any one of these characteristics can be viewed as hindering the functioning ability of the individual, thus leaving the person incapable of coping with life's daily routines and expectations. This definition provides a global understanding of what is entailed in abnormal behavior. By using it as a springboard, one can gain further insights into the realm of mental illness by exploring contributing factors and the specific classifications of some of the more predominant disorders.

Factors That Contribute to Abnormal Behavior

Abnormal behavior has been examined in light of biological, psychological, and sociocultural factors, as well as a combination of these three components. Those adhering to a biological approach embrace the medical model, wherein mental disorders are viewed as medical diseases with a biological origin. Genetics as well as brain processes are considered, and those afflicted are most frequently treated in mental hospitals by doctors.

Abnormal behavior has also been attributed to psychological factors, including distorted thoughts, emotional turmoil, inappropriate learning, and troubled relationships. When examining abnormal behavior from this perspective, attention is focused on the psychological problems that may have occurred in association with social learning and early childhood experiences. In particular, those events and occurrences that may have been stressful are examined as contributing to the present state of the individual.

Although the majority of mental health professionals concur that many psychological disorders are universal, the frequency and intensity of abnormal behavior varies across cultures. According to Draguns (1990), these variations are related to social, economic, technological, and religious aspects of cultures. Those socioeconomic factors that can influence mental disorders include socioeconomic status and neighborhood quality (Brown & Adler, 1998). Research conducted by Grizenko (1998) indicates that people from low-income minority neighborhoods have the highest rates of mental disorders, with socioeconomic status having the strongest influence.

While some mental disorders can be primarily attributed to heredity or poverty, others are influenced by a combination of biological, psychological, and sociocultural factors. When viewed through this perspective, it is believed that the interaction between these three factors contributes to the manifestation of abnormal behavior. The term "interactionist" or "biopsychosocial" approach is frequently applied when these three factors are considered in tandem (Evans, 1998).

Classifying Abnormal Behavior

The scientific study of abnormal behavior in the United States can be traced to the 1840s, when one category was established to identify all types of mental disorders. This category included both the mentally retarded and the insane. From this rudimentary beginning the American Psychiatric Association (APA) developed the first major classification system of mental disorders in this country. Referred to as the Diagnostic and Statistical Manual of Mental Disorders (DSM), this volume provided a much better classification of mental disorders. First published in 1952, it was later revised in

1968 as the DSM-II. This edition received more systematic assistance from expert diagnosticians. Since that time it has undergone three additional revisions. The current edition, the DSM-IV, was published in 1994 and emphasizes refined empirical support for the diagnostic categories (Santrock, 2000, p. 452).

The DSM-IV contains 18 major classifications and describes more than 200 specific disorders. Based on a multiaxial system, it classifies individuals on the basis of five dimensions, or "axes," that reflect the individual's history and highest level of functioning in the last year. Furthermore, it ensures that the individual will be characterized in terms of a number of clinical factors described in the various axes. Table 10.1 provides a brief description of each of the five axes. Through this comprehensive classification system the various clinical and personality disorders can be examined and discussed.

According to the American Psychiatric Association (APA), the DSM-IV is designed to provide diagnostic criteria for mental disorders that can be useful as guidelines when making diagnoses. However, in order for these criteria to be used properly, they must be employed by clinicians that have undergone specialized training. Furthermore, although the DSM-IV is designed to provide information on the various mental disorders, it is by no means comprehensive and should not be viewed as such.

TABLE 10.1   *The DSM-IV Multiaxial System*

Axis	Description
I	Clinical disorders first diagnosed in infancy or adolescence, excluding mental retardation or personality disorders (examples: anxiety disorders, schizophrenia, mood disorders, eating disorders, sleep disorders)
II	Personality disorders: mental retardation; may also be used for noting prominent maladaptive personality features and defense mechanisms (examples: borderline personality disorders, mental retardation, obsessive-compulsive personality disorder)
III	General medical conditions that are particularly relevant to understanding and managing the individual's mental disorder (examples: diseases of the circulatory system, skin, and subcutaneous tissue; congenital anomalies)
IV	Psychosocial and environmental problems: life events that may have a negative effect on the individual (examples: educational problems, housing problems, problems related to the social environment)
V	Global assessment of functioning, for the clinician to report his or her judgment of the individual's overall level of functioning

These brief descriptions of the five axes are taken from the classifications found in the fourth edition of the Diagnostic and Statistical Manual of Mental Disorders.

The following sections outline some of the major areas of mental illness that are discussed in the DSM-IV and explain the distinguishing characteristics of these mental disorders.

Anxiety Disorders

In the face of threatening or stressful situations almost all individuals feel anxious and tense, and these feelings are thought to be normal reactions. However, these same feelings can be considered abnormal when they occur in response to everyday situations that most people can handle with little difficulty. Anxiety disorders tend to run in families. According to Carey and Gottesman (1981), approximately 15 percent of parents and siblings of people who have anxiety disorders are similarly affected.

Anxiety disorders include a group of disorders in which anxiety is either the main symptom (generalized anxiety and panic disorders) or is experienced when the individual attempts to control certain maladaptive behaviors (phobic and obsessive-compulsive disorders) (Atkinson, Atkinson, Smith, & Bem, 1990). Generalized anxiety and panic disorders, phobias, and obsessive-compulsive disorders are all included in this category.

Generalized Anxiety and Panic Disorders.   Generalized anxiety disorders are characterized as persistent, pervasive anxiety that is ongoing for at least a month. Throughout this time the individual is unable to specify the reasons for the anxiety. People who experience this disorder feel nervous the majority of the time; they may tend to overreact to mild stresses and complain of disturbed sleep, fatigue, headaches, dizziness, and rapid heart rate.

In addition, they may experience panic attacks, episodes of acute and overwhelming apprehension or terror. These attacks can occur suddenly and without warning. During a panic attack the individual may have a sense of impending doom, accompanied by shortness of breath, heart palpitations, chest pains, trembling, and dizziness. Those affected by panic disorders frequently feel that something will happen to them that is out of their control (Asnis & Van Praag, 1995).

Phobias.   Those experiencing phobic disorders differ from individuals identified as having a generalized anxiety disorder. In contrast to the vague apprehension characteristic of generalized anxiety disorders, where the individual cannot pinpoint the cause of his or her anxiety, those experiencing phobic disorders are acutely aware of what is responsible for generating the specific feeling of fear. In these instances, the individual has an irrational, overwhelming, persistent fear of a particular object or situation. Although the person generally recognizes that his or her fear is irrational, the fear is still real, and the only way it can be alleviated is by avoiding the feared object or situation. The DSM-IV groups phobias into three broad categories: agoraphobia, specific phobia (formerly simple phobia), and social phobia (social anxiety disorder).

Agoraphobia is the most common phobia among people seeking professional help; it is also the most disabling (Atkinson, Atkinson, Smith, & Bem, 1990). It appears in early adulthood, affecting approximately 2.5 percent of the American population. The majority of those who experience agoraphobia are females. It is defined as intense fear of entering crowded public places, of traveling away from home (especially by public transportation), of feeling confined or trapped, and of being separated from a person or place associated with safety. According to the DSM-IV, agoraphobia can occur with or without panic attacks (Thorpe, 1998).

Specific phobias involve the individual's irrational, overwhelming, persistent fear of a particular object or situation. Some of the more common ones include a fear of height (acrophobia), dogs (cynophobia), flying (aerophobia), and spiders (arachnophobia). In contrast, social phobias entail experiencing an intense fear of being humiliated or embarrassed in social situations. In its mildest form it may inhibit individuals from speaking up in conversations or giving speeches. However, when it becomes intense, it can severely restrict the individual's social life and contribute to feelings of loneliness (Schneider & et al., 1992).

Obsessive-Compulsive Disorder.   This disorder is characterized by anxiety-provoking thoughts that will not dissipate (obsession) and by urges to perform repetitive, ritualistic behaviors to produce some future situation (compulsion). Individuals with obsessive-compulsive disorders repeat and rehearse normal doubts and daily routines, sometimes hundreds of times a day (Frost & Steketee, 1998). According to the DSM-IV, in order for behaviors to be considered obsessive-compulsive, they must occur for more than one hour a day. Furthermore, they must cause marked distress and be excessive or unreasonable. The most common obsessions are repeated thoughts about contamination, and repeated doubts as questions continually recur regarding the completion of specific tasks, such as locking a door or turning off a stove.

Compulsive activities are engaged in for the sake of preventing anxiety or distress; their goal is not to produce pleasure or enjoyment. The most common compulsions involve "washing and cleaning, counting, checking, requesting or demanding assurances, repeating actions, and ordering" (p. 418). Although adults may realize that their behaviors are excessive or unreasonable, they are unable to control their actions when forced to confront their fears on a daily basis.

Mood Disorders

Mood disorders encompass wide emotional swings ranging from deep depression to extreme euphoria and agitation. Although depression can occur in isolation, it can also be coupled with mania, an overexcited, unrealistically optimistic state, as in bipolar disorders (Robins & Register, 1991). Mood disorders can be caused by biological as well as psychosocial factors and can be discussed in terms of major depressive, dysthymic, and bipolar disorders.

Major Depressive Disorders.   According to Munoz (1998), when individuals experience major depressive episodes they are depressed, lethargic, and possess a heightened sense of helplessness for a period of at least two weeks or longer. Furthermore, they must exhibit five of the nine symptoms that are characteristic of a major depressive disorder, which include a depressed mood for the majority of the day, reduced interest or enjoyment of most activities, and a significant weight loss or weight gain corresponding with fluctuations in appetite. In addition, they must experience difficulty sleeping or engage in excessive sleeping. Furthermore, there may be evidence of psychomotor agitation or retardation, fatigue or loss of energy, feelings of worthlessness or guilt in an excessive or inappropriate manner, problems involving concentrating or decision making, or recurrent thoughts of suicide and death.

Dysthymic Disorder.   Individuals diagnosed with dysthymic disorders exhibit fewer symptoms than those who experience major depressive disorders. These individuals reflect a depressed mood for most days for a minimum of two years as an adult, or at least one year as a child or adolescent. Furthermore, before a person is classified as dysthymic, he or she must experience depression throughout a two-year period that has not been broken by a normal mood that has lasted more than two months. In addition, the person must display evidence of four of the following six symptoms: poor appetite or overeating, sleep problems, low energy or fatigue, low self-esteem, poor concentration or difficulty making decisions, and feelings of hopelessness (Munoz, 1998).

Bipolar Disorder.   A bipolar disorder is a mood disorder characterized by extreme mood swings that include one or more episodes of mania (Coryell et al., 1999). These individuals may experience multiple cycles of depression interspersed with mania. During manic episodes people feel as if they are "on top of the world." Then as their manic episode unfolds they enter a state of panic and eventually depression. In essence a manic episode is the equivalent of the inverse of a depressive episode (DeBattista, Solvason, & Schatzberg, 1998). During these times individuals may act impulsively, they display tremendous energy, and rarely sleep. In some instances the person alternates between depressive episodes and manic episodes so swiftly that there is only a brief return to normality in between.

Bipolar disorders are relatively rare, affecting less than 1 percent of the adult population. In reported cases there appears to be an equal representation of both males and females. Those experiencing manic episodes project energetic and enthusiastic behaviors. However, unlike normal elation, manic behavior has a driven quality and is often expressed through hostility rather than elation (Atkinson, Atkinson, Smith, & Bem, 1990).

Schizophrenia

The term *schizophrenia* is derived from the Latin words *schizo*, meaning "split," and *phrenia,* meaning "mind." This severe and debilitating psychological disorder usually develops in late adolescence or early adulthood and requires psychiatric treatment. Current estimates reveal that approximately half of all patients in mental hospitals are classified with schizophrenia as their primary diagnosis.

Schizophrenia is characterized by distorted thoughts and perceptions, odd communication, inappropriate emotion, abnormal motor behavior, and social withdrawal. Differing from the exhibition of multiple or split personalities, schizophrenia involves a split of an individual's personality from reality. This disturbance lasts for a minimum of six months with at least one month of active phase symptoms that include delusions, hallucinations (often in the form of voices), disorganized speech, grossly disorganized or catatonic behavior, negative symptoms, and occasional bizarre motor behaviors.

The disorganized thought processes and irrelevant or idiosyncratic associations that are characteristic of schizophrenia make it difficult to understand what the individual is trying to say. This is evident in the person's use of *neologisms* (new words that have meaning only to the schizophrenic), *tangential thought* (one idea or phrase can spark an entirely different stream of conversation), and *loose associations* (thoughts are illogically connected). Furthermore, there may be evidence of *clang associations* (wrong word usage based on how the word sounds) and *word salad* (a jumble of unrelated words with no meaning).

Most schizophrenics show lack of insight, and when questioned as to why they are hospitalized seem to have no appreciation of their condition and virtually no realization that their behavior is unusual. Additionally, they usually fail to exhibit normal emotional responses and are frequently withdrawn and unresponsive in situations that should make them sad or happy.

Occasionally, the schizophrenic patient expresses emotions that are inappropriately linked to the situation or the thought being expressed. They struggle as they attempt to perform daily living routines, and when they experience schizophrenic episodes they tend to withdraw from others and become absorbed in their inner thoughts and fantasies (Atkinson, Atkinson, Smith, & Bem, 1990).

In acute cases of schizophrenia, withdrawal from reality is temporary. However, in chronic cases withdrawal may progress to the point where the individual is completely unresponsive to external events. During these schizophrenic episodes the person may remain silent and must be cared for like an infant. According to the DSM-IV (APA, 1994), there are five main subtypes of schizophrenia: disorganized, catatonic, paranoid, undifferentiated, and residual (p. 273).

Disorganized Type.   Individuals fitting this classification exhibit disorganized speech, disorganized behavior, and flat or inappropriate affect. The individual may withdraw from human contact and regress to a level of silliness indicative of childlike behavior. If delusions and hallucinations are present, they are fragmented and not organized into a coherent theme, thus they have little if any recognizable meaning.

Catatonic Type.   Marked psychomotor disturbances characterize the catatonic type of schizophrenia. In this type the individual may display motoric immobility, peculiarities of voluntary movement, or excessive motor activity. Additionally, one can observe bizarre rigid postures that are maintained against all attempts to move them. When individuals are in this state, they are conscious of what is happening around them.

Furthermore, while in a catatonic state, in the event someone moves the person's arm and it is allowed to fall, it will assume the new position. This phenomenon is described as displaying a waxy flexibility.

Paranoid Type.   Paranoid schizophrenics experience delusions or auditory hallucinations. Their delusions are typically persecutory or grandiose or both, but delusions with other themes are also common. Although the delusions may be multiple they are usually grouped around a coherent theme. Hallucinations are also typically related to the content of the delusional theme.

Delusions generally form a complex system based on a complete misunderstanding of an actual event. In these instances it is common for the individual to feel special and singled out for attention (delusion of reference). Second, they believe they have been singled out because they are special (delusion of grandeur), and third, they determine that others are jealous and therefore are out to hurt them (delusion of persecution).

Undifferentiated Type.   This type of schizophrenia is characterized by disorganized behavior, hallucinations, delusions, and incoherence. Individuals who have symptoms that do not fit into the other categories are placed here.

Residual Type.   The residual type of schizophrenia is used to classify an individual who has had at least one episode of schizophrenia but currently is without prominent psychotic symptoms. In the event delusions are evident, they are not prominent and are not accompanied by strong affect.

Personality Disorders

Personality disorders are usually recognizable by the time of adolescence. Characterized by chronic, maladaptive cognitive-behavioral patterns, they are thoroughly integrated into the individual's personality. These patterns of behavior are usually not as bizarre as schizophrenia and do not entail the intense fear often exhibited in those with anxiety disorders. However, these behavior patterns are troublesome to others since those exhibiting personality disorders generally draw their enjoyment from illegal or harmful sources (Meyer, Wolverton & Deitsch, 1998).

According to the DSM-IV there are three clusters of personality disorders: the odd/eccentric cluster, the dramatic/emotionally problematic cluster, and the chronic fearfulness/avoidant cluster. Paranoid, schizoid, and schizotypal disorders are located within the odd/eccentric cluster; histrionic, narcissistic, antisocial, and borderline disorders are included in the dramatic/emotionally problematic cluster; and avoidant, dependent, obsessive-compulsive, and passive-aggressive are included in the chronic fearfulness/avoidant cluster.

Antisocial Personality Disorder.   Of all of the clusters of personality disorders, the most problematic for society is the antisocial personality disorder that is found in the dramatic/emotionally problematic cluster. Characterized as irresponsible and self-in-dulgent, these individuals frequently resort to a life of crime and violence.

People diagnosed with this disorder were formerly referred to as psychopaths or sociopaths. More common in men than in women, it is evident before the age of 15 and continues into adulthood. These individuals are guiltless, exploitive, irresponsible, and extremely difficult to treat. Although they represent a very small percentage of the population, they commit a disproportionately large percentage of violent and property crimes (Meyer, Wolverton, & Deitsch, 1998).

Mental Status Exam

Individuals experiencing symptoms of mental illness may find that their disorders prevent them from participating in normal daily activities or that their behaviors are deemed unacceptable by society. In these instances they may become recipients of mental health services. Some teenagers and adults access services through self-referrals, schools, law enforcement, and the courts. In addition, family members are also responsible for referring individuals of all ages for treatment.

When individuals arrive at mental health facilities, highly skilled practitioners interview them. Psychiatrists, psychologists, and other mental health professionals traditionally conduct a mental status exam (MSE) to determine if the person is rooted in reality and if he or she is oriented to time, place, and person. Although the MSE may vary in depth and methodology, it generally involves questions and observations that pertain to a hierarchy of mental, emotional, and psychological functions.

During the interview process, mental health professionals compile a psychosocial history, note their observations, and determine the individual's fund of information. Furthermore, they assess general cognition and affect, and decide what psychological tests are appropriate for a comprehensive evaluation. Based on these findings a treatment plan is devised that frequently includes the dispensing of medications. (Refer to Chapter 8 for additional information regarding the interview process.)

What effect, if any, does deafness have on the mental status exam? Is there evidence of mental illness among deaf and hard-of-hearing individuals? If so, do they exhibit similar symptoms as those who can hear? What are the major pitfalls of identifying mental illness in those who cannot hear?

Identifying Mental Illness in Deaf and Hard-of-Hearing Individuals

Deaf and hard-of-hearing individuals comprise a heterogeneous constituency that experiences the same range of mental disorders and problems as those encountered by the general population. According to Goulder (1977) more than 40,000 deaf Americans suffer from serious mental illness, and when the hard-of-hearing population is included, the incidence rate increases to in excess of 2,000,000 (Trybus, 1987). However, according to Vernon (1983), only 2 percent of deaf people with serious mental illness are actually thought to receive treatment.

Those seeking treatment are frequently referred to mental health agencies where they encounter hearing professionals unfamiliar with the ramifications of deafness. These professionals may rely on spoken communication to interact with their deaf clients, and when and if they fail to understand "deaf speech" they may resort to written exchanges to gather pertinent information. Often, these clinicians fail to recognize that deaf individuals may possess a substandard command of the English language (vocabulary and syntax) and therefore express themselves differently than their hearing clients. As a result, when clinicians attempt to decipher their deaf clients' written responses they may compare these written exposes to similar writing samples of those who can hear and thus misdiagnose their deaf clients as being mentally retarded, psychotic, aphasic, or exhibiting other related serious mental disorders (Pollard, 1998). Therefore, from the onset misinformation can contaminate the critical evaluative phase of treatment as both parties attempt to comprehend what the other is saying.

Some deaf and hard-of-hearing individuals seeking mental health services prefer an oral mode of communication, while others are fluent in American Sign Language (ASL). In contrast, several have been exposed to a smattering of all types of communication and have not developed a proficiency in any one mode. Each of these groups of individuals presents specific challenges to the hearing practitioner who has not received formal training in deafness. Although sign language interpreters are frequently employed in clinical settings to facilitate communication for those who sign, additional factors must be considered when diagnosing and providing services to this population.

Conducting Mental Status Exams with Deaf Clients

When initiating an interview with deaf and hard of hearing clients it is critical to become familiar with the cause of the individual's hearing loss. Because many deafness etiologies are associated with additional physical and neurological impairments, being familiar with the degree, type, cause, and age of onset of the hearing loss can provide valuable information.

Several of the primary causes of deafness are also etiologies of brain damage. Therefore, it is essential that when possible the cause is established early in the evaluative process. While some hereditary conditions, such as Usher's syndrome, may be confused with schizophrenia (Misiaszek et al., 1985), other causes of deafness, such as encephalitis resulting from meningitis, can directly contribute to brain syndromes that in and of themselves cause psychosis (Vernon & Andrews, 1990). Furthermore, when maternal rubella is cited as the cause of deafness, there may be additional hand-icapping conditions. In these instances, impulsive behavior may be evident and is therefore attributed to the factors associated with deafness, rather than to the deaf-ness itself (Chess & Fernandez, 1980).

Before engaging in the interview process, it is imperative that the clinician obtains a clear understanding of the etiology of the client's hearing loss. Based on this information, mental retardation can be considered or possibly eliminated as a potential contributing factor in the diagnosis. Furthermore, by securing this type of background information, diagnostic errors can be avoided.

Throughout the interview process, the clinician assesses general intelligence, fund of information, and overall communication skills. According to Pollard (1998), these abilities cannot be gauged reliably through an interview with deaf or hard-of-hearing individuals unless the clinician is specifically trained in deafness. Although many deaf individuals acquire a normal fund of information, due to the social, cul-tural, and communication differences, others may project deficiencies in this area as well as in intelligence when compared with the standards established for those who can hear.

It is well documented in the literature that intelligence is distributed normally in the deaf population. However, clinical interviews often reveal limitations in fund of information. This is a reflection of experiential deprivation and is not the result of cognitive limitations or psychopathology. Rather, it is a manifestation of being denied access to auditory information that is derived from movies, radio, and secondary or overheard conversations, and from being raised from childhood in environments that lack stimulating communication and therefore abate the development of critical think-ing skills (Braden, 1994; Schlesinger, 1992). It is imperative that clinicians are cog-nizant of these differences when rendering a diagnosis.

Furthermore, within the initial interview hearing clinicians unfamiliar with sign language may misconstrue what they see as an indication of "mania, disinhibition, lability, or other problems of excess." In contrast, active signing behavior can mislead clinicians to overlook depressed affect (Pollard, 1998).

Sign language relies on sign variation and facial expressions to convey inflec-tion. While those who can hear express their emotions through the pitch, intensity, and speed of their delivery, those who are deaf convey similar feelings through signs that may appear to be larger, more intense, and delivered at a rapid pace. In these instances, inflection can be misunderstood as agitation.

Moreover, when mental health professionals encounter deaf individuals who prefer to use speech as their primary mode of communication, they may be faced with vocalizations that are incomprehensible. This is particularly evident in individuals with severe to profound losses who experienced their hearing loss at birth or during the first three years of life. Unable to hear what they say, they draw from years of speech training to monitor their voices. Although some speak clearly, many others have speech characterized by words that are not pronounced clearly. As a result, understanding their speech and comprehending their message becomes a formidable task. When this occurs, clinicians must recognize that the quality of the person's speech is not indicative of his or her intellectual or psychological functioning ability.

When qualified professionals conduct the mental status exam with deaf individuals, it is possible to obtain accurate diagnoses of the various classifications of mental illness. However, when practitioners are unaware of the ramifications of deafness, diagnostic errors are made that lead to the irresponsible characterizations of deaf people (Lane, 1992).

Prevalence of Mental Illness within the Deaf Population

Very few empirical studies have explored incidence rates concerning the various types of psychopathology evident in the deaf population. However, research conducted by Pollard (1994) in 18 public mental health agencies in New York indicates that for the most part deaf individuals reflect the same diagnostic rates for adjustment disorders, mood disorders, organic disorders, anxiety disorders, and personality disorders as those reflected in hearing individuals. Additional studies have focused on specific disorders, including depression, behavior disorders, obsessive-compulsive disorders, psychosis, and in particular schizophrenia.

Depression

There is some controversy regarding the rate of clinical depression among deaf people (Vernon & Andrews, 1990). Research conducted by Altshuler (1971) indicates that there is less depressive illness in the deaf population, while other researchers, such as Grinker (1969), report that there are no differences either quantitatively or qualitatively within the deaf population. According to Altschuler and Abdullah (1981), depression, when present, manifests itself somewhat differently in those who are deaf.

Hearing patients diagnosed with clinical depression frequently experience feelings of guilt, reproach, and other forms of self-deprecation and self-hate. However, when the same diagnosis is evident in those who cannot hear, it is typically characterized by agitation with projective hostile and aggressive feelings. These differences may be attributed in part to the relationship established between children and their parents that begins in infancy. Raised with parental expectations that are conveyed through spoken exchanges, hearing children are well versed in what is considered appropriate behavior. Therefore, in the event that they fail to meet these expectations they may experience feelings of guilt and remorse.

However, deaf and hard-of-hearing children are often isolated from both social and parental expectations due to their hearing loss. Unaware of their parents' expectations, they may be oblivious to the fact that they have failed to meet specific standards. Therefore, unlike their hearing peers who feel remorse because they have failed, those who are deaf may have a different perception of the standard.

In essence, in order to experience any feelings of remorse, children must internalize parental expectations and then recognize that they have failed. In the event that these preconceived expectations are not internalized, this process cannot take place. This in turn may be one of the primary reasons that clinical depression in deaf adults is expressed differently (LeBuffe & LeBuffe, 1979; Rainer, Altshuler, & Kallman, 1969). Further indications of clinical depression in deaf patients indicate that they tend to exhibit activity levels that are near or above normal, accompanied by frequent somatic bodily preoccupations (Altshuler & Abdulla, 1981).

Obsessive-Compulsive Disorder

Deaf children born to hearing parents frequently find themselves raised in homes where communication is strained and behaviors are learned through role modeling rather than through explanations. In these settings, children rely on their visual perception to interpret social expectations while they attempt to model appropriate behaviors. Furthermore, because parents and later teachers typically do not possess the skills to communicate fluently with those who are deaf, they consistently structure their directives and adhere to a daily routine. As a result, deaf children are often raised in structured environments that leave little room for variations in the scheduling of activities or in the development of independent decision-making skills.

Learning atmospheres that foster critical thinking skills, flexibility, and the development of an internal locus of control are conducive to healthy personality development. However, when children are nurtured in rigid environments that stifle exploration and creativity, they tend to reflect rigidity, concrete thinking, lack of insight, projection of responsibility onto others, and impulsive behaviors (Altshuler, 1971).

Within the deaf population these behaviors can be attributed to enculturation, and when observed by untrained practitioners, can be mistaken for personality disorders. According to Misiaszek and his colleagues (1985), while deaf adults may exhibit the "obsessive-compulsive characteristics of rigidity, obstinacy, and dampening of emotional display, they lack the same, guilt, rumination, and anxiety present in obsessive-compulsive individuals" (p. 514). Therefore, although some of the traits frequently associated with this personality disorder are evident in deaf adults they do not reflect the full spectrum of the traits required for a diagnosis to be made. As a result, although there is evidence of several deaf adults projecting some of these behaviors, documentation of bona fide cases of deaf individuals who can be accurately diagnosed with the illness are rare. In fact, the rate of prevalence for deaf adults is no higher than the number of cases reported for the general hearing population (Lesser & Easser, 1972).

Schizophrenia

Schizophrenia is characterized by breaks with reality, hallucinations, delusions, and disorganized thoughts. It strikes equal numbers of deaf and hearing individuals, accounting for half the patients in mental hospitals. Although both populations receive treatment in mental health facilities, due to the difficulty in the diagnosis of deaf clients, these patients tend to be more chronic than what is indicative in individuals who can hear (Vernon & Andrews, 1990).

Clinicians unfamiliar with deafness are responsible for evaluating the majority of deaf and hard-of-hearing individuals referred for psychological evaluations. Unprepared to make an accurate diagnosis, these professionals may respond in one of two ways, either overlooking indicators that signify schizophrenia, or confusing behaviors characteristic of deafness and therefore inappropriately label deaf individuals (Evans & Elliott, 1981).

According to Strauss, Carpenter, and Bartko (1974), manifestations of schizophrenia in hearing clients can be categorized into three groups: positive symptoms or active processes, including hallucinations and delusions; negative symptoms (the absence of normal functions), including poor insight, poverty of content, and vagueness; and disorders of personal relationships, typified in poor rapport. However, when these categories are applied to deaf clients, misdiagnoses may occur.

Those familiar with the ramifications of deafness recognize that those factors contained in the second category (poor insight, poverty of content, and vagueness) can be viewed as secondary characteristics of deafness and have no bearing on mental illness. Poor insight can be attributed to lack of knowledge or experiential deprivation that results from depressed communication exchanges. Although these factors can be present in psychotic deaf patients, they may also be characteristic of those who are nonpsychotic. Thus, many deaf adults lacking fluent communication skills may be inadvertently labeled with a mental illness that they in fact do not have.

A study conducted by Evans and Elliott (1974) identified nine primary symptoms of schizophrenia in deaf patients that can be useful when making a diagnosis: loss of ego boundaries, delusional perception, restricted affect, illogicity, abnormal explanations, hallucinations, inappropriate affect, remoteness from reality, and ambivalence. Five additional common symptoms may also be present in both psychotic as well as nonpsychotic patients: poor insight, lability of affect, poverty of content, poor rapport, and inability to complete a course of action.

Auditory hallucinations are frequently observed in hearing patients who have schizophrenia. However, there is conflicting research regarding the incidence rates of auditory hallucinations in deaf patients. While Evans and Elliott (1981) have identified differences in frequency patterns, Rainer, Abdullah, and Altshuler (1970) have reported similar incident rates in both hearing and deaf populations. According to Pollard (1998), limited research is available concerning the reporting of auditory hallucinations in deaf patients. However, when it is reported it usually occurs in patients with partial hearing or those who have experienced late-onset deafness.

Further research indicates that although some hallucinations experienced by deaf patients may be visual, these are generally rare. Although Vernon and Andrews (1990) have noted that some patients report that "God signs to them," limited examples of this type of visual hallucination are reported in the literature. In contrast, it is very common to see psychotic deaf persons signing to themselves as they experience psychotic episodes.

Additional psychotic symptoms have been observed in the sign communication of some deaf patients who express themselves through sign neologisms, word salad, and clang associations. In these instances, there is an apparent break in the fluency of American Sign Language (ASL), followed either by the production of signs that don't exist in ASL or by the delivery of signs that when presented in sequence fail to reflect any coherent thought pattern.

Although limited research is available in this area, there is the possibility that this disruption in sign communication may be indicative of similar fragmented speech patterns exhibited by hearing individuals experiencing psychotic episodes. However, because research in this area is so meager, it is critical to note that although sign dysfluency may reflect psychopathology, in most cases it is an outgrowth of educational and experiential limitations and should be viewed as such (Thacker, 1994).

Paranoid Disorders

Of all of the myths and misconceptions that have been formulated regarding deafness, perhaps one of the oldest beliefs is that deaf people are paranoid. Recurring in the literature, professionals within the fields of both psychology and psychiatry have been indoctrinated to believe that one term is synonymous with the other. Contrary to popular belief, research indicates that there is no greater incidence of paranoia or paranoid schizophrenia in deaf individuals that there is among those who can hear (Stinson, 1993).

Surdophrenia

Although surdophrenia, also referred to as primitive personality, is not a form of mental illness, it merits discussion as it can be misunderstood by clinicians unfamiliar with deafness. Labeled originally by Rainer and his colleagues (1963) and further defined by Basilier (1964), the term is used to identify deaf patients who have extreme educational deprivation, virtually no understanding of language, limited socialization, and in essence, a psychologically barren life.

These individuals have normal intellectual potential but may exhibit a combination of depression and aggression and reflect severely limited communication skills. Furthermore, they may be particularly susceptible to stress and may grossly overreact to mundane events in their lives (Misiaszek et al., 1985).

Although most of these individuals are not psychotic, many of them require mental health services. In these instances long-term treatment is usually required as efforts are made to provide them with information and social skills needed to raise their overall level of functioning. Unlike forms of mental illness that are treated by returning the patient to previous levels of functioning, the goal for these individuals is to assist them in developing beyond any stage that they have previously experienced (Vernon & Andrews, 1990).

Interpreting during the Mental Status Exam

Hearing clinicians unfamiliar with the field of deafness frequently find themselves challenged when they are asked to conduct a mental status exam on a deaf client. Potentially confronted with individuals from a different language and cultural background, they encounter deaf children and adults who may or may not exhibit signs of mental illness. Characterized by various language and communication backgrounds, cognitive abilities, intellectual functioning levels, and social experiences, these individuals arrive for their appointment with varying degrees of trepidation.

While some clinicians will attempt to rely on paper and pencil to converse with these clients, others will request the services of a sign language interpreter to be available during their initial session. When employed, these professionals serve as facilitators of communication and equalize communication between both the hearing clinician and the deaf consumer.

Interpreting in the mental health setting can be particularly challenging. In these settings, interpreters are confronted with deaf individuals who may manifest their psychotic symptoms in dysfluent sign communication. When this occurs their sign proficiency is typically grossly poorer than their educational and social history would suggest (Pollard, 1998). In these instances, interpreters may have a difficult time understanding or voicing for the deaf consumer. Consequently, they may attempt to "make sense" of what they have seen and thus normalize the individual's responses, skewing the results of the exam.

Interpreters may blame themselves for communication impasses, failing to recognize that the signing being displayed is indicative of an individual with psychosis. However, as they learn to identify invented signs, interpreters gain further insights into mental illness and can begin to differentiate these signs from those attributed to home signs or regional differences. This in turn allows them to ascertain when they are experiencing difficulty due to fatigue or unfamiliarity with the client, or if the sign presentation is not being produced in a comprehensible manner. When interpreters are capable of making this distinction, they provide a very valuable link in the communication process. In these instances, the interpreter is able to confer privately with the clinician, verifying that although signs were produced, the manner in which they were expressed provided no meaning.

Interpreters are also responsible for relaying the affect that is expressed by the deaf consumer. It is critical that this is expressed clearly, especially for clinicians who may have preconceived concepts of deafness. With an accurate interpretation, the mental health professional is better equipped to provide an accurate diagnosis.

Summary

Mental illness finds its way into the lives of deaf people, just as it permeates the lives of hearing individuals. It manifests itself in behavior that is maladaptive or deviant, and interferes with the person's ability to live a normal life. It requires treatment in the form of therapy, medication, and sometimes hospitalization in order for the person to cope with demands of daily living.

When it becomes apparent that an individual is in need of psychological or psychiatric services a referral is generally made, a mental status exam is conducted, and treatment is prescribed. When deaf individuals are referred for services the process becomes more complex. Reflecting years of development in environments that are not conducive to visual communication, depressed social and English-language skills may become tangled in symptoms of mental illness, thus affecting the outcome of the mental status exam. Consequently, deaf individuals may be misdiagnosed and undergo treatment that is counterproductive.

Deafness does not cause mental illness; rather, some of the symptoms associated with mental illness can be exacerbated by the ramifications of deafness. When deaf individuals are treated by clinicians who have received specialized training in deafness, they are afforded the opportunity to receive an accurate diagnosis and be treated for symptoms that do in fact exist.

The field of mental health is slowly adding qualified professionals trained to work with the deaf to its fold. Although there is a great deal of research left to be done in this area, strides are being made to improve mental health services for deaf consumers.

11

Crisis and Intervention

Annually more than one million American children experience some significant form of maltreatment involving physical assault; disregard of their basic needs, including medical, educational, and nutritional neglect; sexual exploitation; drug or alcohol abuse; and emotional deprivation. According to the American Association for Protecting Children (1986), 20 percent of the reported cases of abuse involve abuse alone, 46 percent neglect alone, 23 percent both abuse and neglect, and 11 percent sexual abuse. Of these cases, 11 percent suffer life-threatening, disabling injuries, and 90 percent suffer temporary physical injuries. In addition, although physical injuries are not necessarily prevalent among neglected children, they frequently experience extensive, long-term psychological harm.

Children with disabilities are particularly vulnerable to maltreatment and forms of abuse. Preliminary research indicates that low-birthweight infants are at special risk for child abuse because their care is particularly stressful. Infants born with low birthweights comprise only 10 percent of the newborn population, yet these children represent approximately 20 to 25 percent of those who are physically abused (Solomons, 1979). Studies conducted by Gil, Chotiner, and Lehr (1976) reveal that of the children who are exploited or victimized, between 30 and 70 percent have pre-existing handicaps and developmental disabilities. These children are at greater risk for abuse from surrogate caretakers, including stepparents, foster parents, babysitters, single mothers' boyfriends, and personnel employed in residential settings (Lightcap, Kurland, & Burgess, 1982). Research conducted by Brookhouser, Sullivan, and Scanlon (1986) further indicates that male caretakers, including the biological father, are more likely than female caretaker to abuse a disabled child. In addition, studies reveal that between 60 and 90 percent of these abusers have histories of having been abused during childhood.

What factors contribute to the maltreatment of children with disabilities? How prevalent is abuse among deaf and hard-of-hearing children? What types of behaviors are indicative of abused children? Once identified, what types of treatment programs are available to those who are deaf and hard of hearing?

The Multifaceted Nature of Abuse: Contributing Factors

According to Field (2000), child abuse is a diverse condition that is usually mild to moderate in severity, and is only partially caused by the individual personality characteristics of parents. The most common kind of abuse is inflicted not by a raging, uncontrolled abuser but rather by an overwhelmed single mother living in poverty who neglects the child. In these instances the mother may be lacking the social as well as the financial support she needs.

Furthermore, when parents inflict abuse on their disabled child, it can be partially attributed to their lack of knowing how to be empathetic, or because they find that they are confronted with children with whom they struggle to communicate. In addition, they may find themselves caught in a spiral of interaction patterns that create withdrawal or escalation as conflicts appear. These factors can be further exacerbated when compounded with feelings of isolation, and can ensue as parents attempt to cope with the daily demands of living without support from family and friends.

Community support systems have been found to be extremely beneficial in alleviating stressful family situations, thereby helping reduce the number of children who experience abuse. A study conducted by Garbarino (1976) has revealed a direct relation between the availability of formal community support systems such as crisis centers and counseling services and the reduction in child abuse. Furthermore, these agencies frequently provide instruction in positive parenting techniques, thus educating caregivers in nonviolent disciplinary techniques.

Abusive parenting styles are often the result of learned behaviors. According to Cicchetti and Toth (1998), approximately one-third of the parents who abuse their children come from families in which physical abuse was administered. These parents are locked into an intergenerational transmission of abuse.

While some parents have been raised to be abusive, others model what they observe in the media to structure their discipline techniques. Bombarded with routine violence on television, some mirror the assertion of power that they observe. Oblivious to other disciplinary techniques, they resort to what they interpret to be culturally acceptable. A clear reduction in abusive behavior frequently occurs when parents are provided with alternative discipline techniques.

Abuse can erupt into physical violence, verbal insults, and emotional trauma. It can also become a manifestation of power imbalances between adults and children and older and younger children in the form of sexual abuse. This form of abuse is the most prevalent type of maltreatment endured by children with identified disabilities (Sullivan et al., 1991). This is in contrast to nondisabled children, who endure physical abuse and neglect more often than sexual abuse (Sullivan, 1993).

Sexual Abuse and Children

Child sexual abuse has been defined as "the sexual exploitation of a child under age 18, who is not developmentally capable of understanding or resisting sexual contact, or who may be psychologically, physically, or socially dependent upon the offender. The sexual contact ranges from body exposure to penetration. Victims can be both male and female" (O'Day, 1983). By definition, child-adult sexual interactions involve coercion because children are not legally capable of giving informed consent to sexual activity. This is based on the premise that children and young adolescents generally do not have a clear understanding of sexuality and the possible consequences related to a specific sexual action (Allgeier & Allgeier, 2000).

Sexual activity between a child and an adult is considered a crime in every state. Furthermore, when it involves two people who are related to each other it is defined as incest. All professionals who work with children are legally required to report all suspected cases of the sexual abuse of children.

Prevalence of Sexual Abuse

Prior to the 1990s, estimates of child sexual abuse were based on information provided by the Federal Bureau of Investigation and surveys conducted by the National Committee for the Prevention of Child Abuse. Data from the FBI indicated that as many as 60,000 to 100,000 children are abused annually with only 20 percent of the crimes being reported. Statistics compiled by the U.S. Department of Health and Human Services (1999) indicate that over 200,000 cases of sexual abuse were made.

In an attempt to determine the prevalence of sexual abuse in the United States, Finkelhor, Hotaling, Lewis, and Smith (1990) conducted a nationwide telephone survey with adults. During this interview they inquired about past experiences (occurring at age 18 or under) with what the individuals might now consider in retrospect to be sexual abuse. Their questions focused on four topics: attempts of others to touch them sexually, initiation of sexual acts including intercourse, requests to photograph them in the nude, and requests for them to exhibit themselves or perform sex acts in their presence. Of the respondents, 27 percent of the women and 16 percent of the men answered affirmatively to one of the questions.

More recent surveys conducted by Lauman and colleagues (1994) indicate that 17 percent of women and 12 percent of men were touched sexually during childhood. Furthermore, research conducted by Gorey and Leslie (1997) reflects a prevalence rate of sexual abuse of 14.5 percent for women and 7.9 percent for males. The difference between these figures is a result of the methodological variations and differences in how sexual abuse has been defined.

Further review of the literature reveals that most children who have been sexually abused or adults who remember being sexually abused as children cite heterosexual men as their perpetrators. Statistics indicate male perpetrators in 95 percent of the cases of sexual abuse of girls and 80 percent of the cases of sexual abuse of boys (Finkelhor & Russell, 1984). Additional findings reflect that sexual abusers are not generally violent (Okami & Goldberg, 1992). Based on the national survey conduced by Finkelhor and his colleagues (1990), physical force was used in only 19 percent of incidents involving girls and 15 percent of episodes involving boys. Recent research has also revealed that children, like women, are more likely to be sexually abused by acquaintances, relatives, siblings, family friends, and neighbors than by strangers (Finkelhor et al., 1990; Laumann et al., 1994).

Although child sexual abuse occurs at all socioeconomic levels, in general it appears that children in disrupted, isolated, and economically poor families are at a higher risk than youngsters in more stable middle-class families (Wood & Wood, 2002). Additionally, risk factors have been identified for males and females. The two factors cited for males are living with their mothers alone or living with two nonbiological parents. For females the four risks are having an unhappy family life, living without a biological parent, having inadequate sex education, and region of residence (Allgeier & Allgeier, 2000).

Sexual Abuse of Children with Disabilities

Although many states do not compile statistics on special needs populations when reporting the prevalence of sexual abuse, it is generally acknowledged that this population is very vulnerable. Research based on deaf children and adults receiving clinical treatment provide statistics on the clinical population. Even though this data cannot be directly applied to the general population, it does provide some insights into the magnitude of the problem.

Recent data compiled at the Center for Abused Handicapped Children at Boys Town Research Hospital in Nebraska reveal that 53.4 percent of deaf and hard-of-hearing children who receive services have been sexually abused (Sullivan et al., 1991). Furthermore, the percentages of those who are receiving clinical services at the National Technical Institute for the Deaf reveal that 25 percent have been sexually abused (Elder, 1993).

Sexual abuse is inflicted in a multitude of settings. While family members and acquaintances are frequently cited as perpetrators, deaf individuals may further identify employees of residential programs as the instigator of their abuse. An epidemiological study conducted throughout a 10-year period (1982–1992) by the Boys Town National Research Hospital (BTNRH), the Nebraska Central Registry (NDSS), the Foster Care Review Board (FCRB), and police databases reflects that 88 percent of child maltreatment occurred in the child's own home. Of the 12 percent who were not abused in the home, 4 percent were abused in the perpetrator's home, while only 1 percent indicated they were abused within some type of school setting (Sullivan & Knutson, 1998).

Findings of this report also illustrated that the majority of reported maltreatment cases that were reported cited parents and extended family members as the primary perpetrators. However, extrafamilial abuse constituted approximately 40 percent of the reported cases. Included in this category were babysitters, members of the clergy, van drivers, care attendants, older students, peers, and neighbors. Stranger abuse was noted as accounting for only 7 percent of extrafamilial sexual abuse (Sullivan & Knutson, 1998).

Reports periodically surface reflecting sexual abuse of deaf children by older children in dormitory settings. Furthermore, these reports also cite houseparents and other service workers employed in the residential setting as being sexual perpetrators. In these settings children may be taken advantage of through the use of trickery, emotional pressure, or physical coercion. Children in residential settings are dependent on adults for their basic survival needs. As a result, many adult perpetrators take advantage of the child's dependency role.

When cases of abuse are reported, especially those occurring in any residential setting, the response from society is one of outrage coupled with the urging by legislators to close the school. When incidents of abuse are reported involving schools for the deaf, the controversy regarding school closure assumes an added dimension. Because residential schools are considered to be "cradles of Deaf culture," members of the Deaf community often become adamant when school closures are discussed (Pollard, 1993). Although Deaf professionals frequently mirror the same feelings of outrage when sexual abuse allegations are directed at the schools, in contrast to the general public's view of school closure, they look for ways to resolve the problem within the residential setting.

What are some of the warning signs that indicate a child may have experienced abuse or may currently be residing in an abusive situation? What forms of treatment are available to those who have been abused? What are some of the ramifications of sexual abuse, especially in the event that it is not treated?

Identifying Signs of Sexual Abuse

Due to the ramifications of deafness, deaf and hard-of-hearing children may lack the verbal skills needed to report that they have been victimized. Furthermore, some may remain silent because they assume that what has happened to them routinely happens to all children. Some report feeling "chosen" or "special" by a teacher or a houseparent who sexually abused them. They never considered this relationship abusive; only later, in professional settings, did they realize that this behavior was not appropriate (LaBarre, 1998). Others may sense that the sexual activity they have been subjected to is wrong and thus experience feelings of self-blame, guilt, and embarrassment. Consequently, they may choose not to report these episodes.

Frequently professionals must rely on external behaviors to identify possible signs of abuse. Many of the characteristics displayed by deaf children are similar to those experienced by hearing children. They can include:

- School-related problems including failing grades, absenteeism, truancy, and discipline problems

- Inappropriate play with others or with toys, including sexually related behavior, precocious sex play, knowledge of sexual acts, or compulsive masturbation
- Sleep disturbances, including fear of the dark
- Depression, including feelings of low self-esteem, crying episodes, change in eating or sleeping habits, and poor personal hygiene
- Withdrawal from others or engagement in fantasy or infantile, regressive behavior including bedwetting or encopresis (fecal soiling)
- Suicidal feelings and/or substance abuse, including suicidal gestures or attempts
- Lack of trust in others they have previously viewed as protecting them
- Manifestation of new fears, including the fear of being alone, of going to school, or of staying home
- Direct statement that he or she has been sexually assaulted by a parent, caretaker, older child, or other perpetrator (LaBarre, 1998; Brookhouser et al., 1986)

Sexual abuse is traumatic for those being victimized. While some experience only one encounter, others less fortunate are subjected to prolonged periods of abuse. In these instances the effects of the abuse are long-term and can manifest into a post-traumatic stress disorder.

Post-Traumatic Stress Disorder

Post-traumatic stress disorder is a mental disorder that develops through exposure to a traumatic event, including war; severe abuse, as in rape; natural disasters, such as floods; and accidental disasters, such as plane crashes. The disorder is characterized by anxiety symptoms that may immediately follow the trauma; however, the symptoms may be delayed by months or even years before becoming apparent (Ford, 1999; Ursano et al., 1999).

Although the symptoms vary they can include flashbacks, difficulties with memory and concentration, feelings of apprehension, impulsive outbursts, and a constricted ability to feel emotions. Not every individual exposed to the same situation will develop post-traumatic stress disorder. However, some experts consider sexual abuse and assault victims to be the single largest group of post-traumatic stress disorder sufferers (Koss & Boeschen, 1998). Victims of sexual abuse can develop this disorder regardless of the number of times they have been victimized (Sullivan & Scanlan, 1990).

A growing body of research indicates that the effects of sexual abuse are long-term, and if left untreated can result in adverse consequences for the victim (Kendall-Tackett, Williams, & Finkhor, 1993). Findings indicate that those suffering this form of abuse may become disordered because of the initial stressor. Furthermore, studies indicate that the effects of the trauma can permeate other aspects of the person's life (Saunders et al., 1992).

Finkelhor and Browne (1985) have developed four traumagenic dynamics to explain the effects of child sexual abuse. The first is identified as traumatic sexualization, which refers to a process whereby the child's sexuality is shaped in a developmentally inappropriate and dysfunctional fashion. The second dynamic is betrayal, which results when the child recognizes that someone previously trusted and depended on has caused him or her harm. The third dynamic focuses on feelings of powerlessness whereby the child feels he or she has no power over the situation. In these instances the child may unsuccessfully attempt to halt the abuse, and when the attempts fail the feeling of powerlessness is exacerbated. The fourth dynamic is identified as stigmatization, which refers to the negative connotations that are frequently conveyed to the child regarding the sexual activity. These feelings of shame and guilt can further be assimilated into the child's self-image.

Sexual abuse is multifaceted. Its victims represent a heterogeneous group of individuals who have diverse needs. Recognizing the gravity of the problem, several programs have been established that focus on prevention as well as on treatment. While some are school and community based, others are being initiated in private treatment facilities.

Prevention Programs: Providing Children with Strategies

Within the last two decades a proliferation of childhood sexual abuse programs (CSAP) have been introduced into the schools. These programs are designed to enable children to identify and avoid sexual abuse. Young children are taught to recognize physical contact that is good for them (good touch) and contact that they want to avoid (bad touch). Emphasis is also placed on defining confusing touch, which may start out good and end up feeling bad. The second key element contained in this program is the concept of empowerment. This segment of the program addresses how children can play an active role in avoiding sexual abuse.

Critics of childhood sexual abuse programs note that care must be taken when implementing these programs. They stress that it is critical that information be presented at a developmentally appropriate level. Children must be taught to realize what is abusive behavior; however, they must also recognize that on occasion they may be powerless to stop the unwanted sexual advance. If this concept is not conveyed, if and when abuse occurs, children may develop feelings of guilt, assuming that they are responsible for not halting the activity (Westerlund, 1990).

When programs are implemented for deaf and hard-of-hearing children, curricular modifications are usually required. Materials generally need to be made less wordy and more visual. Furthermore, additional time may need to be invested in providing definitions for terms that may be common knowledge within the hearing community.

Specific instruction frequently includes labeling body parts and providing children with correct terminology. Other program content focuses on teaching children ways to stay safe, how to distance themselves from people, how to say no, and how to yell for help. When engaging in programs of this nature, role-plays and repetition are critical and key concepts are conveyed. When implementing programs of this nature it is beneficial to adapt the content to reflect Deaf culture, and those modifications that are required to meet the specific needs of deaf children.

Prevention programs are beneficial for deaf and hard-of-hearing children when they teach them to identify body parts, recognize what is and isn't considered abusive behavior, and provide them with strategies for survival. Furthermore, these programs serve a very useful function when they provide children and adolescents with guidelines for reporting sexual abuse.

Although an increased emphasis has been placed on preventive measures, abuse continues to be problematic for school-aged children (preschoolers through adolescents). Deaf and hard-of-hearing children frequently find they are in need of counseling services to cope with the abuse. Some require only short-term counseling, while others find themselves in need of long-term treatment programs.

Surviving Sexual Abuse: Providing Treatment for Deaf and Hard-of-Hearing Individuals

Children and adults arriving for therapy may lack a common base of sexual vocabulary or knowledge of their own sexuality. As a result, deaf individuals may misunderstand terms that are frequently used by counselors and therapists. Therefore, from the onset it is critical to determine that a mutual understanding of the terminology exists. Furthermore, concepts of maleness and femaleness may need to be examined. Because these concepts are primarily based on what we see and hear, deaf individuals' perceptions of these gender differences may be inaccurate. In these instances, it may be necessary to answer questions and provide general information before specific abuse issues can be confronted (LaBarre, 1998).

Some of the most extensive work in therapeutic treatment of sexually abused deaf and hard-of-hearing children has been conducted at the Center for Abused Handicapped Children at the Boys Town National Research Hospital. To date this facility has provided therapeutic services to over 600 children with disabilities (Sullivan & Scanlan, 1990). Based on each child's case history, an individual treatment plan is outlined that includes specific goals and objectives. According to Sullivan and Scanlan (1987), typical goals that are frequently included in the psychotherapy treatment plans include:

- Working with children to alleviate guilt that has been engendered by the sexual abuse
- Assisting children to regain trust in peers and adults
- Treating depression, including sleep and eating disorders and sometimes suicidal thoughts
- Providing information on anger management whereby children are taught how to express their anger at being victimized in appropriate and productive ways

- Addressing sexual preference issues, when appropriate, and facilitating gender identity formulation
- Providing children with self-protection techniques, including sexual abuse laws and reporting agencies, as well as what to do when someone well known to them attempts to abuse them
- Instructing children in the development of an effective vocabulary to label emotions and feelings whereby they develop the terminology to adequately express how they feel
- Assisting children to develop a personal value system and to establish of a meaningful and stable identity
- Providing treatment of secondary behavioral characteristics that may be associated with sexual abuse

Once these goals are identified, specific counseling techniques are implemented to insure the goals can be achieved. This center relies on an eclectic approach and draws from numerous counseling techniques to meet the needs of clients. These include behavior therapy, psychodrama, and role-playing.

Sexual abuse can lead to additional forms of abuse, such as eating disorders, substance abuse, and alcohol abuse. Furthermore, these forms of abuse can occur independently of other forms and thus have no relationship to sexual abuse. However, when they develop they have the potential to place the individual in a crisis situation that requires intervention.

Eating Disorders and the Deaf and Hard-of-Hearing Population

Although symptoms of post-traumatic stress disorder can manifest in the form of eating disorders, they can also be attributed to perceptions of body image. Two eating disorders that may appear in adolescence are anorexia nervosa and bulimia nervosa. There is a paucity of research studies related to deafness and eating disorders; however, both can and do affect deaf individuals, who may require therapy for these disorders.

Anorexia nervosa is an eating disorder that involves the continuous pursuit of thinness through starvation. Serious in nature, it can eventually lead to death. According to Davison and Neale (2000), there are three main characteristics of persons with anorexia nervosa. The first entails weighing less than 85 percent of what is considered normal for the person's age and height. The second characteristic involves having an intense fear of gaining weight that does not diminish as the person loses weight. The third characteristic is related to body image. Individuals who are anorexic may perceive that they are fat even when they are very thin. They usually weigh themselves frequently and take their body measurements on a regular basis.

Anorexia nervosa typically begins during the middle teenage years. The onset may be triggered by an episode of dieting and the occurrence of some type of life stress (Abood & Chandler, 1997). Although it can occur in males, it is 10 times more likely to occur in females. However, when diagnosed in males the causes and symptoms are usually similar to those reported by females (Olivardia, Pope, Mangweth, & Hudson, 1995).

The majority of those with anorexia are white adolescent or young females from well-educated middle- or upper-class families. Their parents frequently set high standards for them, thus creating stressful situations. Concerned about how they will be perceived if they fail, some turn to their weight as something they feel they can control (Stiegel-Moore, Silberstein, & Rodin, 1993).

Bulimia nervosa is an eating disorder characterized by binge-and-purge eating patterns. The individual consumes large quantities of food and then purges by self-induced vomiting or by using a laxative. Most of these individuals are in their late teens or their early twenties. They are concerned with becoming overweight and may be depressed or anxious (Davison & Neale, 2000). Bulimia can go undetected due to the fact that many of these women remain within a normal weight range (Mizes & Miller, 2000; Orbanic, 2001). In order to attach a diagnosis of bulimia nervosa the individual must have bulimic episodes at least twice a week for three months (Schwitzer, Rodriguez, Thomas, & Salam, 2001).

Very little written in the literature pertains to deaf individuals and eating disorders. One of the most noted research projects is described in a study conducted by Hills, Rappold, and Rendon (1991). Focusing on binge eating and body image in a sample of deaf college students, they conducted a survey that was twofold in nature. First, they wanted to determine if the incidence of binge eating in deaf college students was as prevalent as that found among hearing college students. Second, they wanted to compare perceptions of body image between deaf and hearing women and determine if there were any differences.

Results of their study revealed that 17 percent of the deaf college students surveyed reported current binge eating. Furthermore, 46 percent of the female students overestimated their body size. Based on its findings, this study determined that eating disorders have made inroads into the Deaf community (Hills, Rappold, & Rendon, 1991).

An additional study conducted by Fletcher (1993) has provided a comparison between hearing and deaf and hard-of-hearing women in respect to their eating and dieting behaviors. Survey questions examined the participants' feelings concerning their bodies, dieting, and eating. Results of this study further support the earlier findings of Hill and her colleagues. There appeared to be no difference between the two groups in their attitudes toward food and dieting.

All respondents in the study expressed concern regarding their personal appearance. Of those responding, 50 percent of the deaf and hard-of-hearing group and 70 percent of the hearing group reported that they spent "a lot of the day" or "most of the day" thinking about food and what their body image is." In addition, both groups indicated equal usage of diet pills, skipping meals, relying on liquid dieting, and binge eating to control their weight (Fletcher, 1993, p. 5).

Eating disorders have recently been recognized as a problem experienced by adolescent and college-aged women. Although there are limited studies regarding the deaf population, those that do exist indicate that women who are deaf or hard of hearing experience the same concerns regarding body image and eating disorders as those who can hear. Additional research into this area needs to be conducted to insure that appropriate therapeutic techniques can be developed.

Alcohol and Substance Abuse and Deafness

Other forms of abuse that are prevalent in the Deaf community are substance and alcohol abuse. Like eating disorders, these can become an outward manifestation of sexual abuse; they can also develop as independent forms of abuse. Regardless of the cause, both are problematic areas that can escalate to a crisis stage and require intervention.

Throughout the 1960s and 1970s Americans experienced a period of marked increase in the use of illicit drugs. Responding to the social and political unrest evident at that time, many adolescents and young adults found refuge in marijuana, stimulants, and hallucinogens (Robinson & Green, 1988). Although this country has entered a new era, the use of psychoactive drugs continues to be prevalent among teenagers.

Psychoactive drugs act on the nervous system. They can alter the individual's state of consciousness, modify perceptions, and produce mood-altering effects. Furthermore, they can provide the person with pleasure-eliciting feelings of inner peace, joy, relaxation, kaleidoscopic perceptions, surges of exhileration, and prolonged heightened sensations (Hales, 1999).

There are three main types of psychoactive drugs: depressants, stimulants, and hallucinogens. While depressants slow down mental and physical activity, stimulants increase the central nervous system's activity. Hallucinogens modify a person's perceptual experiences and produce visual images that are not real.

Depressants include alcohol; barbiturates, such as sleeping pills; and tranquilizers, such as Valium and Xanax, which are used to reduce anxiety and induce relaxation. Other depressants include opiates, which depress the central nervous system's activity.

Of all the forms of stimulants, one of the most widely used are found in amphetamines, frequently prescribed in diet pills. Referred to as "uppers" or "pep pills," they increase activity levels and pleasurable feelings when consumed. Other stimulants include cocaine and crack, an intensified form of cocaine that is usually smoked.

Hallucinogens include marijuana and LSD (lysergic acid diethylamide). The psychological effects of marijuana include a mixture of excitatory, depressive, and mildly hallucinatory characteristics, making it a difficult drug to classify. In contrast, LSD even in low doses produces striking perceptual changes. Objects change their shapes and glow, marvelous images unfold, and bizarre scenes may appear. While these images may be pleasurable they can occasionally become grotesque (Santrock, 2000).

Beginning in 1975 at the Institute of Social Research at the University of Michigan, Lloyd Johnson, Patrick O'Malley, and Gerald Bachman began monitoring drug use by U.S. high school seniors enrolled in a wide variety of public and private high school programs. Their research reflects that although drug use in U.S. secondary school students declined in the 1980s, it increased in the early 1990s, reaching a peak in the mid 1990s (Johnson, O'Malley, & Bachman, 2000). Results of their survey further reveal that adolescent use of inhalents, hallucinogens (such as LSD), marijuana, and amphetamines reached peak levels in the mid-1990s. Additionally, their data revealed that in both 1999 and 2000 there was a drop in the use of crack cocaine among adolescents.

Although the use of some drugs has decreased, others have increased in popularity. Referred to as "club drugs" due to increased use in nightclubs and all-night dance parties also known as raves, Ecstasy and Rohyponol use has increased significantly among adolescents (Johnson, O'Malley, & Bachman, 2000). Ecstasy is a metamphetamine with hallucinogenic properties. Rohypnol, also known as a date rape drug, can induce amnesia of events that occur while under its influence.

Individuals experiment with drugs for a variety of reasons. For some it originates out of curiosity; for others it becomes a way of adapting to the daily stresses encountered in their environment. Still others feel compelled to use drugs because of peer pressure.

The use of psychoactive drugs for personal gratification and temporary relief of stress can quickly develop into drug dependence, personal and social disorganization, and a predisposition to serious and sometimes fatal diseases (Goldberg, 2000). When this occurs relationships can be destroyed and psychological and physical damage can develop, leading to major depression.

Prevalence of Alcohol and Substance Abuse

Of all of the drugs, alcohol is the most widely used by adolescents in our society. Furthermore, alcoholism is noted as the third leading killer in the United States, with more than 13 million people classified as alcoholic. Described as a disorder, alcoholism involves long-term, repeated, compulsive, and excessive use of alcoholic beverages that impair the drinker's health and social relationships (Santrock, 2000). Family studies conducted by Hannigan and colleagues (1999) report a high frequency of alcoholism in first-degree relatives of alcoholics. Additional research by Grant (1992) postulates that 9.6 percent of men and 3.2 percent of women in the United States will become alcohol dependent at some time in their lives, and many more will exhibit drinking behavior that can be classified as alcohol abuse.

Statistics produced by the National Household Survey on Drug Abuse (1992) indicate that more than 74 million Americans have used alcohol and drugs. Studies conducted by Johnson and Lock (1978) indicate that the prevalence of alcohol and drug use among deaf and hard of hearing individuals is comparable to that reported in the larger hearing community. According to McCrone (1983), there may be as many as 73,000 deaf alcoholics, 8,500 heroin users, 14,700 cocaine users, and 10,000 deaf people who use marijuana on a regular basis.

What are some of the characteristics of substance abuse? What do clinicians use to determine that an individual has transitioned from being a "casual user" to an "abuser," whereby he or she has become chemically dependent? Once these symptoms are identified, what treatment options are made available to them?

Characteristics of Chemical Dependency

The diagnostic criteria used to identify chemical dependency may include several or all of the following: loss of control, blackouts, increased tolerance to use, continued use despite negative consequences, preoccupation with use, intoxication throughout the day, and repeated attempts to quit or control use without success. When a person becomes dependent, drugs and alcohol become significantly more important than interpersonal relationships, performance at school or work, physical health, and the establishment of any and all life goals. Initially the person may use chemicals with few consequences; however, as time progresses use may increase, thus exacerbating existing problems. Considered a lifelong, chronic disease, it can be treated but not cured.

According to Guthman and Sandberg (1998), four characteristics can be attributed to chemical dependency. First, it is viewed as a primary disease that can contribute to physical illness, depression, and unresolved grief, all symptoms that cannot be treated until the person refrains from using mood-altering chemicals. Second, it is a progressive disease that when left untreated always becomes worse. Third, it is considered a chronic disease; therefore there is no cure. And fourth, it is a fatal disease, meaning that the person will die prematurely if it is not treated.

Research conducted by Schaefer (1996) indicates that the average life span of an alcoholic is 10 to 12 years shorter than someone who is not alcoholic. Furthermore, he posits that people with alcoholism are 10 times more likely to die from fires and five to 13 more times likely to die from falls. Also, when compared to nonalcoholics, they are six to 15 times more likely to commit suicide.

Substance abuse of any kind can have significant consequences for the person who is struggling with addiction. The far-reaching negative effects permeate all of the major life areas. According to Guthmann and Sandberg (1998), life areas particularly vulnerable to these adverse effects are the family structure, work/school environments, social interactions, physical illness, financial problems, and legal issues. Within these areas, several warning signs can be potential indicators of substance abuse, including:

- Failure to attend family functions
- Neglecting responsibilities
- Unexplained school or work absences
- Isolation, lack of friends, or change in friends
- Problems with teachers or students

- Arriving at school, home, or job under the influence of chemicals
- Frequent and unexplained illnesses
- Memory loss, blackouts, and hangovers
- Borrowing or stealing money
- Sudden weight loss or gain (Guthmann & Sandberg, 1998, p. 16)

Individuals exhibiting signs of alcohol or substance abuse are frequently referred to professionals for treatment. While some receive services in residential treatment facilities, others attend programs housed in community-based outreach centers. Although the approach to treatment may vary among programs, they all share in the common goal of rehabilitating the client. What types of treatment facilities are available to deaf consumers? What barriers, if any, do they face when entering treatment?

Treatment Strategies and Programs

Treatment programs specifically designed to accommodate deaf and hard-of-hearing consumers have only recently come to the forefront. According to Boros (1983), the first treatment program targeting the needs of the deaf population opened in 1973. Over the next decade additional programs were added. However, as of 1983 the total number of substance abuse treatment services in the United States for deaf clients was listed at 10 (Watson, 1983). Although the country has experienced a growth in additional service programs, those designed to specifically meet the needs of this population are scarce.

Programs cited in the literature reflect a diverse range of services. While some programs, such as AID (Addiction Intervention for the Deaf) in Ohio primarily supply interpreting services for area hospitals, other programs, such as CCAIRU (Cape Cod Alcoholism Intervention and Rehabilitation Unit) Project for the Deaf, provide deaf consumers with a residential and an outpatient unit on Cape Cod. Here alcoholics who are deaf have the opportunity to participate in a program with their peers, confront their alcoholism, and potentially resolve any issues they have related to their deafness (Rothfield, 1981). Through individual counseling sessions and opportunities to attend AA meetings with hearing residents, this program is designed to prepare participants so they can transition back into their communities as self-sufficient, functioning individuals.

Additional programs, such as the St. Paul-Ramsey Hospital Mental Health Hearing-Impaired Program and the Minnesota Chemical Dependency Program for Deaf and Hard of Hearing Individuals (MCDPDHHI), provide inpatient services as a key function of their treatment programs. The program in Minnesota was established in 1989 and has served over 375 clients. Several articles have appeared in the literature regarding the extensive services that are provided on a daily basis.

Fostering a multidisciplinary approach, the MCDPDHHI utilizes the 12-step AA model as its therapeutic foundation. From the onset of the program, various assessments are conducted and a treatment plan is developed. Throughout the course of the treatment residents participate in chemical dependency education, coping and decision-making skills, individual and group therapy, occupational and recreational therapy, family therapy, and aftercare planning. In addition, deaf and hard-of-hearing residents have the opportunity to attend outside AA/NA meetings. Staff members involved with the program are fluent in American Sign Language (ASL) and are respectful of Deaf culture (Guthmann, 1999).

This program has been modified to meet the needs of the deaf population. A visual approach to learning and counseling is emphasized, and all information, therapeutic interaction, and other activities are adapted to meet the individual needs of the consumer. The 12-step model is built into the program thus providing the foundation for follow-up meetings that are routinely scheduled in communities throughout the country.

These programs, coupled with other interpreter services, have provided substance abusers who are deaf with some inroads into treatment programs throughout the nation. What are some of the barriers to recovery? How successful are these programs? What can be done to help reduce the prevalence of substance abuse within the Deaf community?

Barriers to Recovery

One of the most noticeable barriers to recovery is the small number of treatment centers that are equipped to treat deaf individuals with substance abuse. Although a few quality programs do exist, they are in the minority. This shortage of programs is not limited to small towns or rural areas. Frequently deaf individuals living in large cities may find that treatment programs in their geographic areas are also virtually nonexistent. Forced to drive considerable distances to access services, many give up before they have a chance to develop the required support system to remain drug free. A study conducted by the California Department of Alcohol and Drug Programs has indicated that 50 percent of deaf and hard-of-hearing persons were unable to find alcohol and other drug treatment services (Erickson & Lowe, 1998). According to Lane (1989) the deaf and hard-of-hearing population is scattered throughout the country, making it difficult to establish programs that will meet the needs of large groups of consumers.

A second barrier to recovery involves the limited number of professionals who are trained in deafness as well as in the treatment of substance abuse. Lacking cultural knowledge and communication skills, these professionals are unable to make spontaneous comments or engage in "spur of the moment" conversations without the use of an interpreter. This stymies many of the informal interactions that are often critical in any treatment program. Furthermore, these treatment programs are traditionally provided in the English language. Verbal sessions start early in the day and may continue late into the evening. Even when interpreting services are available, these sessions can be visually draining for the deaf consumer.

A third barrier stems from within the Deaf community. Within this community substance abuse is frequently viewed as a "moral weakness" rather than as a disease that requires treatment. As a result, the community rarely provides a supportive network to assist the deaf person who is an alcoholic or is addicted to drugs to further cope with the problem. Additionally, Deaf individuals may protect those who have an abuse problem and thus allow them to remain isolated within the community. In these instances denial may be prevalent and may hamper recovery efforts (Rendon, 1992).

A fourth barrier involves a trust issue. Many deaf and hard-of-hearing individuals have been either ignored, neglected, or patronized by their families and later by friends and professionals. Consequently they may be skeptical of dealing with hearing clinicians (Adler, 1983) and may avoid treatment altogether.

Success Rates of Treatment Programs

Very little has been published in the literature regarding the degree of success achieved at treatment programs for deaf substance abusers. Of the two published studies that address success rates, one indicates that deaf alcoholics recover at a higher rate than hearing alcoholics, with a 70 percent recovery rate in contrast to a 40 percent among hearing alcoholics (Hetherington, 1979). An additional study by Boros (1983) confirms similar findings. In order for treatment programs for deaf and hard-of-hearing individuals to be successful, it is critical that:

- Instructional materials are written on a level these individuals can comprehend.
- Materials are enhanced with visual illustrations as frequently as possible.
- Instruction allows them to assimilate the information, master the vocabulary, and then master the sign vocabulary that relates to the spoken message (Wentzer & Ohir, 1986).
- Individuals are given more time to assimilate all the information.
- Cross-cultural counseling techniques are provided.
- Individuals are allowed to focus on present issues rather than on childhood experiences, abstract thoughts, or hearing loss (Cassell & Darmsted, 1986).
- Services are conveyed through qualified interpreters who are perceptive to the differences between nonmanual markers (an important grammatical feature of ASL) and body language.
- Programs are sensitive to the communities where recovering alcoholics will be residing after treatment to further assist individuals in securing an appropriate living environment.

Although this list is not comprehensive, it presents some of the key components that may be beneficial to treatment programs.

Prevention: Taking Steps to Reduce Drug and Alcohol Abuse

Deaf individuals are as vulnerable as hearing individuals are to developing substance abuse problems. While some professionals have placed their energies into recovery programs, others are focusing their attention on preventative measures. Although these programs may vary in nature, the majority of the contemporary treatment programs focus on three goals: primary, secondary, and tertiary prevention. The greatest emphasis is targeted at primary and tertiary prevention.

Primary prevention attempts to stop people from taking drugs by helping them not to start. These programs are initiated with elementary school children to encourage children to abstain from using drugs. Respected role models are used to advocate for abstinence and children are taught how to resist peer pressure (Pentz, 1994).

Secondary prevention works with high school students in an attempt to minimize the harm that is caused by drug use. Targeted individuals are those who may be involved with experimental or occasional use of illicit drugs. These programs also emphasize the hazardous consequences of drinking and driving. Secondary prevention programs further provide crisis counseling and drug abuse counseling for individuals whose drug use has gone beyond experimental or occasional use.

Tertiary prevention consists of the treatment for people who abuse drugs. These programs focus on medical treatment, residential facilities, and rehabilitation. At this level many of the treatment programs previously discussed are employed.

According to Steitler (1984), a variety of steps can be taken to work toward the prevention of substance abuse among deaf persons. Through identification of potential abusers at an early age, preventive measures can be instigated, thus allowing educators and counselors to intervene.

On a tertiary level Rothfield (1983) recommends that deaf counselors be hired at treatment centers for deaf substance abusers. By fostering ease in communication and providing consumers with positive role models, counseling can become more effective. Frequently, deaf substance abusers label themselves as failures and thus sever ties with the community. Increased feelings of self-worth can help the client develop enhanced feelings of self-confidence and self-competence.

Summary

Sexual, drug, and alcohol abuse can strike at the heart of any community, affecting individuals from all walks of life and all socioeconomic backgrounds. Influenced by cultural, social, and psychological factors, some individuals seem to be more susceptible to abuse than others. Although some individuals recognize they have a problem and actively seek help, others remain in denial for extended periods of time and only receive services when family members or legal entities mandate that they receive therapy.

For many, counseling services are extremely beneficial and the person learns how to cope with the ramifications of abuse. However, for others, such as members of the Deaf community, services may be limited or nonexistent, thus minimizing the opportunities for recovery to occur. When services do exist, available professionals may be ill equipped to meet the needs of this population.

As more quality programs are developed, more deaf and hard-of-hearing individuals will have the opportunity to receive services. Furthermore, with these services in place, accessibility will become a reality instead of a rarity. These services, coupled with the elimination of the denial barriers established in the Deaf community, will allow for entry and effective treatment programs to be initiated.

12

Community Mental Health Agencies: Providing Services to Those Who Are Deaf

The delivery of mental health services has changed substantially since the early 1960s. Prompted by the Community Mental Health Center Act of 1963, the nation began to change its focus from providing long-term inpatient services to community-based facilities that stress outpatient care. This has been possible through the development of new medications that are effective in treating schizophrenia, and the funding of community mental health agencies.

Under the 1963 act, funds were allocated for the establishment of one mental health facility for every 50,000 individuals in the nation. These centers were designed to meet two basic goals: first, to provide community-based mental health services, and second, to commit resources to help prevent mental disorders as well as to treat them. Since their inception they have successfully helped large numbers of people with psychiatric problems, especially those living in low-income neighborhoods. (Seidman & French, 1998).

These centers have become part of the deinstitutionalization movement. Although some professionals voice support of this movement and of the centers in general, others view the situation less favorably. They contend that patients may be discharged too early from mental institutions, and that once released they frequently do not receive the psychotherapy they need. Furthermore, critics of the community-based model claim that some therapists limit their services to "young, attractive, verbal, intelligent, and successful clients (called YAVISes) rather than quiet, old, institutionalized, and different clients (called QUOIDs)" (Santrock, 2000). Although some mental health professionals have become sensitive to this problem, it has not been entirely solved.

Additional concerns related to the issue of deinstitutionalization have focused on the transitional period that occurs once the patient leaves the hospital setting. Some

270

mental health professionals contend that a number of patients are discharged too early from the hospital. They further note that they frequently do not have a place to go once they leave the institution and are therefore forced to join the ranks of the homeless.

What effect if any has this trend had on the provision of mental health services for persons who are deaf or hard of hearing? What types of treatment facilities have traditionally been available to this population? What modifications are necessary when designing the delivery of program services for those who can't hear? What standards should be maintained in order to insure the effective provision of mental health services?

A Brief Historical Overview

Prior to the 1950s deaf and hard-of-hearing individuals relied on a network of friends to discuss and find resolutions for mental health issues. Based on affiliations formed in schools for the deaf, Deaf clubs, and associations made at deaf athletic events, and through other social activities, a network was established through a mutual understanding of communication.

Individuals needing mental health services would frequent their churches if there was a minister who could sign, centers for independent living, vocational rehabilitation agencies, and specialized service centers for the deaf and hard of hearing. They would search for individuals who could communicate with them and who would understand their needs. Within these settings lay counselors and professionals trained in other fields of deafness provided them with some form of counseling services. According to Wax (1990), these professionals acted as a "bridge" to mental health services for this population.

As a result, few if any voluntarily sought out services from the mental health system. This was due in part to the services provided by these lay counselors, but also due to the grave misunderstandings that frequently existed when they attempted to communicate with professionals outside the field of deafness. Subjected to multiple barriers to communication, they quickly discovered that when they attempted to express their needs they were frequently misunderstood.

Reports reflecting the mislabeling or institutionalizing of deaf and hard-of-hearing individuals due to misunderstandings based on communication differences are prevalent in the literature. Furthermore, it is not uncommon to read anecdotes of deaf and hard-of-hearing people who have been mistakenly diagnosed as mentally retarded or mentally ill based on evaluations conduced by unskilled professionals (Myers, 1993).

Not until 1955 was a formal attempt was made to alleviate this problem. Under the direction of Dr. Franz Kallmann, the New York Psychiatric Institute initiated a program to serve the needs of deaf and hard-of-hearing consumers. Originating in 1955, the program served over 200 patients with varying degrees of hearing loss within a 10-year period. This initial work was followed in 1963 by the establishment of a new program housed in Washington, DC.

Originating under the guidance of Dr. Luther Robinson and under the direction of two psychiatrists, John Rainer and Kenneth Altshuler, a three-year pilot program was initiated at St. Elizabeth's Hospital in Washington, DC. The focus of this project was to provide comprehensive mental health services for deaf consumers on a regional basis.

A third program that merits mentioning began providing services specifically designed for the deaf and hard of hearing in 1967. At this time the Center on Deafness at the University of California, San Francisco, under the direction of Hilde Schlesinger, began providing outpatient services for persons who were deaf and hard of hearing.

These three programs were instrumental in setting the stage for the establishment of future mental health services. As a result, a number of other states began to set up programs and by 1976, 13 state hospitals were serving deaf and hard-of-hearing patients (Goulder, 1977). Although there continues to be an insurgence of programs designed to serve the needs of this population, significant gaps in services remain. According to Steinberg (1991), mental health services provided to deaf consumers are sparse, and in most areas the mental health service needs of U.S. deaf people remain profoundly underserved. Furthermore, the development of services is frequently delayed based on the low incidence of deaf and hard-of-hearing people in most geographic locations.

Statistics reported by Nickless (1993) indicate that there are approximately 3,500 chronically mentally ill deaf individuals and 212,000 hard-of-hearing mentally ill individuals residing in our country. However, only 15 percent of them receive treatment in psychiatric facilities (Shadish, 1989). Further estimates indicate that it is a probability that there are approximately 3,000 deaf mentally ill and approximately 180,200 hard-of-hearing mentally ill living in our communities. Of this total, it is estimated that only 2 percent receive any type of mental health services (Gerstein, 1988).

According to Myers (1993), there is tremendous variability in both the quality and the quantity of services provided throughout the states. Upon surveying all the mental health centers in one state, McEntee (1993) discovered that 29 percent of the 28 respondents directly indicated that they were not accessible to deaf people. In addition, 39 percent stated that they did not provide interpreters, even though 72 percent of the agencies indicated that they had served deaf individuals; of the 72 percent, only 25 percent employed certified interpreters.

Although federal legislation is in effect today through Section 504 of the Rehabilitation Act of 1973 and Title II of the 1990 Americans with Disabilities Act, mandating that all states provide the same mental health services to all people, they do not specify what equal mental health services are. Therefore, many agencies remain inaccessible to deaf and hard-of-hearing consumers. Of those that do provide services, several do not meet the standards set forth in the *Standards of Care for the Delivery of Mental Health Services to Deaf and Hard of Hearing Persons* outlined by Myers

(1993). What do these standards entail? Where should they be implemented? Why do agencies fall short of meeting the standards?

Standards of Care Recommendations for Accessibility

When designing mental health programs for deaf and hard-of-hearing consumers or when adapting existing programs to meet the special needs of this population, three broad areas should be examined: communication accessibility, familiarity with cultural differences, and technological availability. Each of these components merits further discussion.

Communication Accessibility

Ideally, when designing programs to meet the needs of this diverse group of individuals, it is essential to consider the wide wage of communication techniques embraced by the deaf and hard-of-hearing population. Once identified, appropriate strategies can be implemented to insure these needs are met.

Communication accessibility includes hiring administrative assistants and trained professionals in the mental health field who are sensitive to the speech patterns of the oral deaf and who are also fluent in American Sign Language (ASL), the various sign systems, home signs, and regional sign dialects. These professionals serve a dual role: they are knowledgeable in their field and they are also qualified to meet the specific communication needs of deaf and hard-of-hearing consumers.

When mental health professionals do not possess these communication skills the services of a sign language or an oral interpreter may be needed. A directory of certified interpreters can be obtained by contacting the National Registry of Interpreters for the Deaf. These professionals are trained to facilitate communication between deaf and hearing consumers. Furthermore, they are skilled in assessing the client's communication needs and adjusting their communication style to meet the client's preferences (Leigh et al., 1996). Certified interpreters are bound by a code of ethics whereby they maintain confidentiality and professional standards.

In addition to the individual's interpreting credentials it is beneficial if the interpreter has previously been employed in mental health settings. Those unfamiliar with the mental health process may find it advantageous to work with the therapist prior to the scheduled session to discuss mental health paradigms and expectations.

Clinicians should avoid relying on family members for interpreting services. In the event family members are used in this capacity the psychologist runs the risk of critical information being misconstrued or eliminated. Furthermore, it places the client in an awkward position since he or she may not be comfortable discussing sensitive topics in the presence of family members.

Communication accessibility also entails becoming familiar with the ramifications of deafness and recognizing functional reading and writing levels for what they represent. It is well documented in the literature that the average reading level of those who cannot hear is well below that of hearing individuals. It is critical to keep in mind that the individual may possess a wide range of English skills; however, these skills are not necessarily indicative of functional literacy and should thus be treated accordingly (Marschark, 1993).

Additionally, mastery of written skills should be viewed as a separate entity. Although some deaf and hard-of-hearing clients prefer to speak for themselves and have relatively good speech, they may not necessarily have a command of the other forms of the English language. Caution should be taken when encountering these individuals. The clinician should always bear in mind that although some clients present themselves effectively in a conversational domain, these skills have not automatically transferred into the literate domain.

Cultural Differences

By developing a comprehensive understanding of the cultural characteristics and social differences of Deaf individuals, the clinician can incorporate effective strategies into his or her treatment plan. These characteristics include the use of eye contact and physical proximity, attention-getting maneuvers, and greeting and parting rituals.

Furthermore, there is evidence to suggest that cultural differences exist within the area of privacy and confidentiality. The view that Deaf community members maintain regarding what are considered appropriate behaviors may differ significantly from behaviors that are ingrained in mainstream U.S. culture (Steinberg, 1991). Additionally, culture is reflected in communication preference and educational background (residential versus mainstreamed and included programs.)

Those exploring cultural differences must also investigate whether the individual has hearing or deaf parents. Keeping in mind that this is a heterogeneous group, and that the origins of our culture stem from out parents, those with deaf parents will in all likelihood identify with the Deaf community and will have established a Deaf identity. However, deaf children who have hearing parents may or may not develop an affiliation with the Deaf community and may therefore be oblivious to the cultural expectations of this community. Therefore, it is essential to determine if the deaf client has established a primary identity with the hearing community or if he or she has developed a Deaf identity.

When designing quality programs it is critical that cultural norms found within both hearing and deaf communities are recognized. Furthermore, it is essential to become cognizant of how these cultural norms and behaviors interact. Cultural awareness involves being sensitive to the differences between Deaf and Hearing communities. It also entails becoming aware of the ethnic differences that may be present. Ethnicity plays a central role in cultural development and frequently falls in the shadow of deafness. It is imperative that these differences are recognized because they also play an integral role in social and cultural development. In essence, the deaf individual can be characterized as reflecting tricultural behaviors that represent all three of the various cultural groups of which they are part (ethnicity, Deaf culture, and U.S. culture). Concomitantly, these are interwoven into one total composite that must be acknowledged before appropriate services can be administered.

Technological Accessibility

Treatment facilities designing programs to meet the needs of deaf and hard-of-hearing consumers should become cognizant of the technology that is available to this population. This is particularly critical in residential care facilities where lighting systems are required to inform residents of impending emergencies.

Lights incorporated into smoke detectors serve as warning devices and thus alert deaf individuals of potential fires. Lights are also used in conjunction with doorbells, telephones, and alarm clocks, providing a visual representation of auditory sounds. This equipment affords deaf individuals the opportunity to function independently within the confines of residential settings.

In addition, it is critical that both state-supported hospitals and community-based mental health agencies purchase telecommunication devices for the deaf. Commonly referred to as TTY, by the Deaf community and TDD by the hearing community, these telephones allow deaf consumers to have equal access to telephone capabilities.

The nationwide 24-hour-a-day telecommunications relay service came into existence in 1993. Through this service teletext users are able to contact nonteletext users through statewide relay services. Mandated by the Americans with Disabilities Act (ADA) in 1990, public agencies receiving federal funds were required to purchase equipment to enable them to provide this accommodation.

Telecommunication devices serve a vital role for patients residing in institutional settings, allowing them to remain in contact with their families and friends. Furthermore, they provide deaf and hard-of-hearing consumers in community-based mental health programs with a mechanism whereby they can call and schedule appointments or talk to clinicians.

While some hard-of-hearing individuals rely on a TTY for communication purposes, others require an amplified handset. By enabling the individual to adjust the volume control, those who have mild losses as well as some of those with moderately severe losses can frequently converse on the phone through this type of equipment. Amplified handsets as well as TTYs should be purchased by agencies serving this population.

Hearing professionals working with deaf and hard-of-hearing individuals should also become familiar with cochlear implants and other hearing aid technology. By developing an awareness of what an implant or an aid can and cannot do, the clinician can establish realistic expectations not only about the equipment but also the individual who is wearing it.

Occasionally when mental health personnel observe a hearing aid, they assume that the individual can hear through the aid and that all that is required is that they speak louder. They fail to recognize that some individuals with profound hearing losses wear hearing aids solely to alert them to loud environmental sounds. In these instances it is critical that professionals recognize the function of these hearing aids. They do not serve to amplify speech, and therefore the barriers to spoken communication still remain.

Regardless of the type of setting where mental health services are provided, it is essential that trained professionals in the field of deafness be employed to meet the needs of the deaf. When qualified personnel provide these services, deaf and hard-of-hearing individuals have an optimum opportunity to experience growth and become psychologically healthy individuals.

What typically happens in community-based mental health agencies when deaf consumers attempt to access services? How do hearing professionals respond? Are the needs of the deaf individuals generally met?

Community-Based Mental Health Agencies and Deaf Consumers

Community mental health centers are designed to provide a wide array of services. Generally staffed by mental health professionals, including social workers, counselors, itinerant psychiatrists, and psychologists, these individuals work directly with those requiring services. Clientele served at community agencies include individuals who have been released from inpatient programs as well as community members who require counseling and therapy.

While some agencies provide classes in anger management and conflict resolution, others provide group counseling sessions for victims of domestic violence and sexual abuse, as well as sessions for those struggling with issues related to drug and substance abuse. Furthermore, these agencies offer case management services, whereby they coordinate existing services within their agency with those provided by other agencies.

Some individuals frequent mental health centers on a monthly basis. During their scheduled appointment they may have their medication levels checked and their prescriptions refilled. Other clients arrive at the center on a daily basis. In addition to receiving counseling, they participate in day programs that emphasize the development of basic life skills. These individuals may participate in treatment for an extended period of time.

According to Dickens (1985), there is a fundamental barrier in place for persons who are deaf and are in need of mental health services. It centers on difficulties in communication and affects the clinician as well as the deaf consumer. In some respects, hearing clinicians who lack a basic understanding of this heterogeneous population create this. Furthermore, professionals reporting that they do not possess sign communication skills frequently exacerbate it. Conjuring up feelings of inadequacy, they may feel uncomfortable dealing with these individuals.

These feelings of inadequacy may manifest into what Schlesinger and Meadow (1972) have referred to as "shock-withdrawal-paralysis." In these instances highly qualified professionals may feel that their training is useless when they encounter deaf clients. Overwhelmed by a sense of powerlessness due to the barriers to communication, they forget they have been trained to deal with a variety of different populations. This prevents them from delivering the high-caliber services that they are fully competent of administering.

This barrier to communication is also cited as one of the primary reasons deaf consumers avoid treatment provided by community mental health agencies. Due to previous experiences many deaf consumers have developed a basic sense of distrust of hearing clinicians who cannot communicate with them through American Sign Language. Based on years of experience revolving around misunderstandings and breakdowns in communication, these individuals may be skeptical of working with hearing professionals. Furthermore, they may sense that their prior experiences with mental health professionals have been less than satisfactory.

A study conducted by Pollard (1994) determined that even when deaf and hard-of-hearing patients were served by community mental health centers, they had significantly less access to assessment and therapy. Instead they were provided with a disproportionate amount of case management and continuing treatment services. Pollard further indicates that a possible explanation for this emphasis rests with the fact that assessment and therapy are more communicatively demanding than case management and continuing treatment. As a result, even when the services have been made available, many of the programs remain inaccessible due to language and communication barriers (Gore & Critchfield, 1992).

A second barrier to treatment exists when mental health professionals overly depend on the hearing family of a deaf or hard-of-hearing client for assessment and direction (Dickens, 1985). Because most hearing clinicians lack information regarding the ramifications of deafness they may look to immediate family members for information. However, the majority of these families also lack this information. Therefore, the therapist may receive misinformation about the deafness as well as about available resources.

A third barrier that may prevent the delivery of successful counseling services can be attributed to the initial meeting between the therapist and the client. Deaf consumers frequently arrive for their first session unaware of why they have been referred and of what they can hope to accomplish. Hearing therapists may assume the deaf client has the same working knowledge as their hearing clients and therefore proceed with the session based on these beliefs. The deaf consumer may leave this initial meeting feeling confused, frustrated, and questioning why he or she was referred for services. Often these feelings culminate in a decision to refrain from returning and the therapeutic value of the counseling process is ended before it actually begins.

A variety of techniques can be incorporated to overcome these communication barriers. First and foremost, it is essential that an accurate assessment of the client's linguistic and abstraction skills be ascertained. Deaf consumers, like their hearing counterparts, vary in their knowledge base, capacity for insight, and abstractive abilities (DiFrancesca, 1972). Once this knowledge base is established, counselors can implement certain guidelines to enhance effective treatment strategies, including:

• Obtain feedback from the client on the reception of messages. This can be accomplished by asking the client to retell the information that has just been transmitted. Based on the client's rendition of the information the counselor can determine if the source message was indeed understood in the target message. Retelling is preferred over inquiring if the person understood. In these instances a "yes/no" response may follow. Often the deaf or hard-of-hearing individual will feign understanding to avoid embarrassment and will therefore agree to understandings that in reality do not exist. Deaf consumers may assume that all hearing people understand the information that is being presented and will therefore not want to admit they don't understand, thus risking the appearance of being "dumb or stupid."

• Use open-ended as well as close-ended questions. Some clients may have limited communication experience and questions such as "How do you feel about that?" may be met with by puzzled expressions and inappropriate responses. However, when mental health professionals offer some possibilities that reflect potential feelings (happy, angry, upset, sad, hurt, and so on), the client may be able to respond more clearly.

• Pay particular attention to facial expressions. It is critical that mental health professionals recognize that deaf consumers frequently rely on affirmative head nods as an attending behavior rather than as an indication of confirmation to the topic being discussed. Mental health workers should not assume that the client is understanding or is in agreement based on this communication behavior.

• Guard against inappropriate nonverbal responses. Practicing clinicians occasionally will laugh out of their own embarrassment when breakdowns in communication occur. These outbursts should be avoided because deaf clients may misinterpret the laughter as mockery about what they have said or how they have presented their ideas. Clinicians should also be aware of their facial expressions in general. Abrupt changes in expressions may need to be explained to the deaf consumer. Unlike those who can hear and can relate the inflection of the voice to the expression that is exhibited, deaf clients are restricted to their visual field. Therefore persons who are deaf or hard of hearing may need to receive an explanation for sudden changes in emotion.

• Avoid the use of slang, idioms, and clichés. Although some deaf clients will be very knowledgeable about these phrases, many more will not. When used on a repeated basis they serve to confuse and can create unnecessary misunderstanding. Furthermore, typical phrases that include the use of idioms and metaphors designed to increase the impact of a counseling interchange may not be understood. In these instances the effectiveness of the interchange is diminished. In addition, routine phrases such as "I know where you're coming from" and "I hear what you're saying" should also be omitted (Madanes, 1984).

- Agree to rewrite clinical forms, tests, and other written items that may present difficulties for the deaf consumer. When this is not possible, allow the interpreter to interpret the information to the client.
- Recognizing that the presence of an interpreter will change some of the dynamics of the counseling process will help clinicians adjust to this added dimension. The fact that eye contact will be maintained between the deaf consumer and the interpreter rather than between the deaf person and the clinician may cause some consternation on the part of the therapist. Accustomed to maintaining eye contact with the client, therapists may find it difficult to relinquish eye contact to another individual (Farrugia, 1989).

Deaf and hard-of-hearing consumers can also follow communication guidelines that will aid in the facilitation of services. Clients should be reminded of their communication rights as they enter therapeutic settings. This will enable them to request appropriate services and reap maximum benefit from therapeutic sessions. These rights include:

- Alert the mental health professional to their preferred mode of communication. Clinicians should be sensitive to the fact that some deaf and hard-of-hearing consumers who have excellent speech do not possess speechreading abilities. These are separate entities and must be considered as such. Deaf individuals who lose their hearing after speech is developed may be able to express themselves clearly when interacting with those who can hear. However, these same individuals may lack the ability to understand the hearing counselor and may need the services of an interpreter to equalize communication. Requests of this nature should be respected and an interpreter should be hired to facilitate communication between the therapist and the client.
- Inform practitioners of preferences for interpreting services. Although deaf consumers may not be able to select the interpreter of their choice, they should be aware that they should inform the clinician if they are uncomfortable with the interpreter who is selected. When sensitive issues are being discussed, it can be challenging to work through an interpreter; this can become a virtual impossibility if the consumer is not comfortable with the interpreter who has been hired. Although the person's skills may be excellent, if the consumer is uncomfortable with the individual, he or she may withhold critical information to the counseling process.
- Inform practitioners when they do not comprehend information.
- Make sure they, as deaf consumers, understand the nature of the problem that has been diagnosed and clearly understand the recommendations that are being made for their care.
- Develop a clear understanding of the medication they have been given and the potential side effects of the prescribed medications.

The more knowledgeable deaf and hard-of-hearing consumers are regarding their existing condition, the more active role they can play in the treatment process. Those who arrive for treatment with an understanding of their problems and an awareness of the counseling process are better equipped to benefit from the experience.

Recognizing Traditionally Underserved Persons Who Are Deaf

Within the population of deaf and hard-of-hearing people a group referred to as the traditionally underserved may request mental health services. Previously referred to as "low functioning, minimally language skilled, developmentally delayed deaf, lower achieving, and multiply handicapped" (Dowhower & Long, 1992), these individuals comprise a significant portion of the congenitally deaf population (Nash, 1991).

These individuals are characterized as exhibiting severe communication deficits in all modalities (sign, reading, writing, speech, and speechreading). Furthermore, they are perceived as having concomitant deficits in the areas of "vocational readiness, independent living, social skills, and academic achievement" (Long, 1995). Unable to obtain or maintain competitive employment without assistance, they are frequently unemployed. They may experience difficulty carrying out daily living tasks independently, while exhibiting poor social skills including aggressive and impulsive behavior, a low frustration level, and below average problem-solving skills.

Traditionally underserved persons who are deaf frequently drop out of high school or complete their course of study with a certificate of attendance rather than a high school diploma. Nash (1991) conducted a review of demographic studies and discovered that deaf youths drop out of school twice as often as their hearing peers. His review indicted that the dropout rate for deaf students was between 28 and 32 percent. Studies conducted by Harnisch, Lichtenstein, and Langford (1986) indicate that 19 percent of deaf students exited high school with a certificate of completion and not a diploma. They further reported that only 52 percent of this population left high school with a diploma.

Similar findings have been reported from the Commission on Education of the Deaf (COED, 1988). The commission has estimated that over 60 percent of deaf students leaving high school do not possess the skills or the abilities they need to succeed at the postsecondary level. They estimate that this number increases by approximately 2,000 individuals annually with the matriculation of deaf high school students.

These individuals frequently enter the mental health system and request services. A survey of social service agencies in the Pacific Northwest revealed that 90 percent of deaf persons being served within the mental health settings were identified as low achieving (Mathay & Lafayette, 1990). These individuals have special needs that must be considered prior to establishing effective mental health services. They present a particular challenge to professionals and they strive to provide appropriate services for them.

Providing Services

Clients who are characterized as being part of the traditionally underserved population present further communication challenges to the clinician. In addition to employing a skilled interpreter to facilitate communication, practitioners may find themselves in need of a Certified Deaf Interpreter (CDI). These individuals are deaf and are fluent in a variety of visual/gestural modes of communication as well as American Sign Language. They serve as intermediary or relay interpreters and work in conjunction with other hearing interpreters who are nationally certified. Through this team approach a more accurate exchange of information may be possible.

These clients may have minimal insights into their needs and may rely on clinicians to provide them with goal setting and a course of action. Professionals working with this population may find that it is beneficial to observe the client within his or her environment. By gaining an understanding of the specific skills that are required for daily living experiences, a treatment plan can be devised to cover these objectives.

Psychologists, psychiatrists, and other mental health workers should be sensitive to the limited effectiveness of paper-and-pencil inventories and projective personality tests. These instruments are difficult to administer to this population and frequently do not elicit accurate results.

According to Long (1995), recommended assessment activities for the traditionally underserved population include following a highly functional and ecologically based model. Once specific goals are delineated a team of professionals including educators, vocational rehabilitation counselors, and independent living specialists may need to collaborate with mental health providers to insure that an appropriate treatment plan can be designed. (See Chapter 8 for an in-depth discussion of assessment.)

Contemporary Problems of Service Delivery

Community mental health centers are established to serve geographic catchment areas. Thus, individuals living within the confines of a particular region are expected to access services in their area. According to Vernon and Andrews (1990), this concept works in direct opposition to best practices when meeting the needs of deaf and hard-of-hearing consumers. They cite three reasons why regional centers are counterproductive for this population.

First, community mental health centers tend to isolate deaf patients from one another. Due to a general lack of knowledge, deaf and hard-of-hearing individuals may feel they are the only individual with a hearing loss who experiences any form of mental illness. Recognizing that other individuals with a loss are capable of feeling the way they do can alleviate some of these feelings of isolation.

The second reason cited for these agencies being counterproductive is that they periodically require deaf and hard-of-hearing clients to frequent agencies where there might not be adequate services. The third reason these centers may fail to meet the deaf consumers' needs is that Deaf individuals may view the Deaf community as their primary means of support and thus gravitate to ministers and vocational rehabilitation counselors for mental health services.

Some community mental health centers have made a concerted effort to meet the specific needs of this population and have designed specialized programs that focus on specific areas of treatment. These programs employ professionals who are qualified to serve deaf clients. Furthermore, if those providing direct mental health services do not possess the communication skills they need to interact freely, the services of an interpreter are obtained. Although these programs serve a vital role in the provision of outpatient services, they can become a catchment center for deaf individuals who display various mental health needs.

It should be noted that even when certified interpreters are employed, very few of them have received formal training for specific work in mental health settings. Therefore, it is imperative that other members of the mental health team provide them with background information that will further assist them in facilitating communication.

According to Pollard (1994), deaf patients may be sent to community agencies where the communication barrier has been eliminated. However, little regard is given to the deaf client's mental health needs and to whether the agency is designed to meet these needs. Rather, communication takes precedence over the preexisting mental health condition and deaf and hard-of-hearing clients may find themselves in treatment programs that are not applicable to their needs. Because deaf individuals experience the same array of mental health needs as hearing individuals, they should be treated in programs that are designed to meet their specific forms of mental illness.

Although some deaf and hard-of-hearing clients accessing services at community mental health centers are there because they have been referred by professionals in the community, others arrive for follow-up services after being discharged from residential treatment programs. Upon exiting inpatient programs many will return to their families. While this is a positive arrangement for some, for others it may prove less than satisfactory.

Faced with communication difficulties that are often exacerbated by mental illness, a number of these deaf individuals may find that they need to secure an alternative living environment. In the process of locating new living arrangements these individuals may find that they are homeless. In a study of the available services for deaf and hard-of-hearing clients in South Carolina, Gore and Critchfield (1992) discovered that the numbers of deaf and hard-of-hearing individuals who are also homeless is on the increase. Faced with a limited number of housing options, many find they cannot afford housing while seeking mental health treatment. This presents an added dimension that must be considered when establishing programs for this population.

Mental Health Service Delivery Systems

During the past two decades there has been a proliferation of articles dealing with mental illness and the mental health needs of deaf and hard-of-hearing individuals. Within this body of literature several service delivery systems for providing different types of programs have been delineated. These services were grouped into three models at the first national Mental Health/Deaf Services State Coordinator conference in 1994. The three models were defined as follows:

- **Level I (basic access) capability.** Services provided at this level are basic in nature. Although TDD/TTY accessibility is in place, specialized services are available on contract and primarily include interpreters and communication specialists. The primary staff working at these facilities is responsible for activating support services.
- **Level II (basic access with signing staff support) capability.** Services provided at this level include all services from Level I with the addition of mental health and deaf service professionals being employed by the agency.
- **Level III capability.** This level includes all of the services of Level I and Level II plus full communication and cultural access. At this level all staff persons possess cultural knowledge and sign language skills that have been determined to be at and intermediate or an advanced level.

Future Directions: Focusing on Program Implementation

The mental health needs of deaf and hard-of-hearing individuals parallel the needs of those who can hear. The basic principles of therapy remain the same—there are only differences in the method of implementation, primarily due to the manner whereby deaf and hard-of-hearing individuals receive and conceptualize information (Anderson & Watson, 1985; Patterson & Stewart, 1971).

Although there has been an improvement in mental health services since the 1950s, there remain areas that need modification in order that they can be fully accessible. What can be done to improve community-based mental health services for deaf and hard-of-hearing consumers? What strategies can be implemented that will further equalize and enhance services? Several recommendations for the improvement of service delivery are:

- Provide the deaf community with general information regarding mental health issues and treatment options. Frequently, these individuals are unaware of what constitutes a problem and, once the problem is identified, where to go for help.
- Dispell the myth that surrounds mental illness in the deaf community, thus actively working to eliminate stigmas associated with diagnoses.
- Train crisis intervention team members and first responders to the specific needs of this population.
- Install TTY equipment and train staff on how to use telecommunication devices for the deaf so they can interact with deaf consumers.
- Provide in-service training for agency personnel so they have a heightened awareness as to the needs of this heterogeneous population.

- Provide community-based mental health agencies with interpreting services and itinerant mental health professionals to meet the scheduled needs of deaf and hard-of-hearing consumers.
- Design early intervention programs for families with deaf children, thus reducing the need for inpatient services at a later date.
- Acquaint practitioners with the complexities of American Sign Language and the cultural patterns of those who embrace the language.
- Refer deaf and hard-of-hearing clients to treatment centers that have programming to meet their specific mental health needs, rather than programs that have individuals who can communicate with them.
- Promote the training of more deaf mental health professionals to work within this field.
- Remove catchment restrictions, allowing deaf and hard-of-hearing consumers to take advantage of specialized programs that will meet their needs.
- Establish and deliver mental health services out of deaf service centers to make them more culturally accessible.
- Provide in-service training in ethnic diversity and the ramifications of deafness to insure that both contingencies are considered when designing treatment plans.
- Educate mental health professionals to the qualifications and benefits of employing sign language interpreters.
- Develop interagency collaborative agreements to assist in the diagnosis and assessment of deaf and hard-of-hearing clients.
- Provide life skills training for those requesting mental health services in conjunction with other therapeutic services.

Summary

Deaf and hard-of-hearing individuals arrive at the doors of community mental health agencies in need of a wide variety of program services. Although some receive quality services, others are confronted with communication barriers and a staff that is ill-equipped to meet their needs. Met by hearing clinicians who are unfamiliar with their language and culture, they may quickly develop feelings of distrust, thus establishing another barrier to treatment.

Strides are being made to improve existing services and establish treatment programs as states gain insights into the unique cultural and communication needs of this population. Furthermore, deaf individuals are enrolling in graduate counseling programs, thus preparing them to become future clinicians. All of these factors are working in tandem to improve the overall mental health services for deaf and hard-of-hearing persons.

References

Abood, D.A., & Chandler, S.B. (1997). Race and the role of weight, weight change, and body dissatisfaction in eating disorders. *American Journal of Health Behavior, 21,* 21–25.

Adler, E.P. (1983). Vocational rehabilitation as an intervenor in substance abuse services to deaf people. In D. Watson, K. Steitler, P. Peterson, & W. Fulton (Eds.), *Mental health substance abuse and deafness.* Silver Spring, MD: ADARA.

Ainsworth, M.D. (1979). Infant-mother attachment. *American Psychologist, 34,* 932–937.

Aitken, S. (Ed.). (2000). *Teaching children who are deafblind: Contact, communication and learning.* London: David Fulton.

Allen, T.E. (1986). Patterns of academic achievement among hearing-impaired students. In A.N. Schildroth & M.A. Karchmer (Eds.), *Deaf children in America* (pp. 161–206). Austin, TX: Pro-Ed.

Allen, T.E. (1989). *Deaf students and the school-to-work transition.* Baltimore: P.H. Brookes.

Allen, T.E. (1994). *Who are the deaf and hard of hearing students leaving school and entering postsecondary education?* Paper submitted to Pelavin Research Institute as part of the project. A comprehensive evaluation of the postsecondary educational opportunities for students who are deaf and hard of hearing funded by the U.S. Office of Special Education and Rehabilitative Services.

Allen, T., & Osborn, T. (1984). Academic integration of hearing-impaired students: Demographic, handicapping, and achievement factors. *American Annals of the Deaf, 129,* 100–113.

Allgeier, E.R., & Allegeier, A.R. (2000). *Sexual interactions.* Boston: Houghton Mifflin.

Allport, G.W. (1955). *Becoming basic considerations for a psychology of personality.* New Haven: Yale University Press.

Allport, G.W. (1965). *Pattern and growth in personality.* New York: Holt, Rinehart, & Winston.

Allport, G. (1985). The historical background of social psychology. In L. Gardner (Ed.), *Handbook of social psychology,* Vol. 1. New York: Random House.

Altman, E. (1988). *Talk with me: Giving the gift of language and emotional health to the hearing impaired child.* Washington, DC: AGB Association for the Deaf.

Altshuler, K.Z. (1971). Studies of the deaf: Relevance to psychiatric theory. *American Journal of Psychiatry, 127,* 1521–1526.

Altshuler, K.Z. (1974). The social and psychological development of the deaf child: Problems, their treatment and prevention. *American Annals for the Deaf, 119,* 365–376.

Altshuler, K.Z., & Abdullah, S. (1981). Mental health and the deaf adult. In L. Stein, E. Mindel, & T. Jabaley (Eds.), *Deafness and mental health.* New York: Grune & Statton.

American Association for Protecting Children. (1986). Highlights of official child neglect and abuse reporting: 1984. Denver: American Human Association.

American Psychiatric Association. (1994). *Diagnostic and statistical manual of mental disorders* (4th ed.). Washington, DC: Author.

Anastasi, A., & Urbina, S. (1997). *Psychological testing.* Upper Saddle River, NJ: Prentice Hall.

285

Anderson, R., & Sisco, F. (1997). *Standardization of the WISC-R performance scale for deaf children* (Series T, No. 1). Washington, DC: Gallaudet College Office of Demographic Studies.

Anderson, G., & Watson, D. (Eds.). (1985). *Counseling deaf people: Research and practice.* Little Rock: University of Arkansas, Arkansas Rehabilitation Research & Training Center on Deafness & Hearing Impairment.

Andrews, J.F. (1984). *How do young deaf children learn to read? A proposed model of deaf children's emergent reading behaviors.* Technical Report No. 329. Champaign: University of Illinois: Center for the Study of Reading (ERIC Document Reproduction Service No. ED 250674).

Andrews, J.F., & Mason, J. M. (1991). Strategy usage among deaf and hearing readers. *Exceptional Children, 57,* 536–545.

Ansuinic, R. Fiddler-Woite, J., & Woite, R. (1996). The source, accuracy, and impact of initial sexuality information on lifetime wellness. *Adolescence, 31,* 283–289.

Antia, S.D. (1982). Social interaction of partially mainstreamed hearing-impaired children. *American Annals of the Deaf, 127,* 18–25.

Antia, S.D., & Dittillo, D.A. (1998). A comparison of the peer social behavior of children who are deaf/hard of hearing and hearing. *Journal of Children's Communication Development, 19*(2), 1–10.

Antia, S.D., & Kreimeyer, K.H. (1997). The generalization and maintenance of the peer social behaviors of young children who are deaf or hard of hearing. *Language, Speech and Hearing Services in Schools, 28,* 59–69.

Antia, S.D., Kreimeyer, K.H., & Eldridge, N. (1994). Promoting social interaction between young children with hearing impairments and their peers. *Exceptional Children, 60,* 262–275.

Armstrong, D.G., Henson, K.T., & Savage, T.V. (1997) *Teaching today: An introduction to teaching* (5th ed.) New York: Macmillan.

Asante, M.K., & Davis, A. (1989). Encounter in the interracial workplace. In M.K. Asante & W.K. Gudykunst (Eds.), *Handbook of international and intercultural communication* (pp. 374–391). Beverly Hills, CA: Sage Publications.

Asch, S., & Nerlove, H. (1960). The development of double function terms in children: An exploratory investigation. In B. Kaplan & S. Wapner (Eds.), *Perspectives in psychological theory: Essays in honor of Heinz Werner,* (pp. 47–60). New York: International Universities Press.

Asher, S.R. (1976). Children's ability to appraise their own and another person's communication performance. *Developmental Psychology, 12,* 24–32.

Asnis, G.M., & VanPraag, H.M. (1995). *Panic disorder.* New York: Wiley.

Atkinson, R.L., Atkinson, R.C., Smith, E.E. & Bem, D.J. (1990). *Introduction to Psychology* (10th ed.). New York: Harcourt, Brace, Jovanovich.

Baldwin, J. (1894/1968). *Mental development in the child and the race: Methods and processes.* New York: Kelley.

Bandura, A. (1965). Influences of models' reinforcement contingencies on the acquisition of imitative responses. *Journal of Personality and Social Psychology, 1,* 589–596.

Bandura, A. (1986). *Social foundations of thought and action.* Englewood Cliffs, NJ: Prentice-Hall.

Bandura, A. (1998). Self-efficacy. In H.S. Friedman (Ed.), *Encyclopedia of mental health* (Vol. 3). San Diego: Academic Press.

Bandura, A. (2000). Self-efficacy. In A. Kazdin (Ed.) *Encyclopedia of psychology.* Washington, DC, & New York: American Psychological Association & Oxford University Press.

Barnhartt, S.N., & Christiansen, J.B. (1996). Into their own hands. In L. Bragg (2001), *Deaf world.* New York: New York University Press.

Barres, B. (1992). Facing AIDS, parts I & II. *Hearing Health, 8*(2), 8(3).

Basilier, T. (1964). Surdophrenia: The psychic consequences of congenital or early acquired deafness. *Acta Psychiatrica Scandihavica, 40,* 362–372.

Bat-Chava, Y. (1993). Antecedents of self-esteem in deaf people: A meta-analytic review. *Rehabilitation Psychology, 38*(4), 221–234.

Bates, E., Bretherton, I., Beeghley-Smith, M., & McNew, S. (1982). Social bases of language development: A reassessment. In H.W. Reese & L.P. Lipsett (Eds.), *Ad-*

vances in child development and behavior. (Vol. 16, pp. 7–75). New York: Academic Press.

Battle, D. (1998). *Communication disorders in multicultural populations* (2nd ed.). Boston: Butterworth-Heinemann.

Baugh, R. (1984) Sexuality education for the visually and hearing impaired child in the regular classroom. *JOSH, 54*(10), 407–409.

Bearison, D.J., & Levy, L.M. (1977). Children's comprehension of referential communication: Decoding ambiguous messages. *Child Development, 48,* 716–720.

Beazley, S. (1995). *Deaf children, their families and professionals: Dismantling barriers.* London: David Fulton Publishers.

Becker, R., Heimberg, R. & Bellack, A. (1987). *Social skills training: Treatment for depression.* New York: Pergamon Press.

Bell, A.R., Weinberg, M.S., & Hammersmith, S.K. (1981). *Sexual preference: Its development in men and women.* Bloomingham: Indiana University Press.

Bellenir, K. (2000). *Mental health disorders sourcebook.* Detroit: Omnigraphics.

Benderly, B.L. (1980). *Dancing without music.* Garden City, NY: Doubleday.

Bennett, L., Jr. (1966). *Before the Mayflower.* Baltimore: Penguin Books.

Bergin, D. (1988). Stages of play development. In D. Bergin (Ed.), *Play as a medium for learning and development.* Portsmouth, NH: Heinemann.

Bernal, G. (1982). Cuban families. In M. McGoldrick, J. Pearce, & J. Giordano (Eds.), *Ethnicity and family therapy,* pp. 187–207.

Berndt, T.J., & Perry, T.B. (1990). Distinctive features and effects of early adolescent friendships. In R. Montemayor (Ed.), *Advances in adolescent research.* Greenwich, CT: JAI Press.

Bernstein, D.K., & Tiegerman-Farber, E. (1997). *Language and communication disorders in children.* Boston: Allyn & Bacon.

Bienvenue, M.J., & Colonomos, Betty (1992). *An introduction to American Deaf culture, rules of social interaction workbook.* Riverdale, MD: Bicultural Center.

Bierstedt, R. (1963). *The social order.* New York: McGraw-Hill.

Billingsley, A. (1968). *Black families in white America.* Englewood Cliffs, NJ: Prentice-Hall.

Billingsley, A. (1974). *Black families in white America* (2nd ed.). Englewood Cliffs, NJ: Prentice-Hall.

Blackwell, P., Engen, E., Fischgrund, J., & Zarcadoolas, C. (1978). *Sentences and other systems: A language and learning curriculum for hearing-impaired children.* Washington DC: National Association of the Deaf.

Blennerhasset, L. (1990). Intellectual assessment. In D.F. Moores & K. Meadow-Orlans (Eds.), *Educational and developmental aspects of deafness* (pp. 255–280). Washington, DC: Gallaudet University Press.

Bloch, S. (1999). *Understanding troubled minds: A guide to mental illness and its treatment.* New York: New York University Press.

Bloom, L., & Lahey, M. (1978). *Language development and language disorders.* New York: Wiley.

Bochner, J. (1982). English in the deaf population. In D. Sims, G. Walter, & R. Whitehead (Eds.), *Deafness and communication.* Baltimore: Williams & Wilkins.

Bodner-Johnson, B., & Sass-Leher, M. (1996). *Concepts and premises in family school relationships. Pre-college national missions programs.* Washington, DC: Gallaudet University.

Bolander, A.M. (2000). *I was number 87: A deaf woman's ordeal of misdiagnosis, institutionalization, and abuse.* Washington, DC: Gallaudet University Press.

Borke, H. (1971). Interpersonal perception of young children: Egocentrism or empathy? *Developmental Psychology, 5*(2), 263–269.

Boros, A. (1983). Issues in treating deaf alcoholics within hospitals. In D. Watson, K. Steitler, P. Peterson, & W. Fulton (Eds.), *Mental health, substance abuse and deafness.* Silver Spring, MD: ADARA.

Bowers, L. (1998). *The social nature of mental illness.* London, New York: Routledge.

Bozik, J.M. (1985). *A study of egodevelopment and psychosocial adjustment in mainstreamed hearing impaired adolescents.* Unpublished doctoral dissertation, University of Pittsburgh.

Brackett, D., & Donnelly, J. (1982). *Hearing impaired adolescents' judgment of appropriate conversational entry points.* Paper presented at the American Speech-Language-Hearing Association Convention, Toronto.

Braden, J.P. (1994). *Deafness, deprivation, and IQ.* New York: Plenum Press.

Bradley-Johnson, S., & Evans, L. (1991). *Psychoeducational assessment of hearing-impaired students infancy through high school.* Austin TX: Pro-Ed.

Bragg, B. (1973). Amelish—Our American heritage: A testimony. *American Annals of the Deaf, 118,* 672–674.

Brauer, B. (1978). *Mental health and deaf persons: A status report.* Gallaudet Today.

Bretherton, I. (1991). Intentional communication and the development of an understanding mind. In D. Grye & C. Moore (Eds.), *Children's theories of mind.* Hillsdale, NJ: Lawrence Erlbaum Associates.

Brinton, B., Fujiki, M., Loeb, D., & Winkler, E. (1986). Development of conversational repair strategies in response to requests for clarification. *Journal of Speech and Hearing Research, 29,* 75–81.

Brody, L., & Harrison, R. (1987). Developmental changes in children's abilities to match and label emotionally laden situations. *Motivation and Emotion, 11,* 347–365.

Bronfenbrenner, U. (1986). Ecology of the family as a context for human development: Research perspectives. *Developmental Psychology, 22,* 723–742.

Bronfenbrenner, U. (1995, March). *The role research has played in Head Start.* Paper presented at the meeting of the Society for Research in Child Development, Indianapolis.

Brookhouser, P.E., Sullivan, P., & Scanlon, J.M. (1986). Identifying the sexually abused deaf child: The otolaryngologist's role. *Laryngoscope, 96,* 152–158.

Brown, H.D., & Adler, N.E. (1998). Socioeconomic status. In H.S. Friedman (Ed.), *Encyclopedia of mental health* (Vol. 3). San Diego: Academic Press.

Brown, L. (1995). Lesbian identities: Concepts and issues. In A. D'Augelli & C. Patterson (Eds.), *Lesbian, gay, and bisexual identities over lifespan: Psychological perspec-* tives (pp. 3–23). New York: Oxford University Press.

Brown, R. (1973). *A first language: The early stages.* Cambridge, MA: Harvard University Press.

Bruner, J. (1986). *Actual minds, possible worlds.* Cambridge, MA: Harvard University Press.

Buhrmester, D. (1996). Need fulfillment, interpersonal competence, and the developmental contexts of early adolescent friendships. In W.M. Bukowski, A.E. Newcomb, & W.W. Hartup (Eds.), *The company they keep: Friendship during childhood and adolescence* (pp. 158–185). New York: Cambridge University Press.

Byrne, D., & Schulte, L. (1990). Personality dispositions as mediators of sexual responses. *Annual Review of Sex Research, 1,* 93–117.

Byrne, M.R. (1998). Diversity within deaf or hard of hearing population: wisdom from seeing the whole. *Early Childhood Development and Care, 147,* 55–70.

CADS (1992–1993). *Inclusion statistics: 1992–1993.* Annual Survey. Website Center for Assessment and Demographic Studies. Washington, DC: Gallaudet University.

Calderon, R., Bargones, J.Y., & Sidman, S. (1998). Characteristics of hearing families and their young deaf and hard of hearing children: Early intervention follow-up. *American Annals of the Deaf, 143,* 347–362.

Cambra, C. (2000). A comparative study of personality descriptors attributed to the deaf, the blind, and individuals with no sensory disability. *American Annals of the Deaf, 141*(1), 24–28.

Campbell, R. (1992). *Mental lives: Case studies in cognition.* Oxford, UK & Cambridge, MA: Blackwell Publishers.

Cangelosi, J.S. (1997). *Classroom management strategies: Gaining and maintaining students' cooperation* (3rd ed.). White Plains, NY: Longman.

Canter, L., & Canter, M. (1976). *Assertive discipline: A take charge approach for today's educator.* Seal Beach, CA: Lee Canter & Associates.

Canter, L., & Canter, M. (1992). *Assertive discipline: Positive behavior management for today's schools* (rev. ed.). Santa Monica, CA: Lee Canter & Associates.

Carey, G., & Gottesman, I.I. (1981). Twin and family studies of anxiety, phobic, and obsessive disorders. In D.F. Klein & J. Rabkin (Eds.), *Anxiety: New research and changing concepts.* New York: Haven Press.

Carey, S. (1977). The child as a word learner. In M. Halle, J. Bresman, & G.A. Miller (Eds.), *Linguistic theory and psychological reality.* Cambridge, MA: MIT Press.

Carmel, S.J., & Monagham, L.F.(1991). Studying Deaf culture. An introduction to ethonographic work in deaf communities. *Sign Language Studies, 73,* 411–421.

Casby, M., & McCormack, S. (1985). Symbolic play and early communication development in hearing-impaired children. *Journal of Communication Disorders, 18,* 67–78.

Casillo, R. (1997). *Culture and mental illness: A client centered approach.* Pacific Grove: Brooks/Cole Publisher.

Cassell, J., & Darmsted, N. (1986). Signs for drug and alcohol use. In D. Watson, K. Steitler, P. Peterson, & W. Fulton (Eds.), *Mental health, substance abuse and deafness.* Silver Spring, MD: ADARA.

Cates, D.S., & Shontz, F.C. (1990). Role-taking ability and social behavior in deaf school children. *American Annals of the Deaf, 135,* 217–221.

Cates, J.A. (1991). Self-concept in hearing and prelingual, profoundly Deaf students. *American Annals of the Deaf, 136,* 354–359.

Cazden, C. (1998). *Classroom discourse: The language of teaching and learning.* Portsmouth, NH: Heinemann.

Center for Assessment and Demographic Studies. (1994). *Annual survey of deaf and hard of hearing youth, 1993–1994.* Washington, DC: Gallaudet University.

Centers for Disease Control and Prevention. (1997). *HIV/AIDS Surveillance Report, 9*(2), 1–43.

Centers for Disease Control and Prevention. (1998). *HIV/AIDS Surveillance Report, 9*(2), 5–43.

Chan, S. (1986). Parents of exceptional Asian children. In M.K. Kitano & P.C. Chinn (Eds.), *Exceptional Asian children and youth,* pp. 36–53. Reston, VA: Council for Exceptional Children.

Charles, C.M. (1999). *Building classroom discipline* (6th ed.). New York: Longman.

Cheng, L.L. (2002). Asian and Pacific American cultures. In D.E. Battle (Ed.), *Communication disorders in multicultural populations* (3rd ed.). Boston: Butterworth-Heinemann.

Cheskin, A. (1982). The use of language by hearing mothers of deaf children. *Journal of Communication Disorders, 15,* 145–153.

Chess, S., & Fernandez, P. (1980). Impulsivity in rubella deaf children: A longitudinal study. *American Annals of the Deaf, 125*(8), 998–1001.

Children's Defense Fund. (1994). *The state of America's children yearbook, 1994.* Washington, DC: Author.

Choitiner, N., & Lehr, W. (Eds.). (1976). *Child abuse and developmental disabilities.* A report from the New England Regional Conference.

Christensen, K.M., & Delgado, G.L. (Eds.) (1993). *Multicultural issues in deafness.* White Plains, NY: Longman.

Christopher, F.S., Johnson, D.C., & Roosa, M.W. (1993). Family, individual, and social correlates of early Hispanic adolescent sexual expression. *Journal of Sex Research, 30,* 54–61.

Christopher, F.S., & Roosa, M.W. (1990). An evaluation of an adolescent pregnancy prevention program: Is "Just Say No" enough? *Family Relations, 39,* 68–72.

Cicchetti, D., & Toth, S.L. (1998). Perspectives on research and practice in developmental psychology. In W. Damon (Ed.), *Handbook of child psychology* (Vol. 4). New York: Wiley.

Clark, M. (1989). *Language through living for hearing impaired children.* London: Hodder & Stoughton.

Cloninger, R. (Ed.). (1999). *Personality and psychopathology.* Washington, DC: American Psychiatric Press.

Cofer, C.N., & Appley, M.H. (1964). *Motivation: Theory and research.* New York: Wiley.

Cohen, B.S. (1991). *A comparison of self-concept scores in secondary-aged hearing-impaired students enrolled in mainstreamed and self-contained classes.* Unpublished doctoral dissertation, Pace University, New York.

Coie, J.D., & Dodge, K.A. (1998). Aggression and antisocial behavior. In N. Eisenberg (Ed.), *Handbook of childhood psychology: Vol. 3 Social, emotional, and personality development* (5th ed, pp. 779–862). New York: Wiley.

Coie, J.D., Dodge, K.A., & Copotelli, H. (1982). Dimensions and types of social status: A cross-age perspective. *Developmental Psychology, 18,* 557–570.

Cokely, D. (1983). When is a pidgin not a pidgin? An alternative analysis of the ASL-English contact situation. *Sign Language Studies, 38,* 1–24.

Coleman, L. (1985). Language and the evolution of identity and self-concept. In F. Kessel (Ed.), *The development of language and language research: Essays in tribute to Roger R. Brown.* Hillsdale: Lawrence Erlbaum Associates.

Coles, R. (1977). *Children of crisis: Vol. IV. Eskimos, Chicanos, Indians.* Boston: Little, Brown.

Coley, R.L., & Chase-Landsdale, P.L. (1998). Adolescent pregnancy and parenthood: Recent evidence and future directions. *American Psychologist, 53,* 152–166.

Commission on Education of the Deaf. (1988). *Toward equality: Education of the deaf.* Washington DC: U.S. Government Printing Office.

Conrad, R. (1979). *The deaf schoolchild: Language and cognitive function.* London: Harper & Row.

Cooley, C.H. (1909/1956). *Human nature and the social order.* Glencoe, IL: Free Press.

Coopersmith, S. (1967). *The antecedents of self-esteem.* San Francisco: W.H. Freeman.

Cormier, L.S., & Hackney, H. (1987). *The professional counselor: A process guide to helping.* Englewood Cliffs, NJ: Prentice-Hall.

Corsini, R. (1984). *Current psychotherapies.* Itasca, IL: Peacock Publications.

Corson, D. (1995). Worldview, cultural values, and discourse norms: The cycle of cultural reproduction. Special Issue. *Language, Culture, and Worldview. International Journal of Intercultural Relations, 19*(2), 183–195.

Coryell, W.H., et al. (1999). Polarity sequence, depression, and chronicity in bipolar I disorder. *Journal of Nervous and Mental Disease, 64,* 181–187.

Coyner, L. (1993a). Academic success, self-concept, social acceptance and perceived social acceptance for hearing, hard of hearing and deaf students in a mainstream setting. *JADARA, 27*(2), 13–20.

Coyner, L. (1993b). Comparison the relationship of academic success to the self-concept, social acceptance and perceived social acceptance for hearing, hard of hearing and deaf students in a mainstream setting. *JADARA, 27*(2), 13–20.

Craig, W., & Craig, H. (1987). Directory of services for the deaf. *American Annals of the Deaf, 132,* 81–127.

Critchfield, A.B. (1986). Psychometric assessment. In L.G. Stewart (Ed.), *Clinical rehabilitation assessment and hearing impairment: A guide to quality assurance.* Silver Spring, MD: National Association of the Deaf.

Crocker, J., & McGraw, K.M. (1983). Personal memory and causal attributions. *Journal of Personality and Social Psychology, 44,* 55–56.

Cuellar, I., & Paniagua, F. (Eds.) (2000). *Handbook of multicultural mental health: Assessment and treatment of diverse populations.* San Diego: Academic Press.

Cunningham, C., & Davis, H. (1985). *Working with parents.* Philadelphia: Open University Press.

Czuczka, D. (1999). The twentieth century: An American sexual history. *SIECUS Report, 28*(2), 15–18.

Damon, W. (1977). *The social world of the child.* San Francisco: Jossey-Bass.

Damon, W. (1988). *The moral child.* New York: Free Press.

Damon, W., & Hart, D. (1988). *Self-understanding in childhood and adolescence.* New York: Cambridge University Press.

Daniels, M. (1997). *Benedictine roots in the development of deaf education: Listening with the heart.* Westport, CT: Bergin & Garvey.

Danziger, K. (1971). *Socialization.* Harmondsworth, UK: Penguin.

Dapretto, M. (1999, April). *The development of word retrieval abilities in the second year of life and its relation to early vocabulary growth.* Paper presented at the meeting of the Society for Research in Child Development, Albuquerque.

Davis, J. (1986). Academic placement in perspective. In D. Luterman (Ed.), *Deafness in perspective* (pp. 205–224). San Diego: College Hill Press.

Davis, L.J. (2000). *My sense of silence: Memoirs of a childhood with deafness.* Urbana: University of Illinois Press.

Davis, R.A. (1993). *The black family in a changing black community.* New York: Garland Publishing.

Davison, G.C., & Neale, J.M. (2000). *Abnormal psychology* (8th ed). New York: Wiley.

Day, P. (1986). Deaf children's expression of communicative intentions. *Journal of Communication Disorders, 19,* 367–385.

Day, R.D. (1992). The transition to fast intercourse among racially and culturally diverse youth. *Journal of Marriage and the Family, 54,* 749–762.

DeBattista, C., Solvason, H.B., & Schatzberg, A.F. (1998). Mood disorders. In H.S. Friedman (Ed.), *Encyclopedia of mental health* (Vol. 2). San Diego: Academic Press.

DeBlassie, R.R., & Cowan, M.A. (1976). Counseling with the mentally handicapped child. *Elementary School Guidance and Counseling, 10,* 246–253.

Delgado, M. (1988). Groups in Puerto Rican spiritism: Implications for clinicians. In C. Jacobs & D. Bowels (Eds.), *Ethnicity and race: Critical concepts in social work* (pp. 71–83). Silver Spring, MD: National Association of Social Workers.

Denmark, J. (1994). *Deafness and mental health.* London; Bristal, PA: Jessica Kingsley Publishers.

Desselle, D.D. (1994). Self-esteem, family climate, and communication patterns in relation to deafness. *American Annals of the Deaf, 139,* 322–328.

deVilliers, J., deVilliers, P., Hoffmeister, R., & Schick, B. (1996). *The role of language in the thinking of Deaf children.* Proposal to NIH's national Institute on Deafness and Other Communicative Disorders, Washington, DC.

Diamond, M. (1993). Homosexuality and bisexuality in different populations. *Archives of Sexual Behavior, 22,* 291–310.

Dickens, D. (1985). Problems encountered by clinicians in providing services to deaf psychiatric patients. In G. Anderson & D.

Watson (Eds.), *Counseling deaf people: Research and practice.* Little Rock: University of Arkansas.

Dickinson, D., & Smith, M. (1994). Long-term effects of preschool teachers' book readings on low-income children's vocabulary and story comprehension. *Reading Research Quarterly, 29*(2), 104–122.

DiFrancesca, S. (1972). *Academic achievement test results of a national program for hearing impaired students.* Washington, DC: Office of Demographic Studies, Gallaudet College.

Dillard, J.M., & Reilly, R.R. (1998). Communication skills process approach to interviewing. In J.M. Dillard & R.R. Reilly (Eds.), *Systematic interviewing: Communication skills for professional effectiveness* (36–65). Columbus, OH: Merrill.

Dishon, T.J., & Li, F. (1996, March). *Childhood peer rejection in the development of adolescent problem behavior.* Paper presented at the meeting of the society for research on adolescence, Boston.

Dobosh, P., & Gutman, V. (1998). *Assessment and individual treatment issues with deaf survivors.* Paper presented at the World Conference on Mental Health and Deafness, Gallaudet University Press.

Dolnick, E. (September, 1993). Deafness as culture. *Atlantic Monthly,* 37–53.

Dowhower, D., & Long, N. (1992). What is traditionally underserved? *NIU-RTC Bulletin, 1*(2), 1–7.

Doyle, A.G. (1995). AIDS knowledge, attitudes and behaviors among deaf college students: A preliminary study. *Sexuality and Disability, 13*(2), 107–134.

Draguns, J.G. (1990). Applications of cross-cultural psychology in the field of mental health. In R.W. Brislin (Ed.), *Applied cross-cultural psychology.* Newbury Park, CA: Sage Publications.

Dusay, J.M., & Dusay, K.M. (1984). Transactional analysis. In R. Corsini (Ed.), *Current psychotherapies.* Itasca, IL: Peacock Publishers.

Ebert, M.H., Poosen, P. T., & Nurcombe, B. (2000). *Current diagnosis and treatment in psychiatry.* New York: Lange Medical Books/McGraw-Hill.

Eccles, J.S., Wigfield, A., & Schiefele, U. (1998). Motivation to succeed. In W. Damon (Ed.),

Handbook of child psychology (5th ed., Vol. 3). New York: Wiley.

Ekman, P. Friesen, W., & Ellsworth, R. (1972). *Emotion in the human face.* New York: Pergamon.

Elder, M. (1993). Deaf survivors of sexual abuse: A look at the issues. *Moving Forward Newsjournal, 2*(5). Retrieved 7/10/02 from the Internet: www.moving forward.org/v2n5-cover.html. Retrieved 6/10/01.

Elliott, H., Glass, L., & Evans, J.W. (1987). *Mental health assessment of deaf clients: A practical manual.* Boston: Little, Brown.

Ellis, A. (1984). Rational-emotive therapy. In R. Corsini (Ed.), *Current psychotherapies.* Itasca, IL: Peacock Publishers.

Emerton, R.G. (1996). Marginality biculturalism and social identity of deaf people. In I. Parasnis (Ed.), *Cultural and language diversity and the deaf experience* (pp. 136–145). New York. Cambridge University Press.

Epanchin, B., Townsend, B., & Stoddard, K. (1994). *Constructive classroom management.* Pacific Grove, CA: Brooks/Cole Publishing Company.

Erickson, J., & Lowe, L. (1988). *Summary and recommendations of the alcohol and drug services provided to disable, participants in California, 1988.* Sacramento: State of California Department of Alcohol and Drug Problems.

Evans, J.F. (1998). Changing the lens. *American Annals of the Deaf, 143*(3), 246–254.

Evans, J.W., & Elliott, H. (1981). Screening criteria for the diagnosis of schizophrenia in deaf patients. *Archives of General Psychiatry, 40,* 1281–1285.

Everhart, V.S., & Marschark, M. (1988). Linguistic flexibility in the written and signed/oral language productions of deaf and hearing children. *Journal of Experimental Child Psychology, 46,* 174–193.

Farrugia, D. (1988). Practical steps for access and delivery of mental health services to clients who are deaf. *Journal of Applied Rehabilitation Counseling, 20*(1), 33–35.

Farrugia, D., & Austin G. (1980). A study of the socio-emotional adjustment patterns of hearing-impaired students in different educational settings. *American Annals of the Deaf, 120,* 391–405.

Feinman, S. (1992). In the broad valley: An integrative look at social referencing. In *Social referencing and the social construction of reality in infancy.* New York: Plenum.

Fenson, L., Dale, P., Reznick, J.S., Bates, E., Thal, D., & Pethick, S. (1994). Variability in early communicative development. *Monographs of the Society for Research in Child Development, 59* (5, Serial No. 242).

Fenson, L., Dale, P., Reznick, J., Thal, D., Bates, E., Hartung, J. Pethick, S., & Reilly, J. (1993). *MacArthur communicative development inventories: User's guide and technical manual.* San Diego: Singular Publications.

Fey, M.E., Warr-Lepper, G., Webber, S.A., & Disher, L.M. (1988). Repairing children's repairs: Evaluation and facilitation of children's clarification requests and responses. *Topics in Language Disorders, 8,* 63–84.

Field, T. (2000). Child abuse. In A. Kazdin (Ed.), *Encyclopedia of psychology.* Washington, DC, & New York: American Psychological Association and Oxford University Press.

Finkelhor, D., & Browne, A. (1985). The traumatic impact of child sexual abuse: A conceptualization. *American Journal of Orthopsychiatry, 55*(4), 530–541.

Finkelhor, D., Hotaling, G., Lewis, I.A., & Smith, C. (1990). Sexual abuse in a national survey of adult men and women: Prevalence, characteristics, and risk factors. *Child Abuse and Neglect, 14,* 19–28.

Finkelhor, D., & Russell, D.E.H. (1984). The gender gap among perpetrators of child sexual abuse. In D.E.H. Russell (Ed.), *Sexual exploration: Rape, child sexual abuse, and work place harassment* (pp. 215–231). Beverly Hills, CA: Sage Publications.

Finn, G. (1995). Developing a concept of self. In *Sign language studies.* Silver Spring, MD: Linstock Press.

Fisher, T. (1986). Parent-child communication about sex and young adolescents' sexual knowledge and attitudes. *Adolescence, 21,* 517–527.

Fitz-Gerald, D., & Fitz-Gerald, M. (1976). Sex education survey of residential facilities for the deaf. *American Annals of the Deaf, 121*(5), 480–483.

Fitz-Gerald, D., & Fitz-Gerald, M. (1983). How to develop and implement a comprehensive sex education program for the deaf. *Perspectives for Teachers of the Hearing Impaired, 1*(3), 8–12.

Fitz-Gerald, D., & Fitz-Gerald, M. (1998). A historical review of sexuality education and deafness: Where have we been this century? *Sexuality and Disability 16*(4), 249–268.

Fletcher, M.L. (1993). A pilot study of the eating/dieting behaviors and attitudes of college-aged women who are hearing impaired vs their hearing peers. *JADARA, 27*(2), 1–7.

Flinn, S. (1982). Preparing teachers of the deaf to teach sex education. *Sexuality and Disability, 5*(4), 230–236.

Foley, V.D. (1984). Family therapy. In r. Corsini (Ed.), *Current psychotherapies.* Itasca, IL: Peacock Publishers.

Fong, R., & Mokuau, H. (1994). Not simply "Asian American:" Periodical literature review on Asian and Pacific Islanders. *Social Work, 30,* 289–305.

Ford, J.D. (1999). Disorders of extreme stress following war-zone military trauma: Associated features of posttraumatic stress disorder or comorbid but distinct syndromes? *Journal of Consulting and Clinical Psychology, 67,* 3–12.

Foster, S. (1988). Life in the mainstream: Deaf college freshman and their experiences in the mainstream high school. *JADARA, 22*(2), 27–35.

Foster, S. (1989a). Educational programmers for deaf students: An insider perspective on policy and practice. In L. Barton (Ed.), *Integration: Myth or reality?* (pp. 57–82). London: Falmer Press.

Foster, S. (1989b). Reflections of deaf adults on their experiences in residential and mainstream school programs. *Disability, Handicap and Society, 4*(1), 37–56.

Foster, S. (1996). Communication experiences of deaf people: An ethnographic account. In I. Parasnis (Ed.), *Cultural and language diversity and the deaf experience* (pp. 117–135). New York: Cambridge University Press.

Foster, S. (1998). Communication as social engagement: Implications for interactions between deaf and hearing persons. *Social Audiology, 27* (Suppl. 49), 116–124.

Foster, S., & Brown, P. (1989). Factors influencing the academic and social integration of hearing impaired college students. *Journal of Postsecondary Education and Disability, 7,* 78–96.

Foster, S., & Emerton, G. (1991). Mainstreaming the deaf student: Blessing or curse? *Journal of Disability Policy Studies, 2,* 61–76.

Fox, R. (1995). Bisexual identities. In A. D'Augelli & C. Patterson (Eds.), *Lesbian, gay, and bisexual identities over the lifespan* (pp. 48–86). New York: Oxford University Press.

Frankl, V. (1962). *Man's search for meaning: An introduction to logotherapy.* Boston: Beacon Press.

Freedman, P. (1964). Counseling with deaf clients: The need for culturally and linguistically sensitive interventions. *JADARA, 27*(4), 16–28.

Freeman, H.S. (1993). *Parental control of adolescents through family transitions.* Paper presented at the biennial meeting of the society for research in child development, New Orleans.

Frick, W.B. (Ed.). (1995). *Personality selected readings in theory.* Itasca, IL: F.E. Peacock Publishers.

Fromm, E. (1947). *Man for himself.* New York: Rinehart & Co.

Frost, J.J., & Forrest, D.F. (1995). Understanding the impact of effective teenage pregnancy prevention programs. *Family Planning Perspectives, 27,* 188–195.

Frost, R.O., & Steketee, G. (1998). Obsessive-compulsive disorder. In H.S. Friedman (Ed.), *Encyclopedia of mental health* (Vol. 3). San Diego: Academic Press.

Galda, S. (1981, April). *The development of the comprehension of metaphor.* Paper presented at the Annual Meeting of the American Educational Research Acrosiation, Los Angeles.

Gallaudet Regional Institute. (1998). *Annual Survey of hearing impaired children and youth.* Center for Assessment and Demographic Studies, Washington, DC.

Gallaway, C., & Woll, B. (1994). Interaction and childhood deafness. In C. Gallaway & B. Richards (Eds.), *Input and instruction in language acquisition* (pp. 197–218). Cambridge, UK: Cambridge University Press.

Gannon, C. (1998a). Developing HIV/AIDS resources for the deaf. *SIECUS Report, 26*(2), 19–20.

Gannon, C. (1998b). The deaf community and sexuality education. *Sexuality and Disability, 16*(4), 283–293.

Gannon, J.R. (1991). The importance of a cultural identity. In M.D. Garretson (Ed.), *Perspectives on deafness.* Silver Spring, MD: National Association of the Deaf.

Gans, J. (1995, July). *The relation of self-image to academic placement and achievement in hearing impaired students.* Paper presented at the 18th International Congress on Education of the Deaf, Tel Aviv, Israel.

Garbarino, J. (1976). The ecological correlates of child abuse: The impact of socioeconomic stress on mothers. *Child Development, 47,* 178–185.

Garcia-Preto, N. (1982). Puerto Rican families. In M. McGoldrick, J. Pearce, & J. Giordano (Eds.), *Ethnicity and family therapy* (pp. 164–186). New York: Guilford Press.

Garretson, M. (1977). The residential school. *Deaf American, 29,* 19–22.

Garretson, M. (1991). Deaf adults in society. In M.D. Garretson (Ed.), *Perspectives on deafness.* Silver Spring, MD: National Association of the Deaf.

Garrett, J.F., & Levine, E.S. (1969). Communication difficulties of the deaf. In *Psychological practices with the physically disabled.* New York: Columbia University Press.

Gaustad, M., & Kluwin, T. (1990, April). *Contribution of communication made to the social integration of hearing impaired adolescents.* Paper presented at the annual meeting of the American Educational Research Association, Boston.

Gearhart, B., Mullen, R., & Gearhart, C. (1993). *Exceptional individuals: An introduction.* Pacific Grove, CA: Brooks/Cole Publishing Co.

Geers, A.E., & Lane, H.S. (1984). *CID preschool performance scale.* St. Louis, MO: Central Institute for the Deaf.

Gerstein, A.I. (1988). A psychiatric program for deaf patients. *Psychiatric Hospital, 19*(3), 125–128.

Getch, Y., & Gabriel, K. (1998). A sexuality curriculum for deaf students: A cause for concern and action. *Deaf Worlds, 14*(2), 20–26.

Getch, Y.Q., Young, M., & Denny, G. (1998). Sexuality education for students who are deaf: Current practices and concerns. *Sexuality and Disability, 16*(4), 269–281.

Gil, T., Chotiner, N., & Lehr, S. (1976). Child abuse: Preying on individuals with disabilities. *Ethology and Sociobiology, 2*(3), 51–58.

Gill, D.G. (1970). *Violence against children: Physical child abuse in the United States.* Cambridge, MA: Harvard University Press.

Glasser, W. (1969). *Schools without failure.* New York: Harper and Row.

Glasser, W. (1984). Reality therapy. In R. Corsini (Ed.), *Current psychotherapies.* Itasca, IL: Peacock Publishers.

Glasser, W. (1986). *Control theory in the classroom.* New York: Harper & Row.

Glickman, N.S. (1993). *Deaf identity development: Construction and validation of a theoretical model.* Unpublished doctoral dissertation, University of Massachusetts.

Glickman, N.S., & Carey, J.C. (1993). Measuring Deaf cultural identities: A preliminary investigation. *Rehabilitation Psychology, 38,* 275–283.

Glickman, N.S., & Harvey, M. (Eds.). (1996). *Culturally affirmative psychotherapy with Deaf persons.* Mahwah, NJ: Lawrence Erlbaum Associates.

Glickman, N.S., & Zitter, S. (1989). On establishing a culturally affirmative psychiatric inpatient program for Deaf people. *JADARA, 23*(3), 89–93.

Goffman, E. (1963). *Stigma: Notes on the management of spoiled identity.* Englewood Cliffs, NJ: Prentice-Hall.

Goldberg, R. (2000). *Clashing views on controversial issues in drugs and society* (4th ed). New York: McGraw-Hill.

Goldman, R., & Goldman, J. (1982). *Children's sexual thinking: A comparative study of children aged five to fifteen years in Australia, North America, Britain, and Sweden.* London: Routledge Kegan Paul.

Goleman, D. (1995). *Emotional intelligence.* New York: Basic Books.

Gonsiorek, J. (Ed.) (1995). *Homosexuality and psychotherapy: A practitioner's handbook of affirmative models.* New York: Haworth Press.

Gonzales, R.K., & Luckner, J.L. (1993). No, they're too young: Teaching children about HIV/AIDS. *Perspectives, 12*(2), 120–129.

Gonzalez-Mena, J. (1997). *Multicultural issues in childcare.* Mountain View, CA: Mayfield Publishing Co.

Goodheart, A. (1992). Abstinence ed: How everything you need to know about sex you won't be allowed to ask. *Playboy, 39,* 42–44.

Goodman, K.S., & Goodman, Y.M. (1981). *A whole language, comprehension-centered reading program (Rep. No.1).* Tucson: University of Arizona, Center for Research & Development.

Goodman, M.E., & Beman, A. (1971). Child's-eye-views of life in an urban barrio. In N. Wagner & M. Haug (Eds.), *Chicanos: Social and psychological perspectives* (pp. 109–122). St. Louis: CV Mosley.

Goodman, M.J. (1971). *The deaf student in the hearing class.* Unpublished handbook for instructors. Golden West College, Huntington Beach, CA.

Gordon, R. (1997). *Worldview, self concept, and cultural identity patterns of deaf adolescents: Implications for counseling.* Unpublished dissertation, University of Georgia.

Gore, T.A., & Critchfield, A.B. (1992). A development of a state-wide mental health system for deaf and hard of hearing persons. *JADARA, 26*(2), 1–8.

Gorey, K.M., & Leslie, D.R. (1997). The prevalence of child sexual abuse: Integrative review adjustment for potential response and measurement biases. *Child Abuse and Neglect, 21,* 391–398.

Gottman, J.M., & Parker, J.G. (Ed.) (1987). *Conversations of friends.* New York: Cambridge University Press.

Goulder, T. (1977). Federal and state mental health programs for the deaf in hospitals and clinics. In R.Trybus (Ed.), The future of mental health services for deaf people: Proceedings of the first orthopsychiatric workshop on deafness. *Journal of Mental Health and Deafness,* experimental issue No. 1, 13–17.

Grant, B.F. (1992). DSM-IIIR and proposed DSM-IV alcohol abuse and dependence. United States 1988: A nosological comparison. *Alcoholism: Clinical and Experimental Research, 16*(6), 1068–1077.

Gray, C.D., Hosie, J.A., Russell, P.A., & Ormel, E.A. (2002). Emotional development in deaf children: Facial expressions, display rules, and theory of mind. In M.D. Clark, M. Marschark, & M. Karchmer (Eds.), *Context, cognition, and deafness.* Washington, DC: Gallaudet University Press.

Greenberg, M.T. (1980). Social interactions between deaf preschoolers and their mothers: The effects of communication method and communication competence. *Developmental Psychology, 16,* 463–474.

Greenberg, M. (1985). Problem-solving and social relationships: The applications of a stress and coping model for treating deaf clients. In G. Anderson & D. Watson (Eds.), *Counseling deaf people: Research and practice* (pp. 83–104). Little Rock: University of Arkansas.

Greenberg, M.T., Calderone, R., & Kusché, C. (1984). Early intervention using simultaneous communication with deaf infants: the effect on communication development. *Child Development, 55,* 607–616.

Greenberg, M.T., & Kusche, C.A. (1987). Cognitive, personal and social development of deaf children and adolescents. In M.C. Wang, M.C. Reynolds, & H.J. Walberg (Eds.), *Handbook of special education: Research and practice.* Vol. 3, Low incidence conditions (pp. 95–129). New York: Pergaman Press.

Greenberg, M.T., & Kusche, C.A. (1993). *Promoting social and emotional development in deaf children: The PATHS Project.* Seattle: University of Washington Press.

Greenberg, M., Kusche, C., Gustafson, R., & Calderone, R. (1984). The PATHS project: A model for prevention of psychosocial difficulties in deaf children. In G. Anderson & D. Watson (Eds.), *The habilitation and rehabilitation of deaf adolescents* (pp. 243–263). Proceedings of the National Conference on Habilation and Rehabilitation of Deaf Adolescents, Wagoner, OK.

Greenberg, M.T., & Marvin, R. (1979). Attachment patterns in profoundly deaf preschool children. *Merrill-Palmer Quarterly, 25,* 265–279.

Greenspan, S.L. (1995). *The challenging child.* Reading, MA: Addison-Wesley Publishing Company.

Gregory, S. (Ed.) (1998). *Issues in deaf education.* London: D. Fulton Publishers.

Gregory, S., Bishop, J., & Sheldon, L. (1995). *Deaf young people and their families.* Cambridge, UK: Cambridge University Press.

Gregory, S., & Mogford, K. (1983). The development of symbolic play in young deaf children. In D. Rogers & J. Sloboda (Eds.), *The acquisition of symbolic skills* (pp. 221–231). New York: Plenum.

Griffith, P.L, Johnson, N.A., & Dastoli, S.L. (1985). If teaching is conversation, can conversation be taught? Discourse abilities in hearing impaired children. In D.N. Ripich & F.M. Spinelli (Eds.), *School discourse problems.* San Diego: College Hill Press.

Grinker, R., Sr. (Ed.). (1969). *Psychiatric diagnosis, therapy, and research on the psychotic deaf.* Final report, grant No. R.D. 2407 S. Social & Rehabilitation Service, Department of Health, Education and Welfare.

Grinspoon, L. (1987). Personality and personality disorders—Part I. *Harvard Medical School Mental Health Letter, 4*(3), 1–4.

Griswold, E.L., & Commings, J. (1974). The expressive vocabulary of preschool deaf children. *American Annals of the Deaf, 119,* 16–28.

Grizenko, N. (1998). Protective factors in development of psychopathology. In H.S. Friedman (Ed.), *Encyclopedia of mental health* (Vol. 3). San Diego: Academic Press.

Gross, A.L., & Ballif, B. (1991). Children's understanding of emotion from facial expressions: A review. *Developmental Review, 11,* 368–398.

Grossman, S. (1972). *Sexual knowledge, attitudes and experiences of deaf college students.* Unpublished master's thesis. George Washington University, Washington, DC.

Guthmann, D. (1999). *Is there a substance abuse problem among deaf and hard of hearing individuals?* From: http://home.earthlink.net/drblood/minn/articles/problem_adhtm.

Guthmann, D., & Sandberg, K. (1998). Assessing substance abuse problems in deaf and hard of hearing individuals. *American Annals of the Deaf, 143*(1), 14–21.

Guthmann, D., & Sandberg, K. (2002). Assessing substance abuse problems with deaf and hard of hearing students. From: http://home.earthlink.net/drblood/minn/articles/students_ad.htm. Retrieved 7/10/02.

Haffner, D.W., & deMauro, D. (1991). *Winning the battle: Developing support for sexuality and HIV/AIDS education.* New York: Sex Information and Education Council of the United States.

Hales, D. (1999). *Invitation to health* (8th ed.) New York: McGraw-Hill.

Hammill, D. (Ed.) (1987). *Assessing the abilities and instructional needs of students.* Austin, TX: Pro-Ed.

Hannigan, J.H., Spear, L.P., Spear, N.E., & Goodlet, C.R. (Eds.). (1999). *Alcohol and alcoholism.* Mahwah, NJ: Lawrence Erlbaum Associates.

Harnisch, D.J., Lichtenstein, S.J., & Langford, J.B. (1986). *Digest on youth in transition.* Champaign: Transition Institute at Illinois.

Harper, P. (1983). Understanding deafness. *Perspectives, 3*(2), 17–21.

Harris, J. (1995). *The cultural meaning of deafness.* Brookfield, VT: Ashgate Publishing Co.

Harris, R. (1978). The relationship of impulse control to parent hearing status, manual communication, and academic achievement in deaf children. *American Annals of the Deaf, 123*(1), 52–67.

Harry, B. (1992). An ethnographic study of cross-cultural communication with Puerto Rican-American families in the special education system. *American Educational Research Journal, 29*(3), 471–494.

Harry, J. (1993). Being out: A general model. *Journal of Homosexuality, 26,* 25–40.

Harter, S. (1990). Issues in the assessment of the self-concept of children and adolescence. In A.M. LaGreca (Ed.), *Through the eyes of the child: Obtaining self-reports from children and adolescents* (pp. 292–325). Boston: Allyn & Bacon.

Harmatz, M.G. (1978). *Abnormal psychology.* Englewood Cliffs, NJ: Prentice Hall.

Hartup, W.W., & Stevens, N. (1997). Friendships and adaptation in the life course. *Psychological Bulletin, 121,* 355–370.

Harvey, J., & Siantz, J. (1979). Public education and the handicapped. *Journal of Research and Development in Education, 12*(1), 1–9.

Harvey, M. (1982). The influence and utilization of an interpreter for deaf persons in family therapy. *American Annals of the Deaf, 127,* 821–827.

Harvey, M.A. (1989). *Psychotherapy with deaf and hard-of-hearing persons: A systemic model.* Hillsdale, NJ: Lawrence Erlbaum Associates.

Hayes, W.D., & Shulman, B.B. (1998). *Communication development.* Baltimore: Williams & Wilkins.

Heller, B. (1987). Mental health assessment of deaf persons: A brief history. In H. Elliott et al. (Eds.), *Mental health assessment of deaf clients.* Boston: Little, Brown and Co.

Helms, J.E., & Parham, T.A. (1996). The development of the racial identity attitude scale. In R.L. Jones (Ed.), *Handbook of tests and measurements for black populations* (Vol. 2, pp. 167–174). Berkeley, CA: Cobb & Henry.

Henry, J. (1965). Pathways to madness. New York: Random House.

Henwood, P.G., & Pope-Davis, D.B. (1994, July). Disability as cultural diversity: Counseling the hearing impaired. *The Counseling Psychologist, 22*(3), 489–503.

Hetherington, E.M. (1995, March). *The changing American family and the well-being of children.* Paper presented at the meeting of the society for Research in Child Development, New Orleans.

Hetherington, E.M., & Stanley-Hagan, M.M. (1995). Parenting in divorced and remarried families. In M.H. Bornstein (Ed.), *Children and parenting* (Vol. 4). Hillsdale, NJ: Lawrence Erlbaum Associates.

Hetherington, R. (1979). Deafness and alcoholism. *JADARA, 12*(4), 9–12.

Hewitt, L.E. (1994). Narrative comprehension: the importance of subjectivity. In J. Duchan Hewitt, & L.E. Sonnenmeir (Eds), *Pragmatics from theory to practice.* Englewood Cliffs, NJ: Prentice-Hall.

Higginbotham, D.J., & Baker, B.M. (1981). Social and cognitive play differences in hearing-impaired and normally hearing preschoolers. *Volta Review, 83,* 135–149.

Higgins, P.C., & Nash, J.E. (1996). *Understanding deafness socially.* Springfield, IL: Charles C. Thomas.

Hill, R. (1972). *Strengths of black families.* New York: Emerson Hall.

Hill, R. (1993). *Research on the African American family.* Boston: William Monroe Trotter Institute, University of Massachusetts at Boston.

Hill, R.B., with Billingsley, A. (1993). *Research on the African-American family: A holistic perspective.* Wesport, CT: Auburn House.

Hills, C.G., Rappold, E.S., & Rendon, M.E. (1991). Binge eating and body image in a sample of the deaf college population. *JADARA, 25*(2), 20–28.

Hoffmeister, R.J., Philip, M.J., Costello, P. & Grass, W. (1998). Evaluating American sign language in deaf children: ASL influences on reading with a focus on classifiers, plurals, verbs of motion, and location. In *Deaf studies I: Toward 2000 unity and diversity (pp. 79–106).* Washington, DC: Gallaudet University.

Holcomb, T.K. (1996). Social assimilation of deaf high school students: The role of the school environment. In I. Parasnis (Ed.), *Cultural and language diversity and the deaf experience* (pp. 189–198). Cambridge, England: Cambridge University Press.

Holcomb, T.K. (1997). Development of Deaf bicultural identity. *American Annals of the Deaf, 142*(3), 89–93.

Holloway, J., & Bass, W.K. (1993). *The African heritage of American English.* Bloomington: Indiana University Press.

Holt, J. (1990). Classroom attributes and achievement test scores for the deaf and hard of hearing students. *American Annals of the Deaf, 139,* 430–437.

Hosie, J.A., Russell, C.D., Gray, C., Scott, N., Hunter, J.S., Banks, L. & Macaulay, M.C. (2000). Knowledge of display rules in prelingually deaf and hearing children. *Journal of Child Psychology and Psychiatry and Allied Disciplines, 41,* 389–398.

Howe, G. (1999). *Hospital treatment and care.* London & Philadelphia: Jessica Kingsley Publishers.

Howes, C., & Matheson, C.C. (1992). Sequences in the development of competent play with peers. Social and social pretend play. *Developmental Psychology, 28,* 961–974.

Hulit, L.M., & Howard, M.R. (1993). *Born to talk: An introduction to speech and language development.* New York: Macmillan.

Humphries, T. (1991). An introduction to the culture of deaf people in the United States. *Sign Language Studies, 72,* 209–240.

Isenberg, G. (1996). Storytelling and the use of culturally appropriate metaphors in psychotherapy with Deaf people. In N.S. Glickman & M.A. Harvey (Eds.), *Culturally affirmative psychotherapy with Deaf persons* (pp. 169–183). Mahwah, NJ: Lawrence Erlbaum Associates.

Isselbacher, K.J., Adams, R.D., Braunwald, E., Petersdorf, R.G., & Wilson, J.D. (1980). *Harrison's principles of internal medicine* (9th ed.) New York: McGraw-Hill.

Ivimey, G.P., & Lachterman, D.H. (1980). The written language of young English deaf children. *Language and Speech, 23,* 351–377.

Jacobs, J.L. (1989). *A comparison of deaf pupils in residential and mainstream settings on self-concept.* Unpublished doctoral dissertation, Spalding University, Louisville, Kentucky.

Jacobs, L.M. (1980). *A deaf adult speaks out.* Washington, DC: Gallaudet University Press.

James, W. (1890/1993). *The principles of psychology.* Cambridge, MA: Harvard University Press.

Janos, P.M., & Robinson, N.M. (1985). Psychological development in intellectually gifted children. In F.D. Horowitz & M. O'Brien (Eds.), *The gifted and talented.* Washington, DC: American Psychological Association.

Janowsky, D. (1999). *Psychotherapy indications and outcomes.* Washington, DC: American Psychiatric Press.

Jeanes, R.C., Nienhuys, T.G., & Richards, F.W. (2000). The pragmatic skills of profoundly deaf children. *Journal of Deaf Studies and Deaf Education.* Oxford University Press.

Johnson, B., & Lock, P. (1978). As cited in W.P. McCrone (1982), Serving the deaf substance abuser. *Journal of Psychoactive Drugs, 14,* 199–205.

Johnson, L.D., O'Malley, P.M., & Bachman, J.G. (2000). *The monitoring of the future: National results on adolescent drug use.* Washington, DC: National Institute on Drug Abuse.

Johnson, R.E., & Erting, C. (1989). Ethnicity and socialization in a classroom for deaf children. In C. Lucas (Ed.), *The sociolinguistics of the deaf community* (pp. 41–84). New York: Academic Press.

Johnson, R.E., Liddell, S.K., & Erting, C.J. (1989). *Unlocking the curriculum: Principles for achieving access in deaf education.* Gallaudet Research Institute. Working paper 89-3. Washington, DC: Gallaudet University Press.

Jones, E., & Badger, T. (1991). Deaf children's knowledge of internal human anatomy. *Journal of Special Education, 25*(2), 252–260.

Joe, D., & Malach, P. (1998). Families with Native American roots. In E. Lynch & M. Hanson (Eds.), *Developing cross-cultural competencies: A guide for working with young children and their families.* Baltimore: Paul H. Brookes.

Joiner, L.M., Erickson, E.L., Crittenden, J.B., & Stevenson, V.M. (1966). Predicting the academic achievement of the acoustically impaired using intelligence and self-concept of academic ability. *Journal of Special Education, 3,* 425–431.

Jones, E. (1985). Major development in social psychology during the past five decades. In L. Gardner (Ed.), *Handbook of social psychology,* Vol. 1. New York: Random House.

Joseph, J., Sawyer, R., & Desmond, S. (1995). Sexual knowledge, behavior, sources of information among deaf and hard of hearing college students. *American Annals of the Deaf, 140*(4), 338–345.

Jung, C.G. (1954). *The development of personality.* New York: Pantheon.

Kalichman, S.C. (1995). *Understanding AIDS: A guide for mental health professionals.* Washington, DC: American Psychological Association.

Karchmer, M. (1985). A demographic perspective. In E. Charrow (Ed), *Hearing impaired children and youth with developmental disabilities.* Washington, DC: Gallaudet University Press.

Kaufman, P., Kwan, J., Klein, S., & Chapman, C. (1999). Dropout rates in the United States. *Education Statistics Quarterly.*

Keen, E. (1998). *Drugs, therapy, and professional power: Problems and pills.* Westport, CT: Praeger.

Kegan, R. (1982). *The evolving self: Problem and process in human development.* Cambridge, MA: Harvard University Press.

Kendall-Tackett, K.A., Williams, L.M., & Finkhor, D. (1993). Impact of sexual abuse on children. A review and synthesis of recent empirical studies. *Psychological Bulletin, 113,* 164–180.

Kennedy, S., & Buchholz, L. (1995). HIV and AIDS among the deaf. *Sexuality and Disability, 13*(2), 145–158.

Kestenbaum, R., & Nelson, C.A. (1990). The recognition and categorization of upright and inverted emotional expressions by seven-month-old infants. *Infant Behavior and Development, 13,* 497–511.

King, A.J.C., Beazeley, R.P., Warren, W.K., Hankins, C.A., Robertson, A.S., & Sadford, J.L. (1998). *Canada youth and aids study.* Ottawa: Federal Centre for AIDS Health Protection Branch, Health and Welfare Canada.

Kinsey, A.C., Pomeroy, W.B., & Martin, E.E. (1948). *Sexual behavior in the human male.* Philadelphia: W.B. Saunders.

Kirby, D., Barth, R.P., Leland, N., & Fetro, J.V. (1991). Reducing the risk: Impact of a new curriculum on sexual risk-taking. *Family Planning Perspectives, 23,* 253–263.

Kirby, D., Korpi, M. Barth, R.P., & Cagampang, H.H. (1997). The impact of the Postponing Sexual Involvement Curriculum among youth in California. *Family Planning Perspectives, 29,* 100–108.

Kisor, H. (1990). *What's that pig outdoors?* New York: Hill & Wang.

Kluckhohn, F., & Strodbeck, F. (1961). *Variations in value orientations.* Evanston, IL: Row & Peterson.

Kluwin, T.N. (1989). *Consumer motivated research to development: The rationale for the national research to development network.* Washington, DC: Gallaudet University Research Institute. (Rept. #1 National Research to Development Network for Public School Programs for Hearing Impaired), DHHS, Grant MCJ-110563.

Kluwin, T., Moores, D., & Gaustad, M.G. (1992). *Toward effective public school programs for deaf students.* New York: Teachers College Press.

Kluwin, T.N., & Stinson, M.S. (1993). *Deaf students in local public high schools: Background, experiences, and outcomes.* Springfield, IL: Charles C. Thomas.

Koelle, W.H., & Convey, J.J. (1982). The prediction of achievement of deaf Adolescents from self-concept and locus of control measures. *American Annals of the Deaf, 127,* 769–779.

Koester, L., & MacTurk, R. (1991). *Attachment behaviors in deaf and hearing infants: Mothers and Deaf Infants.* Final report to Maternal and Child Health Research Program, Bureau of Maternal and Child Health and Resources Development, HRSA, PHS.

Kohlberg, L. (1987). *Child psychology and childhood education: A cognitive developmental view.* New York: Langman.

Kornblum, W. (1991). *Sociology in a changing world.* Chicago: Holt, Rinehart & Winston.

Koss, M., & Boeschen, L. (1998). Rape. In H.S. Friedman (Ed.), *Encyclopedia of mental health* (Vol. 3). San Diego: Academic Press.

Kretschmer, R.R., & Kretschmer, L.W. (1978). *Language development and intervention in the hearing impaired.* Baltimore: University Park Press.

Kumabe, K.T., Nishida, C., & Hepworth, D.H. (1985). *Bridging ethnocultural diversity in social work and health.* Honolulu: University of Hawaii, School of Social Work.

Kusche, C.A., Greenberg, M.T., & Garfield, T.S. (1983). Nonverbal intelligence and verbal achievement in deaf adolescents: An examination of heredity and environment. *American Annals of the Deaf, 128,* 458–466.

LaBarre, A. (1998). Treatment of sexually abused children who are deaf. *Sexuality and Disability, 16*(4), 321–324.

LaBruzza, A.L. (1997). *Using DSM-IV: A clinician's guide to psychiatric diagnosis.* Northvale, NJ: J. Aronson.

Ladd, G.W. (1999). Peer relationships and social competence during early and middle childhood. *Annual Review of Psychology, 50.*

Ladd, G.W., Munson, J.L., & Miller, J.K. (1984). Social integration of deaf adolescents in secondary level mainstreaming programs. *Exceptional Children, 50,* 419–429.

Lane, H. (1984). *The deaf experience: Classics in language and education.* Cambridge, MA: Harvard University Press.

Lane, H. (1992). *The mask of benevolence: Disabling the deaf community.* New York: Knopf.

Lane, H. (1995). Constructions of deafness. *Disability and Society, 10*(2), 171–189.

Lane, H., Hoffmeister, R., & Bahan, B., (1996). *A journey into the deaf world.* San Diego: Dawn Sign Press.

Lane, K.E. (1989). Substance abuse among the deaf population: An overview of current strategies, programs and barriers to recovery. *JADARA, 22,* 79–86.

Langholtz, D., & Ruth, R. (1999). Deaf people with HIV/AIDS: Notes on the Psychotherapeutic Journey. In I. Leigh (Ed.), *Psychotherapy with deaf clients from diverse groups.* Washington, DC: Gallaudet University Press.

Larrivee, B. (1999). *Authentic classroom management.* Boston: Allyn & Bacon.

Lasswell, T.E., Burma, J.H., & Aronson, S.H., (1986). *Life in Society.* Chicago: Scott, Foresman & Company.

Laumann, E.O., Gagnon, J.H., Michael, R.T., & Michaels, S. (1994). *The social organization of sexuality: Sexual practices in the United States.* Chicago: Chicago University Press.

LeBuffe, F.P., & LeBuffe, L.A. (1979). Psychiatric aspects of deafness. *Primary Care, 6,* 295–310.

Lederberg, A., & Everhart, V. (1996). *Communicative interactions between deaf toddlers and their hearing mothers.* Manuscript submitted for review.

Lederberg, A.R., & Everhart, V.S. (August 1998). Communication between Deaf children and their hearing mothers: The role of language, gesture, and vocalizations. *Journal of Speech, Language and Hearing Research, 41*(4), 887–1003.

Lederberg, A.R., & Mobley, C.E. (1990). The effect of hearing impairment on the quality of attachment and mother-toddler interaction. *Child Development, 61,* 1596–1604.

Lee, E. (1996). Asian American Families: An overview. In M. McGoldrick, J. Giordano, & J.K. Pearce (Eds.), *Ethnicity and family therapy* (pp. 227–248). New York: Guilford Press.

Leigh, I. (Ed.) (1999). *Psychotherapy with deaf clients from diverse groups.* Washington, DC: Gallaudet University Press.

Leigh, I.W., Corbett, C.A., Gutman, V., & Morere, D.A. (1996). Providing psychological services to deaf individuals: A response to new perceptions of diversity. *Professional Psychology: Research and Practice, 27*(4), 364–371.

Leigh, I.W., & Stinson, M.S. (1991). Social environments, self-perceptions, and identity of hearing-impaired adolescents. *Volta Review, 93*(5), 7–23.

Lesser, S.R., & Easser, B.R. (1972). Personality differences in the perceptually handicapped. *Journal of American Academy of Child Psychiatry, 11,* 458–466.

Letourneau, E.J., & O'Donahue, W. (1997). Classical conditioning of female sexual arousal. *Archives of Sexual Behavior, 26,* 63–78.

LeVay, S. (1996). *Queerscience: The use and abuse of research into homosexuality.* Cambridge, MA: MIT Press.

Levine, E.S. (1981). *The ecology of early deafness.* New York: Columbia University Press.

Levy-Shiff, R., & Hoffman, M. (1985). Social behavior of hearing-impaired and normally-hearing preschoolers. *British Journal of Educational Psychology, 55,* 111–118.

Lewis, K.J.C. (1982, March). Sex education: The role of schools and units for the deaf. *Teacher of the Deaf, 6*(2).

Libbey, S., & Pronovost, W. (1980). Communication practices of mainstreamed hearing impaired adolescents. *Volta Review, 82,* 197–213.

Lightcap, J.L., Kurland, J.A., & Burgess, R.L. (1982). Child abuse: A test of some predictions from evolutionary theory. *Ethology and Sociobiology, 3*(2), 61–67.

Ling, D. (1989). *Foundation of spoken language for hearing-impaired children.* Washington DC: AGB Association for the Deaf.

Locke, D. (1991). The Locke paradigm of cross cultural counseling. *International Journal for the Advancement of Counseling,14,* 15–25.

Loeb, R., & Sarigiani, P. (1986). The impact of hearing impairment on self-perception of children. *Volta Review, 88,* 89–100.

Loera, P.A. (1994). The use and application of cognitive-behavioral psychotherapy with deaf persons. In R.C. Nowell & L.E. Marshak (Eds.), *Understanding deafness and the rehabilitation process.* Boston: Allyn & Bacon.

Long, G. (1995). Providing mental health services to traditionally underserved persons who are deaf. In R. Myers (Ed.), *Standards of* care for the delivery of mental health services to deaf and hard of hearing persons. Silver Spring, MD: NAD.

Lucas, C. (1989). *The sociolinguistics of the Deaf community*. San Diego: Academic Press.

Lucas, C. (1998). Linguistic variation in ASL: An overview. In *Deaf studies V: Toward 2000—unity and diversity* (pp. 163–185). Washington, DC: Gallaudet University.

Luckner, J.L., & Gonzales, R.K. (1993). What deaf and hard of hearing adolescents know and think about AIDS. *American Annals of the Deaf, 138*(4), 338–342.

Luetke-Stahlman, B. (1995). Social interaction assessment and intervention with regard to students who are deaf. *American Annals of the Deaf, 140*(3), 295–305.

Luetke-Stahlman, B., & Luckner, J. (1991). *Effectively educating students with hearing impairments.* New York: Longman.

Luetke-Stahlman, B., Griffiths, C., & Montgomery, N. (1999). A deaf child's language acquisition verified through text retelling. *American Annals of the Deaf, 144*(3), 270–344.

Luterman, D. (Ed.). (1986). *Deafness in perspective.* San Diego: College-Hill Press.

Luterman, D. (1987). *Deafness in the family.* San Diego: College-Hill Press.

Luterman, D. (1997). Emotional aspects of hearing loss. *Volta Review, 99*(5), 75–84.

Luterman, D.M., with Kurtzer-White, E., & Seewald, R.C. (1999). *The young deaf child.* Baltimore, MD: York Press.

Luterman, D.M. & Ross, M. (1991). *When your child is deaf: A guide for parents.* Parkton, MD: York Press.

Lynch, E.W. & Hanson, M.J. (1998). *Developing cross-cultural competence* (2nd ed). Baltimore, MD: Brooks Publishing Company.

Macionis, J.J. (1998). *Society, the basics* (4th ed). Upper Saddle River, NJ: Prentice-Hall.

Madanes, C. (1984). *Beyond the one-way mirror.* San Francisco: Jossey-Bass.

Mahler, M.S., Pine, F., & Bergman, A. (1975). *The psychological birth of the human infant: Symbiosis and individuation.* New York: Basic Books.

Major, J.S. (1989). *The land and people of China.* New York: J.B. Lippincott.

Marion, M. (1995). *Guidance of young children.* Englewood Cliffs, NJ: Merrill.

Marschark, M. (1993). *Psychological development of deaf children.* New York: Oxford University Press.

Marschark, M. (1997). *Raising and educating a deaf child.* New York: Oxford University Press.

Marschark, M., & Clark, D. (Eds.). (1993–1998). *Psychological perspectives on deafness.* Hillsdale, NJ: Lawrence Erlbaum Associates.

Martinez, C., & Silvestre, N. (1995). Self-concept in profoundly deaf adolescent pupils. *International Journal of Psychology, 30*(3), 305–316.

Martin, F. (1987). *Hearing disorders in children: Pediatric Audiology.* Austin, TX: ProEd.

Maslow, A.H. (1954). *Motivation and personality.* New York: Harper.

Mathay, M., & Lafayette, R. (1990). Low achieving deaf adults: An interview survey of service providers. *JADARA, 23*(1), 23–32.

McAdoo, H. (1993). *Family ethnicity: Strength in diversity.* Newbury Park, CA: Sage.

McAdoo, H. (1997). *Black families* (3rd ed.). Beverly Hills: Sage Publications.

McCauley, R.W., & Bruininks, R.H. (1976). Behavior interactions of hearing impaired children in regular classrooms. *Journal of Special Education, 10,* 277–284.

McCay, V. (1990). *The psychology of deafness: Understanding deaf and hard-of-hearing people.* New York: Longman.

McCrone, W.P. (1983). Reality therapy with deaf rehabilitation clients. *JADARA, 17,* 13–15.

McEntee, M.K. (1993). Mental health and crisis intervention service availability for the deaf. *American Annals of the Deaf, 138*(1), 26–30.

Mead, G.H. (1934). *Mind, self and society: From the standpoint of a social behaviorist.* Chicago: University of Chicago Press.

Meador, B.D., & Rogers, C.R. (1984). Person centered therapy. In R. Corsini (Ed.), *Current psychotherapies.* Itasca, IL: Peacock Publishers.

Meadow, K.P. (1969). Self-image, family climate, and deafness. *Social Forces, 47,* 428–438.

Meadow, K.P. (1980). *Deafness and child development.* Berkeley: University of California Press.

Meichenbaum, D. (1977). *Cognitive-behavior modification: An integrative approach.* New York: Plenum Press.

Melick, A.M. (1998). *Deaf identity inquiry.* Unpublished doctoral dissertation, Pennsylvania State University.

Meltzoff, A., & Moore, W. (1977). Imitation of facial and manual gestures by human neonates. *Science, 198,* 75–78.

Mertens, D. (1989). Social experiences of hearing-impaired high school youth. *American Annals of the Deaf, 134,* 15–19.

Meyer, R.G. (1998). Personality disorders. In H.S. Friedman (Ed.), *Encyclopedia of mental health (Vol. 2).* San Diego: Academic Press.

Meyer, R.G., Wolverton, D., & Deitsch, S.E. (1998). Antisocial personality disorder. In H.S. Friedman (Ed.), *Encyclopedia of mental health* (Vol. 2). San Diego: Academic Press.

Miller, M., & Moores, D. (1990). Principles of group counseling and their applications for deaf clients. *JADARA, 23,* 82–87.

Min, P.G. (1995). An overview of Asian Americans. In P.G. Min (Ed.), *Asian Americans: Contemporary trends and issues.* (pp. 10–37). Beverly Hills, CA: Sage Publications.

Mindel, E.D., & Vernon, M. (1987). *They grow in silence.* Boston: College Hill Press.

Misiaszek, J., Dooling, J., Gieseke, M. Melman, H., Misiaszek, J.G., & Jorgensen, K. (1985, November/December). Diagnostic considerations in deaf patients. *Comprehensive Psychiatry, 26*(6), 513–521.

Mizes, J.S., & Miller, K.J. (2000) Eating disorders. In M. Herson & R.T. Ammerman (Eds.), *Advanced abnormal child psychology* (2nd ed.) Mahwah, NJ: Lawrence Erlbaum Associates.

Mohay, H. (1990). The interaction of gesture and speech in the development of two profoundly deaf children. In V. Voltera & C.J. Erting (Eds.), *From gesture to language in hearing and deaf children* (pp. 187–204). Berlin: Springer-Verlag.

Moores, D.F. (1970). An investigation of the psycholinguistic functioning of deaf adolescents. *Exceptional Children, 36,* 645–652.

Moores, D.F. (1982). *Educating the deaf: Principles and practices.* Boston: Houghton-Mifflin.

Moores, D.F. (2001). *Educating the deaf: Psychology, principles and practices.* Boston: Houghton Mifflin.

Moores, D.F., & Meadow-Orlans, K.P. (Eds.) (1990). *Educational and developmental aspects of deafness.* Washington, DC: Gallaudet University Press.

Moreno, Z. (1959). A survey of psychodramatic techniques. *Group Psychotherapy, 12,* 5–24.

Mowrer, D.E. (1988). *Methods of modifying speech behaviors: learning theory in speech pathology* (2nd ed.). Prospect Heights, IL: Waveland Press.

Munoz, R.F. (1998). Depression-applied aspects. In H.S. Friedman (Ed.), *Encyclopedia of mental health* (Vol. 1). San Diego: Academic Press.

Murdoch, H. (1996). Stereotyped behavior in deaf and hard of hearing children. *American Annals for the Deaf, 141*(5), 379–386.

Murphy, J., & Newlon, B. (1987). Loneliness and the mainstreamed hearing-impaired college student. *American Annals of the Deaf, 132,* 21–25.

Myers, D.G. (1987). *Social psychology.* New York: McGraw-Hill.

Myers, P.C., & Danek, M.M. (1989). Deafness mental health needs assessment: A model. *JADARA, 22,* 72–78.

Myers, M.T. (1992). The African American experience with HIV disease. *Focus: A Guide to AIDS Research and Counseling, 7,* 79–82.

Myers, R.P. (1993). Model mental health state plan (MMHSP) of services for persons who are deaf or hard-of-hearing. *JADARA, 28*(4), 19–28.

Myklebust, H. (1964). *The psychology of deafness.* New York: Grune & Stratton.

Naremore, R.C., & Hopper, R. (1997). *Children learning language.* San Diego: Singular Publishing Group.

Nash, K. (1991). Programs and services for the postsecondary deaf: Strategic planning considerations for the 1990s. *JADARA, 25*(2), 29–35.

Nathan, P. (1999). *Treating mental disorder: A guide to what works.* New York: Oxford University Press.

Nathan, P., & Gorman, J.M. (Eds.) (1998). *A guide to treatments that work.* New York: Oxford Press.

National Center for Health Statistics (NCHS). (1990–1991). *Data from the National Health Interview Survey.* Washington, DC: Department of Health and Human Services.

National Household Survey on Drug Abuse. (1992). Rockville, MD: *National Institute of Drug Abuse, United States Department of Health and Human Services.*

Neisser, U. (1993).The self perceived. In U. Neisser (Ed.), *The perceived self: Ecological and interpersonal sources of self knowledge* (pp. 3–21). New York: Cambridge University Press.

Nicholas, J.G. (2000). Age differences in the use of informative/heuristic communicative functions in young children with and without hearing loss who are learning spoken language. *Journal of Speech, Language and Hearing Research, 43*(2), 1–15.

Nicholas, J.G., & Geers, A.E. (1997). Communication of oral deaf and normally hearing children at 36 months of age. *Journal of Speech, Language and Hearing Research, 40,* 1314–1327.

Nicholls, J.G. (1984). Conceptions of ability and achievement motivation. In R.E. Ames & C. Ames (Eds.), *Motivation in education.* New York: Academic Press.

Nickless, C. (1993). Program outcome research in residential programs for deaf mentally ill adults. *JADARA, 27*(3), 42–48.

Nippold, M. (1994). Persuasive talk in social contexts. Development, assessment, and intervention. *Topics in Language Disorders, 14*(3), 1–12.

Nippold, M. (1998a). *Later language development: The school-age and adolescent years.* Austin, TX: Pro-Ed.

Nippold, M. (Ed.). (1998b). *Later language development: Ages nine through nineteen.* Boston: Little, Brown & Company.

Nippold, M. (1998c). The literate lexicon. In M. Nippold (Ed.), *Later language development: Ages nine through nineteen* (pp. 29–48). Boston: Little Brown and Company.

Norton, A.J., & Glick, P.C. (1986). One parent families: A social and economic profile. *Family Relations, 35,* 9–17.

Norton, R. (1978). Reality therapy: A practical approach to troubled youth. In L.S. Stein, E.D. Mindel, & M.A. Jabaley (Eds.), *Deafness and mental health.* New York: Grune & Statton.

Oblowitz, N. Green, L., & Heyns, I. (1991). A self-concept scale for the hearing-impaired. *Volta Review, 93*(1), 19–29.

O'Brien, D. (1987). Reflection-impulsivity in total communication and oral deaf and hearing children: A developmental study. *American Annals of the Deaf, 132*(3), 213–221.

O'Day, B. (1983). *Preventing sexual abuse of persons with disabilities.* St. Paul: Minnesota Program for Victims of Sexual Abuse.

Ogden, P., & Lipsett, S. (1982). *The silent garden: Understanding the hearing impaired child.* Chicago: Contemporary Books.

Okami, P., & Goldberg, A. (1992). Personality correlates of pedeophilia: Are they reliable indicators? *Journal of Sex Research, 29,* 297–328.

Okun, B.F. (1987). *Effective helping: Interviewing and counseling techniques* (3rd ed.) Monterey, CA: Brooks/Cole.

Olivardia, R., Pope, H.G., Mangweth, B., & Hudson, J.I. (1995). Eating disorders in college men. *American Journal of Psychiatry, 152,* 1279–1284.

Orbanic, S. (2001). Understanding bulimia. *American Journal of Nursing, 101,* 35–41.

Ortiz, F. (1998). *Los Negros brujos [The Negro Witches]* Miami: New House Publishing.

Owens, R.E. (1996). *Language development: An introduction* (4th ed.) New York: Merrill.

Padden, C. (1989). The deaf community and the culture of Deaf people. In S. Wilcox (Ed.), *American Deaf culture.* Burtonsville, MD: Linstock Press.

Padden, C., & Humphries, T. (1988). *Deaf in America.* Cambridge, MA: Harvard University Press.

Parasnis, I. (Ed.) (1996). *Cultural and language diversity and the deaf experience.* New York: Cambridge University Press.

Parker, F., & Riley, K. (2000). *Linguistics for non-linguistics.* Boston: Allyn & Bacon.

Parten, M. (1932). Social play among preschool children. *Journal of Abnormal and Social Psychology, 27,* 243–269.

Patel, V. (1998). *Culture and common mental disorders in sub-Saharan Africa.* London & Zimbabwe: Institute of Psychiatry.

Patterson, C.H., & Stewart, L.G. (1971). Principles of counseling with deaf people. In A.E. Sussman & L.G. Stewart (Eds.), *Counseling with deaf people* (pp. 43–86). New York: New York University School of Education, Deafness, Research & Training Center.

Patterson, C.J., & Kister, M.C. (1981). The development of listener skills for referential communication. In W. Dickson (Ed.), *Children's oral communication skills.* New York: Academic Press.

Patterson, O. (1983). The nature, causes, and implications of ethnic identification. In C. Fried (Ed.), *Minorities, community and identity* (pp. 25–50). New York: Springer-Verlag.

Paul, P.V. (1998). *Literacy and deafness: The development of reading, writing, and literate thought.* Boston: Allyn & Bacon.

Paul, P.V., & Jackson, D.W. (1993). *Toward a psychology of deafness: Theoretical and empirical perspectives.* Boston: Allyn & Bacon.

Paul, V., & Quigley, S. (1994). *Language and deafness.* (2nd ed.) San Diego: Singular Publishing Group.

Paul, R. (2001). *Language disorders from infancy through adolescence.* St Louis, MO: Mosby.

Pendergrass, R.A. (1982). A "thinking" approach to teaching responsibility. *Clearing House, 56,* 90–92.

Pentz, M.A. (1994). Primary prevention of adolescent drug abuse. In C. Fisher & R. Lerner (Eds.), *Applied developmental psychology.* New York: McGraw-Hill.

Peter, P.V., & Jackson, D. (1993). *Toward a psychology of deafness: Theoretical and empirical perspectives.* Boston: Allyn & Bacon.

Pflaster, G. (1980). A factor analysis of variables related to academic performance of hearing impaired children in regular classes. *Volta Review, 82,* 71–84.

Phaneuf, J. (1987, March). Considerations of deafness and homosexuality. *American Annals of the Deaf,* 52–55.

Pien, D. (1985). The development of language functions in deaf infants of hearing parents. In D. Martin (Ed.) *Cognition, education and deafness* (Vol. 2, pp. 30–33). Washington, DC: Gallaudet University Press.

Pierangelo, R., & Giuliani, G.A. (2002). *Assessment in special education: A practical approach.* Boston: Allyn & Bacon.

Pollard, R.Q. (1993). One hundred years in psychology and deafness: A centennial retrospective. *JADARA, 26*(3).

Pollard, R.Q. (1994). Public mental health services and diagnostic trends regarding individuals who are deaf or hard of hearing. *Rehabilitation Psychology, 39*(3), 147–161.

Pollard, R.Q. (1998). Psychopathology. In M. Marschark & D. Clark (Ed.), *Psychological perspectives on deafness,* Vol. 2. New Jersey: Lawrence Erlbaum Associates.

Ponterotto, J.G. (1995). *Handbook of multicultural counseling.* Thousand Oaks: Sage Publications.

Prout, T.F. (1998). *The development of self-understanding in deaf children.* Unpublished doctoral dissertation, University of Pittsburgh.

Purkey, W.W., & Schmidt, J.J. (1987). *The inviting relationship: An expanded perspective for professional counseling.* Englewood Cliffs, NJ: Prentice-Hall.

Quigley, S.P., & Kretschmer, R.E. (1982). *The education of deaf children.* Austin, TX: ProEd.

Quigley, S.P., & Paul, P.V. (1984). *Language and deafness.* San Diego: College Hill Press.

Quigley, S., Power, D., & Steinkamp, M. (1977). The language structure of deaf children. *Volta Review, 79,* 73–84.

Raffaelli, M., & Duckett, E. (1989). We were just talking . . . conversations in early adolescence. *Journal of Youth and Adolescence, 18,* 567–581.

Raffini, J. (1993). *Winners without losers.* Boston: Allyn & Bacon.

Rainer, J.D., Abdullah, S., & Altshuler, K.Z. (1970). Phenomenology of hallucinations in the deaf. In *Origins and mechanisms of hallucinations* (pp. 449–465). New York: Plenum Press.

Rainer, J.D., & Altshuler, K.Z. (1966). *Comprehensive mental health services for the deaf.* New York: Psychiatric Institute, Columbia University.

Rainer, J.D., Altshuler, K.Z., & Kallman, F.J. (1969). *Family and mental health problems in a deaf population.* (pp. 179–192). Springfield, IL: Thomas Publishing Co.

Rainer, J.D., Altshuler, K.Z., Kallman, F.T., & Deming, W.F. (Eds.). (1963). *Family and mental health problems in deaf population.* New York: State Psychiatric Institute.

Ramsey, C.L. (1997). *Deaf children in public schools: Placement, context, and conse-*

quences. Washington, DC: Gallaudet University Press.

Reed, V. (1994). *An introduction to children with language disorders* (2nd ed.). New York: Macmillan.

Rendon, M.E. (1992). Deaf culture and alcohol and substance abuse. *Journal of Substance Abuse Treatment, 9,* 103–110.

Rendon, M.E., Hills, C.G., & Rappold, E.S. (1992). Eating and related disorders: Implications for the deaf community. *JADARA, 25*(4), 11–14.

Ritter, E. (1979). Social perspective taking ability, cognitive complexity and listener adapted communication in early and late adolescence. *Communication Monograph, 46,* 40–51.

Robins, L., & Register, D. (Eds.). (1991). *Psychiatric disorders in America.* New York: Free Press.

Robinson, D.P., & Greene, J.W. (1988). The adolescent alcohol and drug problem: A practical approach. *Pedatric Nursing, 14,* 305–310.

Robinson, L.D., & Weathers, O.D. (1974). Family therapy of deaf parents and hearing children. A new dimension in psychotherapeutic intervention. *American Annals of the Deaf, 119,* 235–330.

Rogers, C.R. (1961). *On becoming a person.* Boston: Houghton Mifflin.

Rogers, R. (2000). *Conducting insanity evaluations* (2nd ed.). New York: Guilford Press.

Romaine, S. (1984). *The language of children and adolescence: The acquisition of communicative competence.* New York: Basil Blackwell.

Roosa, M.W., & Christopher, F.S. (1990). Evaluation of an abstinence-only adolescence pregnancy prevention program: A replication. *Family Relations, 39,* 363–367.

Rose, H., & Smith, A. (2000). Sighting sound/ sounding sight: The "violence" of deaf-hearing communication. In D.O. Braithwaite & T.R. Thompson (Eds.), *Handbook of communication and people with disabilities.* Mahwah, NJ: Lawrence Erlbaum Associates.

Rosen, R. (1986). Deafness: A social perspective. In D.M. Luterman (Ed.), *Deafness in perspective.* San Diego: College Hill Press.

Ross, M., & Fletcher, G. (1985). Attribution and social perception. In L. Gardner (Ed.), *Handbook of social psychology,* Vol. 3. New York: Random House.

Rothfield, P. (1981). Alcoholism treatment for the deaf: Specialized services for special people. *Journal of Rehabilitation of the Deaf, 14,* 14–17.

Rothfield, P. (1983). Residential services for deaf alcoholics. In D. Watson, K. Steitler, P. Peterson, & W. Fulton (Eds.), *Mental health, substance abuse and deafness.* Silver Spring, MD: ADARA.

Royce, A.P. (1982). *Ethnic identity: Strategies of diversity.* Bloomington: Indiana University Press.

Rush, P., Blennerhassett, L., Epstein, K., & Alexander, D. (1989). In D. Martin (Ed.), *Advances in cognition.* Washington, DC: Gallaudet University Press.

Russell, J.A., & Bullock, M. (1985). Multidimensional scaling of emotional facial expressions: Similarity from presechoolers to adults. *Journal of Personality and Social Psychology, 48,* 1290–1298.

Rust, P.C. (1993). "Coming out" in the age of social constructionism: Sexual identity formation among lesbian and bisexual women. *Gender and Society, 7,* 50–77.

Rutherford, S. (1988). The culture of American deaf people. *Sign Language Studies, 59,* 129–147.

Ryan, R. (1998). *Intrinsic/extrinsic motivation.* Paper presented at the meeting of the American Educational Research Association. *San Diego Review, 79,* 73–84.

Saarni, C. (1993). Socialization. In M. Lewis & J.M. Haviland (Eds.), *Handbook of emotions* (pp. 435–446). New York: Guilford Press.

Salovy, P., & Mayer, J.D. (1990). Emotional intelligence. *Imagination, Cognition, and Personality, 9,* 185–211.

Santrock, J.W. (1997). *Psychology* (5th ed.). Madison, WI: Brown & Benchmark.

Santrock, J.W. (1999). *Psychology,* Dubuque, IA: Brown and Benchmark.

Santrock, J.W. (2000). *Psychology* (6th ed). Boston: McGraw-Hill.

Santrock, J.W. (2002). *Life-span development* (8th ed.). Boston: McGraw-Hill.

Saunders, B.E., Villeponteaux, L.A., Lipovsky, J.A., Kilpatrick, D.G., & Vernon, L.J. (1992). Child sexual assault as a risk fac-

306 References

tor for mental disorders among women: A community survey. *Journal of Interpersonal Violence, 7,* 189–204.

Schaefer, D. (1996). *Choices and consequences: What to do when a teenager uses alcohol/drugs.* Minneapolis, MN: Johnson Institute.

Scheetz, N. (1993). *Sign communication for everyday use.* Austin, TX: Pro-ed.

Scheetz, N. (2001). *Orientation to deafness.* Boston: Allyn & Bacon.

Schildroth, A.N. (1988). Recent changes in the educational placement of deaf students. *American Annals of the Deaf, 133,* 61–67.

Schildroth, A.N., & Hotto, S.A. (1994). Deaf students and full inclusion: Who wants to be excluded? In R. Johnson & O. Cohen (Eds.), *Implication for deaf students of the full inclusion movement* (pp. 7–30). Washington, DC: Gallaudet University.

Schildroth, A., & Hotto, S. (1995). Race and ethnic background in the annual survey of deaf and hard of hearing children and youth. *American Annals of the Deaf, 140,* 96–99.

Schildroth, A.N., & Hotto, S.A. (1996). Changes in students and program characteristics. 1984–85 and 1994–95. *American Annals of the Deaf, 141,* 68–71.

Schirmer, B. (1989). Relationships between imaginative play and language development in hearing-impaired children. *American Annals of the Deaf, 134,* 219–222.

Schlesinger, H.S. (1992). Elusive X factor: Parental contributions to literacy. In M. Walworth, D.F. Moores, & T.J. O'Rourke (Eds.), *A free hand: Enfranchising the education of deaf children* (pp. 37–64). Silver Spring, MD: T.J. Publishers.

Schlesinger, H.S., & Meadow, K.P. (1972). *Sound and sign: Childhood deafness and mental health.* Berkeley: University of California Press.

Schloss, P.J., & Smith, M.A. (1990). *Teaching social skills to hearing-impaired students.* Washington, DC: Alexander Graham Bell Association for the Deaf.

Schneider, F.R., Johnson, J., Hornig, C.D., Olibowitz, M.R., & Weissman, M.M. (1992). Social phobia: Comorbidity and morbidity in an epidemiologic sample. *Archives of General Psychiatry, 49,* 288–298.

Schowe, B.M. (1979). *Identity crisis in deafness: A humanistic perspective.* Tempe, AZ: Scholars Press.

Schultz, D. (1977). *Growth psychology.* New York: Van Nostrand Reinhold Company.

Schwitzer, A.M., Rodriguez, I.E., Thomas, C., & Salam, H. (2001). The eating disorders NOS profile among college women. *Journal of American College Health, 49,* 157–166.

Scott, E.W., & Adams, D. (1974). *Sex education and drug abuse.* Proceedings of the forty-sixth meeting of the Convention of American Instructors of the Deaf. Washington, DC: Government Printing Office.

Scott, S. & Dooley, D. (1985). A structural family therapy approach for treatment of deaf children. In G.B. Anderson & D. Watson (Eds.), *Counseling deaf people: Research and practice.* Little Rock, AR: Arkansas Rehabilitation Research and Training Center on Deafness and Hearing Impairment.

Seidman, E., & French, S.E. (1998). Community mental health. In H.S. Friedman (Ed.), *Encyclopedia of mental health* (Vol. 1). San Diego: Academic Press.

Seligman, L. (1998). *Selecting effective treatments: A comprehensive, systematic guide to treating mental disorders.* San Francisco: Jossey Bass Publishers.

Seligmann, J. (1989). Variations on a theme. *Newsweek, 22*(2), 38–46.

Sex Information and Education Council of the U.S. (SIECUS). (1991). *Guidelines for comprehensive sexuality education.* New York: SIECUS.

Shadish, W.R. (1989). Private sector care for chronically mentally ill individuals. The more things change, the more they stay the same. *American Psychologist, 44*(8), 1142–1147.

Shapiro, J.P. (1993). *No pity: People with disabilities forging a new civil rights movement.* New York: Times Books.

Shapiro, R.J., & Harris, R. (1976). Family therapy in treatment of the deaf: A case report. *Family Process, 15,* 83–97.

Shaul, S. (1981, June). Deafness and human sexuality: A developmental review. *American Annals of the Deaf,* 432–439.

Shils, E. (1985). Sociology. In A. Kuper & J. Kuper (Eds.), *The social science encyclo-*

pedia. London: Routledge and Kegan Paul.

Shipley, K. (1992). *Interviewing and counseling in communicative disorders*. New York: Macmillan.

Simkin, J.S., & Yontef, G.M. (1984). Gestalt therapy. In R. Corsini (Ed.), *Current psychotherapies*. Itasca, IL: Peacock Publishers.

Singer, M. (1991). *Psychology of language: An introduction to sentence and discourse processes*. Hillsdale, NJ: Lawrence Erlbaum Associates.

Sipes, D.S. (1993). Cultural values and American-Indian families. In N. Chavki (Ed.), *Families and schools in a pluralistic society*. Albany, NY: SUNY Press.

Sisco, F., & Anderson, R. (1980). Deaf children's performance on the WISC-R relative to hearing status of parents and child rearing experiences. *American Annals of the Deaf, 125,* 923–930.

Skarakis, E., & Prutting, C. (1977). Early communication: Semantic functions and communicative intents in the communication of the preschool child with impaired hearing. *American Annals of the Deaf, 122,* 382–391.

Slobin, D. (1972, July). Children and language: They learn the same way all around the world. *Psychology Today,* 71–76.

Snyder, M., & Ickes, W. (1985). Personality and social behavior. In G. Lindzey & E. Aronson (Eds.), *Handbook of social psychology* (3rd ed.). New York: Random House.

Solomons, G. (1979). Child abuse and developmental disabilities. *Dev. Med. Child. Neurol., 21*(1), 101–106.

Sorenson, D.A. (1992). Facilitating responsible behavior in deaf children. *JADARA, 25*(3), 1–7.

Spencer, P.E. (1993a). Communication behaviors of infants with hearing loss and their hearing mothers. *Journal of Speech and Hearing Research, 36,* 311–321.

Spencer, P.E. (1993b). The expressive communication of hearing mothers and deaf infants. *American Annals of the Deaf, 138,* 275–283.

Spencer, P.E., & Deyo, D.A. (1993). Cognitive and social aspects of deaf children's play. In M.

Marschark & M.D. Clark (Eds.), *Psychological perspectives on deafness*. Hillsdale, NJ: Lawrence Erlbaum Associates.

Spencer, P.E., & Lederberg, A.R. (1997). Different modes, different models communication and language of young deaf children and their mothers. In L.B. Adamson & M.A. Romski (Eds.), *Communication and language acquisition* (pp. 203–230). Baltimore, MD: Paul H. Brookes Publishing Co.

Spencer, P.E. & Waxman, R. (1995). Joint attention and maternal attention strategies: 9, 12, 18 months. In *Maternal responsiveness and child competency in deaf and hearing children*. Final Report, Grant H023C10077. Washington, DC: U.S. Department of Education Office of Special Education and Rehabilitation Services.

Spragins, A. (1999). *1997–98 update to the reviews of four types of assessment instruments used with deaf and hard of hearing students: Cognitive assessment, adaptive behavior and social-emotional assessment, academic/readiness assessment*. Retrieved from the Internet on 9/1/00: http://gri.gallaudet.edu/~catraxle/reviews.html.

Stedt, J. (1992). Issues of educational interpreting. In T. Kluwin, D. Moores, & M.G. Gaustad (Eds.), *Toward effective public school programs for deaf students*. (pp. 83–100). New York: Teachers College Press.

Stein, M. (1976). *Role playing and spontaneity in teaching social skills to deaf adolescents*. Unpublished research paper. Saint Elizabeth's Hospital, Washington, DC.

Steinberg, A. (1991). Issues in providing mental health services to hearing-impaired persons. *Hospital and community psychiatry, 42*(4), 380–388.

Steitler, K.L.A. (1984). *Substance abuse and deaf adolescents*. Wagoner, OK: University of Arkansas Rehabilitation Research & Training Center on Deafness & Hearing-Impairment.

Stevenson, M.R., & Black, K.N. (1996). *How divorce affects offspring*. Boulder, CO: Westview.

Stern, D. (1985). *The interpersonal world of the infant: A view from psychoanalysis and developmental psychology*. New York: Basic Books.

Stewart, D., & Kluwin, T.N. (1996). The gap between guidelines, practices, knowledge in interpreting services for deaf students. *Journal of Deaf Studies and Deaf Education, 1,* 29–39.

Stewart, D., & Stinson, M. (1992). The role of sport and extracurricular activities in shaping socialization patterns. In T.N. Kluwin, D.F. Moores & M.G. Gaustad (Eds.), *Toward effective public school programs for deaf students* (pp. 129–148). New York: Teachers College Press.

Stiegel-Moore, R.H., Silberstein, I.R., & Rodin, J. (1993). The social self in bulimia nervosa; Public self-consciousness, social anxiety, and perceived fraudulence. *Journal of Abnormal Psychology, 102,* 297–303.

Stinson, M. (1993). Affective and social development. In R.C. Nowell & L.E. Marshak (Eds.), *Understanding deafness and the rehabilitation process.* Boston: Allyn & Bacon.

Stinson, M., Chase, K., & Bondi-Wolcott, J. (1988). *Use of social activity scale as part of personal social development activities during "Explore Your Future."* Working paper. National Technical Institute for the Deaf, Rochester, NJ.

Stinson, M., Chase, K., & Kluwin, T. (1990). *Self-perceptions of social relationships in hearing-impaired adolescents.* Paper presented at the convention of the American Educational Research Association. Boston.

Stinson, M., & Whitmore, K. (1991). Self-perception of social relationships among hearing-impaired adolescents in England. *Journal of British Association of Teachers of the Deaf, 15,* 104–114.

Stinson, M., & Whitmore, K. (1992). Students' views of their social relationships. In T.N. Kluwin, D.F. Moores, M.G. Gaustad (Eds.), *Toward effective public school programs for deaf students.* (pp. 149–175). New York: Teachers College Press.

Stinson, M. & Foster, S. (2000). *The deaf child in the family and at school: Essays in honor of Kathryn P. Meadow.* Mahwah NJ: Lawrence Erlbaum Associates.

Stinson, M.S. Whitmore, K., & Kluwin, T. (1996). Self-perceptions of social relationships in hearing impaired adolescents. *Journal of Educational Psychology, 88,* 132–143.

Strauss, J. T., Carpenter, W.T. & Bartko, J.J. (1974). Specializations on the processes that underlie schizophrenic symptoms and signs. *Schizophrenia Bulletin, 11,* 61–69.

Strong, M. (Ed.). (1988). *Language learning and deafness.* New York: Cambridge University Press.

Stuart, A., Harrison, D., & Simpson, P. (1991). The social and emotional development of a population of hearing-impaired children being educated in their local mainstream schools in Leicestershire, England. *Journal of the British Association of Teachers of the Deaf, 15*(5), 121–125.

Sue, D.W., & Sue, D. (1981). *Counseling the culturally different: Theory and practice* (2nd ed.). New York: Wiley.

Sullivan, H.S. (1953). *The interpersonal theory of psychiatry.* New York: W.W. Norton.

Sullivan, P.M. (1993). Sexual abuse therapy for special children. *Journal of Child Sexual Abuse, 2*(2), 117–125.

Sullivan, P.M., Brookhouser, P.E., Scanlan, J.M., Knutson, J.F., & Schulte, L.E. (1991). Patterns of physical and sexual abuse of communicatively handicapped children. *Annals of Otology, Rhinology and Laryngology, 100*(3), 188–194.

Sullivan, P.M., & Knutson, J.F. (1998). Maltreatment and behavioral characteristics of youth who are deaf and hard of hearing. *Sexuality and Disability, 16*(4), 295–319.

Sullivan, P.M., & Scanlan, J.M. (1987). Therapeutic issues. In J. Garbarino, P.E. Brookhouser, & K. J. Authier (Eds.), *Special children—special risks: The maltreatment of children with disabilities* (pp. 127–159). New York: Aldine de Gruyter.

Sullivan, P.M., & Scanlan, J.M. (1990). Psychotherapy with handicapped sexually abused children. *Developmental Disabilities Bulletin, 18*(2), 21–34.

Sussman, A. (1992). *Characteristics of well adjusted deaf person or: The art of being a deaf person.* Paper presented at the Statewide Conference on Deafness and Hard of Hearing, April, North Carolina Department of Human Resources, Raleigh.

Sussman, A., & Stewart, L. (1971). *Counseling with deaf people.* New York: New York University.

Swartz, D. (1989). *Perceptual attitudes of male homosexuals from differing socio-cultural and audiological backgrounds.* Unpublished manuscript, Gallaudet University, Washington, DC (ERIC Document Reproduction Service no. ED 408456).

Swartz, D.B. (1993). A comparative study of sex knowledge among hearing and deaf college freshmen. *Sexuality and Disability, 11*(2), 129–147.

Swartz, D.B. (1995a). Cultural implication of audiological deficits on the homosexual male. *Sexuality and Disability, 13*(2), 159–181.

Swartz, D.B. (1995b). Effective techniques in treating survivors of child sexual abuse: Problematic areas in their application to the deaf population. *Sexuality and Disability, 13*(2), 135–144.

Swink, D.F. (1985). Psychodramatic treatment for deaf people. *American Annals of the Deaf, 130,* 272–277.

Swisher, M.V. (1984). Signed input of hearing mothers to deaf children. *Language Learning, 34,* 69–85.

Taylor, I.G. (Ed.). (1987). *The education of the deaf: Current perspectives.* London & New York: Croom Helm.

Taylor, R. (1994). Black American families. In R. Taylor (Ed.), *Minority families in the United States: A multicultural perspective* (pp. 19–46). Englewood Cliffs, NJ: Prentice-Hall.

Te, H.D. (1989). *The Indochinese and their cultures.* San Diego: San Diego State University, Multifunctional Resource Center.

Telljohann, S.K., & Price, J.H. (1993). A qualitative examination of adolescent homosexual life experience: Ramifications for secondary school personnel. *Journal of Homosexuality, 26,* 41–56.

Terrell, S.L., & Jackson, R.S. (2002). African Americans in the Americas. In D.E. Battle (Ed.), *Communication disorders in multicultural populations* (3rd ed.) Boston: Butterworth-Heinemann.

Tessler, R.C. (2000). *Family experiences with mental illness.* Westport, CT: Auburn House.

Thacker, A.J. (1994). Formal communication disorder. *British Journal of Psychiatry, 165*(6), 818–823.

Thomas, A., & Chess, S. (1977). *Temperament and development.* New York: Brunner/Mazel.

Thomas, R. (1994). Bringing up our children to be bilingual and bicultural: A three part presentation. In C.J. Erting, R.C. Johnson, D.S. Smith, & B.D. Snider (Eds.), *The deaf way* (pp. 552–556). Washington, DC: Gallaudet University Press.

Thorpe, G.L. (1998). Agoraphobia. In H.S. Friedman (Ed.), *Encyclopedia of mental health* (Vol. 1). San Diego: Academic Press.

Tripp, A., & J. Kahn (1986). Comparison of the sexual knowledge of hearing impaired and hearing adults. *JADARA, 19*(3-4), 15–18.

Trybus, R. (1978). What the Stanford Achievement Test has to say about the reading abilities of deaf children. In H. Reynolds & C. Williams (Eds.), *Proceedings of the Gallaudet conference on reading in relation to deafness* (pp. 231–221). Washington, DC: Gallaudet College Press.

Trybus, R. (1987). Unpublished manuscript, Washington, DC: Gallaudet University.

Trybus, R., & Buchanan, G. (1973). *Patterns of achievement test performance. Studies in achievement testing, hearing-impaired students. United States, 1971* (Series D., No. 11). Washington, DC: Gallaudet College, Office of Demographic Studies.

Trybus, R., & Karchmer, M.A. (1977). School achievement scores of hearing impaired children: National data on achievement status and growth patterns. *American Annals of the Deaf, Directory of Programs and Services, 122,* 62–69.

Turnball, R., Turnball, A., Shank, M., Smith, S., & Leal, D. (2002). *Exceptional lives.* Upper Saddle River, NJ: Merrill.

Tvingstedt, A. (1993). *Social conditions of hearing-impaired pupils in regular classrooms* (Monograph No. 773). Malmo, Sweden: University of Lund, Department of Education Psychological Research.

Tweney, R., Hoeman, H., & Andrews, C. (1975). Semantic organizations in deaf and hearing subjects. *Journal of Psycholinguistic Research, 4,* 61–73.

Uba, L. (1994). *Asian Americans: Personality patterns, identity, and mental health.* New York: Guilford Press.

Ursano, R.J. et al. (1999). Acute and chronic posttraumatic stress disorder in motor vehicle accident victims. *American Journal of Psychiatry, 156,* 589–595.

U.S. Bureau of the Census. (2000a). *Categories by race for the U.S.* Washington, DC: Author.

U.S. Bureau of the Census. (2000b). *Population by race and Hispanic origin for the U.S.* Washington, DC: Author.

U.S. Department of Education (1989). *Eleventh annual report to Congress on the implementation of the Education of the Handicapped Act.* Washington DC: Author.

U.S. Department of Education. (1999). *Dropout rates in the United States: 1997.* Washington, DC: U.S. Government Printing Office.

U.S. Department of Health and Human Services. (1999). *Health United States 1998–1999 and injury chartbook.* Washington, DC: U.S. Bureau of the Census.

Valenstein, E. (1998). *Blaming the brain: The truth about drugs and mental health.* New York: Free Press.

Valli, C., & Lucas, C. (2000). *Linguistics of American Sign Language.* Washington, DC: Gallaudet University Press.

VanBienna, D. (1994, April 4). AIDS. *Time* 76–77.

Vandell, D.L., & George, L.B. (1981). Social interaction in hearing and deaf preschoolers: Successes and failures in initiations. *Child Development, 52,* 627–635.

VanKleek, A. (1984). Metalinguistic skills: Cutting across spoken and written language and problem solving abilities. In G. Wallach & K. Butler (Eds.), *Language learning disabilities in school age children* (pp. 129–153). Baltimore: Williams and Wilkins.

Vega, W.A. (1990). Hispanic families in the 1980s: A decade of research. *Journal of Marriage and Family, 52,* 1015–1024.

Venn, J. (1987). *Scale of social development.* Tulsa, OK: Modern Education Corporation.

Vernon, M. (1976). Psychologic evaluation of hearing-impaired children. In L. Loyd (Ed.), *Communication, assessment and intervention strategies* (pp. 195–223). Baltimore: University Park Press.

Vernon, M. (1978). Deafness and mental health: Some theoretical views. *Gallaudet Today.*

Vernon, M. (1983). Deafness and mental health: Emerging responses. In E. Petersen (Ed.), *Mental health and deafness: Emerging responses* (pp. 1–15). Silver Spring, MD: American Deafness and Rehabilitation Association.

Vernon, M. (1995). A historical perspective on psychology and deafness. *JADARA, 29,* 8–13.

Vernon, M., & Andrews, J. (1990). *The psychology of deafness.* New York: Longman.

Vernon, M., & Daigle-King, B. (1999). Historical overview of inpatient care mental patients who are deaf. *American Annals of the Deaf, 144,* 51–79.

Vernon, M., & Ottinger, P. (1981). Psychological evaluation of the deaf and hard of hearing. In L.K. Stein, E.D. Mindel, & T. Jabaley (Eds.), *Deafness and mental health* (pp. 49–64). New York: Grune & Stratton.

Vygotsky, L. (1978). Mind in society. *The development of higher psychological processes.* Cambridge, MA: MIT Press.

Walden, T.A. (1993). Communicating the meaning of events through social referencing. In D.B. Gray, A.P. Kaiser (Eds.), *Enhancing children's communication: Research foundations for intervention.* Baltimore: Paul H. Brookes.

Wallman, S. (1983). Identity options. In C. Fried (Ed.), *Minorities: Community and identity* (pp. 69–78). Berlin: Springer-Verlag.

Warner, H.C. (1987). Community service centers for deaf people. Where are we now? *American Annals of the Deaf, 132*(3), 237–238.

Watson, D. (Ed.). (1976). *Deaf evaluation and adjustment feasibility.* New York: New York University, Deafness Research & Training Center.

Watson, D. (1983). Substance abuse services for deaf clients: A question of accessibility. In D. Watson, K. Steitler, P. Peterson, & W. Fulton (Eds.), *Mental health, substance abuse and deafness.* Silver Spring, MD: ADARA.

Wax, T.M. (1990). Deaf community leaders as liaisons between mental health and deaf cultures. *JADARA, 24,* 23–40.

Wedell-Monnig, J., & Lumley, J. (1980). Child deafness and mother-child interaction. *Child Development, 51,* 766–774.

Weinberg, D.H. (2000). *Press briefing on 2000 income and poverty estimates.* Retrieved on the Internet on 7/17/02: http://www.census.gov/hhes./income/income00/prs01asc.html.

Weisel, A. (Ed.) (1998). *Issues unresolved: New perspectives on language and deaf education.* Washington, DC: Gallaudet University Press.

Weismann, M. (2000). *Comprehensive guide to interpersonal psychotherapy.* New York: Basic Books.

Wentzel, K.R., & Asher, S.R. (1995). The academic lives of neglected, rejected, popular, and controversial children. *Child Development, 66,* 754–763.

Wentzer, C., & Dhir, A. (1986). An outline for working with the hearing impaired in an inpatient substance abuse treatment program. *JADARA, 20*(2), 11–15.

Westby, C.E. (1998). Social-emotional bases of communicative development. In W.O. Hayes & B.B. Shulman (Eds.), *Communication development* (pp. 167–204). Baltimore: Williams & Wilkens.

Westby, C., & Vining, C. (2002). Living in harmony: Providing services to native American children and families. In D.E. Battle (Ed.), *Communication disorders in multicultural populations* (3rd ed.) Boston, MA: Butterworth-Heinemann.

Westerlund, E. (1990). Thinking about incest, deafness, and counseling. *JADARA, 23*(3), 105–107.

White, M., & Epston, D. (1990). *Narrative means to therapeutic ends.* New York: W.W. Norton.

Whitmore, K. (2000). Adolescence as a developmental phase: A tutorial. *Topics in Language Disorders, 20*(2), 1–14.

Wiig, E. (1982, May). *Identifying language disorders in adolescents.* LaCross, WI: Oral presentation at Gunderson Clinic.

Wiig, E., & Secord, W. (1992). From word knowledge to world knowledge. *Clinical Connection, 6*(3), 12–14.

Wilbur, R. (1979). American Sign Language and sign systems. Baltimore, MD: University Park Press.

Wilcox, S. (Ed.) (1989). *American Deaf culture.* Burtonsville, MD: Linstock Press.

Williams, S. (1994). The influence of topic and listener familiarity on aphasic discourse. *Journal of Communication Disorders, 27*(3), 207–222.

Willis, W. (1998). Families with African American roots. In E.W. Lynch & M.J. Hanson (Eds.), *Developing cross-cultural competence.* Baltimore, MD: Paul H. Brookes.

Wilson, J.J., Rapin, I., Wilson, B.C., & VanDenburg, V. (1975). Neuropsychologic function of children with severe hearing impairment. *Journal of Speech and Hearing Science, 18,* 634–651.

Winiarski, M.G. (1991). *AIDS related psychotherapy.* New York: Pergamon.

Winick, B.J. (1997). *The right to refuse mental health treatment.* Washington, DC: American Psychological Association.

Wisniewski, A.M., DeMatteo, A.J., Lee, S.M., & Orr, F.C. (1985). Neuropsychological assessment. In L.G. Stewart (Ed.), *Clinical rehabilitation assessment and hearing impairment: A guide to quality assurance.* Silver Spring, MD: National Association of the Deaf.

Wolf-Schein, E.G. & Schein, J.D. (Eds.). (1991). *Postsecondary education for deaf children.* Edmonto: Educational Psychology, University of Alberta.

Wood, D. et al. (Eds.). (1986). *Teaching and talking with deaf children.* Chichester, NY: Wiley.

Wood, S.E., & Wood, E.G. (2002). *The world of psychology.* Boston: Allyn & Bacon.

Yoshinaga-Itano, C. (1986). Beyond the sentence level: What's in a hearing impaired child's story? *Topics in Language Disorders, 6*(3), 71–83.

Yoshinaga-Itano, C. (1994). Language assessment of infants and toddlers with significant hearing loss. *Seminars in Hearing, 15,* 128–147.

Yoshinaga-Itano, C., & Stredler-Brown, A. (1992). Learning to communicate: Babies with hearing impairments make their needs known. *Volta Review, 95,* 107–129.

Zakarewsky, G.T. (1979). Patterns of support among gay and lesbian deaf persons. *Sexuality and Disability, 2*(3), 178–191.

Zakarewsky, G.T. (1982, June). *Social aspects of deafness.* Vol. 3: The deaf community and the deaf population. Collected papers from the conference, Sociology of Deafness. Gallaudet College, Washington, DC.

Ziezula, F.R. (1982). *Assessment of hearing-impaired people: A guide for selecting psychological, educational, and vocational tests.* Washington, DC: Gallaudet University Press.

Ziezula, F., & Harris, G. (1998). National Survey of School Counselors working with deaf and hard of hearing children. *American Annals of the Deaf, 143*(1), 40–45.

Zitter, S. (1996). Report from the front lines: Balancing multiple roles of a deafness therapist. In N.S. Glickman & P. Harvey (Eds.), *Culturally affirmative psychotherapy with deaf persons.* Mahwah, NJ: Lawrence Erlbaum Associates.

Zuckerman, M. (1999). *Vulnerability to psychopathology: A biosocial model.* Washington, DC: American Psychological Association.

Zuniga, M. (1998). Families with Latino roots. In E. Lynch & M. Hanson (Eds.), *Developing cross-cultural competencies: A guide for working with young children and their families.* Baltimore: Paul H. Brookes.

Author Index

Subject Index

Deaf and hard-of-hearing individuals (*cont.*)
    depression, 246–247
    identifying, 243–244
    interpreting during the mental status exam,
        244–246
    obsessive-compulsive disorder, 247
    paranoid disorders, 249
    prevalence, 244–246
    schizophrenia, 247–249
    surdophrenia, 249–250
    sexual abuse treatment, 259–260
    treatment strategies and programs, 265–266
Deaf and hard-of-hearing students, 93–97,
       213–214
    assessing, 182–192
        general assessment tests, 182–187
            Detroit Tests of Learning Aptitude-2, 182
            Gates MacGintie Reading Tests, 182
            Metropolitan Achievement Test, 184
            Stanford Achievement Test, 184
            Test of Nonverbal Intelligence (TONI-3),
                186–187
            Test of Syntactic Abilities, 184–185
            Wechsler Intelligence Scale for Children,
                185
            Wide Range Achievement Tests, 185–186
            Wide Range Achievement Test-3 (WRAT-3),
                186
        projective techniques, 188–190
            Draw-A-Person: Screening Procedure for
                Emotional Disturbance, 189–190
            Goodenough Harris Drawing Test,
                188–189
            House-Tree-Person Projective Technique
                (H-T-P), 190
            Make A Picture Story (MAPS), 189
        special clinical tests, 187–188
            Bender Visual Motor Gestalt, 187
            Benton Revised Visual Retention Test, 187
            Bruininks-Oseretsky Test of Motor
                Proficiency, 188
            Graham-Kendall Memory for Designs
                Test, 188
        vocational interest batteries, 190–192
            Differential Aptitude Test (DAT), 192
            General Aptitude Test Battery (GATB),
                191–192
            Kuder Occupational Interest Inventories,
                191
            Strong-Campbell Interest Inventory,
                190–191
    classroom management approaches, 93–95

    in mainstream classrooms, 94–97
    self-esteem, enhancing, 101–102
    sexual education programs, 121–122
Deaf community, 18–20, 104–122, 154–155, 170,
       172, 274
    HIV/AIDS, 119–121
    sexuality, 104–122
Deaf Cultural Identity Scale (DCIS), 31
Deaf culture, 19–20
Deaf identity, establishing, 20–22, 25–37
    childhood deafness and self-identity, 21–22
    early years, 25–28
    four phases, 33–35
    Glickman's Deaf Identity Model, 20–21
    impact of school settings, 28–29, 35–37
        mainstream, 36
        research, 36–37
        residential, 35–36
    work of Robin Gordon, 31–32
    work of Teresa Prout, 29–31
    works of Amy Melick, 33–35
Deafness, 14–18, 116–118, 130–136, 150–155,
       235–250
    deaf, 17–18
    hard of hearing, 17
    healthy personality, 150–155
    hearing loss, 17
    and homosexuality, 116–118
    and mental illness, 235–250
    social development, 124–141
    socialization process, 132–136
    society's perceptions and expectations,
       130–132
Denver Developmental Screening Test, 178–179
Depression, 246–247
Detroit Tests of Learning Aptitude-2, 182
Diagnostic and Statistical Manual of Mental
       Disorders (DSM-IV), 236, 237
Differential Aptitude Test (DAT), 192
Draw-A-Person: Screening Procedure for
       Emotional Disturbance, 189–190
Dreikurs, Rudolph, 88–89
    approach to classroom discipline, 88–89
Dysthymic disorder, 240

E

Eating disorders, 260–262
Ecological theory, 127–128
Educational domain, 84–102
Education for All Handicapped Children Act, 94
Emotional intelligence, 128
Encephalitis as cause of deafness, 244

English-based signing systems, 170, 210–212
Contact Signing or Pidgin Sign English (PSE), 211
cued speech, 212
Rochester method, 211–212
Seeing Essential English (SEE I), 211
Signing Exact English (SEE II), 211
Ethnic identity, 12–13

F
Families, diversity of, 42–52
African American origins, 45–46
Anglo-European origins, 44–45
Asian origins, 46–47
biracial/bicultural origins, 49
Latino or Hispanic origins, 48–49
Native American origins, 47–48
Family dynamics and deafness, 40–62
Family structures, 40–42, 52, 85–86
augmented extended families, 42
and economic status, 85–86
economic variability, 52
extended families, 41
families with secondary members, 42
single-parent families, 40–41
step- and blended families, 41–42
subfamilies, 42
Family therapy, 227–228
Family unit, 52
economic variability, 52
fostering independence, 57–58
Finn, Gail, 28–29
Foster Care Review Board (FCRB), 255
Frankl, Viktor, 148–149, 159–160
healthy personality theory, 148–149
theory on deafness, 159–160
Freud, Sigmund, 9, 104–106
stages of personality development, 9
views on sexual development, 105–106
Fromm, Eric, 146–147, 158
healthy personality theory, 146–147
theory on deafness, 158

G
Gates MacGintie Reading Tests, 182
Gay identity, 115–116
General anxiety, 238
General Aptitude Test Battery (GATB), 191–192
Gestalt therapy, 230–231
Ginott, Haim, 89–91
theory of classroom communication, 89–91
Glasser, William, 87–88

philosophy of classroom management, 87–88
Glickman's Deaf Identity Model, 20, 28
bicultural, 21
culturally hearing, 20
culturally marginal, 20
immersed, 21
Goodenough Harris Drawing Test, 188–189
Gordon, Robin, work of, 31–32
Deaf Cultural Identity Scale (DCIS), 31–32
Graham-Kendall Memory for Designs Test, 188

H
Hard of hearing, 17
Health and sex education, school-based programs, 110–115
abstinence-only, 111
postponement and protection, 111–113
in residential schools, 113–115
Healthy personality, developing, 143–160
applying theories, 155–160
comparison of perspectives, table, 151
deaf child in Deaf community, 154–155
deaf child in hearing community, 152–154
and deafness, 150–155
theories, 143–150
Allport, Gordon, 144–145, 156–157
Frankl, Viktor, 148–149, 159–160
Fromm, Erich, 146–147, 158
Jung, Carl, 147–148, 158–159
Maslow, Abraham, 149–150, 160
Rogers, Carl, 145–146, 157–158
Hearing loss, 16, 17
categories, table, 16
Hearing parents/deaf children, cultural conflicts, 52–53
HIV (human immunodeficiency virus), 118–119
and the Deaf community, 119–121
Homosexual behavior, 115–116
and deafness, 116–118
House-Tree-Person Projective Technique (H-T-P), 190
Humanistic theory of personality development, 10

I
Identity, 12–14
attribution, 14
ethnic, ethnicity, and ethnocentrism, 12–13
stereotyping, 13–14
Individuals with Disabilities Education Act (IDEA), 94